T0186743

MOTIVATIONAL INTERVIEWING
IN THE TREATMENT
OF PSYCHOLOGICAL PROBLEMS

Applications of Motivational Interviewing

Stephen Rollnick, William R. Miller, and Theresa B. Moyers,
Series Editors

www.guilford.com/AMI

Since the publication of Miller and Rollnick's classic *Motivational Interviewing*, now in its third edition, MI has been widely adopted as a tool for facilitating change. This highly practical series includes general MI resources as well as books on specific clinical contexts, problems, and populations. Each volume presents powerful MI strategies that are grounded in research and illustrated with concrete, "how-to-do-it" examples.

Motivational Interviewing in Health Care:
Helping Patients Change Behavior
Stephen Rollnick, William R. Miller, and Christopher C. Butler

Building Motivational Interviewing Skills:
A Practitioner Workbook
David B. Rosengren

Motivational Interviewing with Adolescents and Young Adults
Sylvie Naar-King and Mariann Suarez

Motivational Interviewing in Social Work Practice
Melinda Hohman

Motivational Interviewing in the Treatment of Anxiety
Henny A. Westra

Motivational Interviewing, Third Edition: Helping People Change
William R. Miller and Stephen Rollnick

Motivational Interviewing in Groups
Christopher C. Wagner and Karen S. Ingersoll, with Contributors

Motivational Interviewing in the Treatment
of Psychological Problems, Second Edition
Hal Arkowitz, William R. Miller, and Stephen Rollnick, Editors

Motivational Interviewing in Diabetes Care
Marc P. Steinberg and William R. Miller

Motivational Interviewing in Nutrition and Fitness
Dawn Clifford and Laura Curtis

MOTIVATIONAL INTERVIEWING
in the Treatment of Psychological Problems

• • • • • •

SECOND EDITION

Edited by

HAL ARKOWITZ
WILLIAM R. MILLER
STEPHEN ROLLNICK

THE GUILFORD PRESS
New York   London

© 2015 The Guilford Press
A Division of Guilford Publications, Inc.
370 Seventh Avenue, Suite 1200, New York, NY 10001
www.guilford.com

Paperback edition 2017

All rights reserved

No part of this book may be reproduced, translated, stored in
a retrieval system, or transmitted, in any form or by any means,
electronic, mechanical, photocopying, microfilming, recording,
or otherwise, without written permission from the publisher.

Printed in the United States of America

This book is printed on acid-free paper.

Last digit is print number: 9 8 7 6 5

The authors have checked with sources believed to be reliable in their efforts to
provide information that is complete and generally in accord with the standards
of practice that are accepted at the time of publication. However, in view of the
possibility of human error or changes in behavioral, mental health, or medical
sciences, neither the authors, nor the editors and publisher, nor any other party
who has been involved in the preparation or publication of this work warrants
that the information contained herein is in every respect accurate or complete,
and they are not responsible for any errors or omissions or the results obtained
from the use of such information. Readers are encouraged to confirm the
information contained in this book with other sources.

Library of Congress Cataloging-in-Publication Data

Motivational interviewing in the treatment of psychological problems / edited
by Hal Arkowitz, William R. Miller, Stephen Rollnick. — Second edition.
        pages cm. — (Applications of motivational interviewing)
    Includes bibliographical references and index.
    ISBN 978-1-4625-2103-6 (hardback)
    ISBN 978-1-4625-3012-0 (paperback)
    1. Interviewing in psychiatry.   I. Arkowitz, Hal, 1941–   II. Miller,
William R. (William Richard)   III. Rollnick, Stephen, 1952–
    RC480.7.M68 2015
    616.89—dc23
                                                          2015015934

*To my grandchildren, Mackenzie, Sarah,
Reya, and Zachary, with love*
—H. A.

*In memory of Carl Rogers, who pioneered
psychotherapy process and outcome research*
—W. R. M.

*In memory of a good friend
and inspired colleague, Dr. Guy Azoulai*
—S. R.

About the Editors

Hal Arkowitz, PhD, until his death in 2019, was Emeritus Associate Professor of Psychology at the University of Arizona. His life's work was dedicated to understanding how people change and why they don't. Dr. Arkowitz published widely in the areas of psychotherapy and motivational interviewing. A scientist–practitioner for his entire career, he was deeply interested in how science can inform practice and how practice can inform science.

William R. Miller, PhD, is Emeritus Distinguished Professor of Psychology and Psychiatry at the University of New Mexico. He introduced the concept of MI as a clinical method in a 1983 article. With over 50 published books and 400 articles and chapters, he has been listed by the Institute for Scientific Information as one of the world's most highly cited scientists over a 25-year span. With Stephen Rollnick, Dr. Miller is coauthor of the classic work *Motivational Interviewing: Helping People Change*, now in its third edition.

Stephen Rollnick, PhD, is Honorary Distinguished Professor in the Department of Primary Care and Public Health at Cardiff University, Wales, United Kingdom. Dr. Rollnick has published widely on MI and behavior change and has a special interest in challenging consultations in health and social care. His books include *Motivational Interviewing in Health Care: Helping Patients Change Behavior* (coauthored with William R. Miller and Christopher C. Butler).

Contributors

Hal Arkowitz, PhD, Department of Psychology, University of Arizona, Tucson, Arizona

Adi Aviram, MA, Department of Psychology, York University, Toronto, Ontario, Canada

Iván C. Balán, PhD, Anxiety Disorders Clinic, New York State Psychiatric Institute, New York, New York

David H. Barlow, PhD, Center for Anxiety and Related Disorders, Boston University, Boston, Massachusetts

Kate H. Bentley, MA, Center for Anxiety and Related Disorders, Boston University, Boston, Massachusetts

James F. Boswell, PhD, Department of Psychology, University at Albany, State University of New York, Albany, New York

Peter C. Britton, PhD, Center of Excellence, Canandaigua VA Medical Center, Canandaigua, New York

Stephanie C. Cassin, PhD, CPsych, Department of Psychology, Ryerson University, Toronto, Ontario, Canada

Suzanne M. Colby, PhD, Center for Alcohol and Addiction Studies, Brown University, Providence, Rhode Island

Katherine M. Diskin, PhD, RPsych, Canadian Forces Health Services Centre, Canadian Forces Base Esquimalt, Victoria, British Columbia, Canada

Michelle L. Drapkin, PhD, Department of Psychology, University of Pennsylvania, Philadelphia, Pennsylvania

Heather Flynn, PhD, Department of Medical Humanities and Social Sciences, Florida State University College of Medicine, Tallahassee, Florida

Josie Geller, PhD, RPsych, Eating Disorders Program, St. Paul's Hospital, Vancouver, British Columbia, Canada

Nancy K. Grote, PhD, School of Social Work, University of Washington, Seattle, Washington

David C. Hodgins, PhD, Department of Psychology, University of Calgary, Calgary, Alberta, Canada

Roberto Lewis-Fernández, MD, Department of Psychiatry, Columbia University Medical Center, Columbia University, and New York State Center of Excellence for Cultural Competence and Hispanic Treatment Program, New York State Psychiatric Institute, New York, New York

William R. Miller, PhD, Departments of Psychology and Psychiatry, University of New Mexico, Albuquerque, New Mexico

Theresa B. Moyers, PhD, Center on Alcoholism, Substance Abuse and Addictions, University of New Mexico, Albuquerque, New Mexico

Sylvie Naar, PhD, Pediatric Prevention Research Center, Wayne State University, Detroit, Michigan

Stephen Rollnick, PhD, Institute of Primary Care and Public Health, Cardiff University, Cardiff, Wales, United Kingdom

Helen Blair Simpson, MD, PhD, Department of Psychiatry, Columbia University Medical Center, Columbia University, New York, New York

Jennifer L. Swan, BA, Department of Psychology, University of Calgary, Calgary, Alberta, Canada

Holly A. Swartz, MD, Western Psychiatric Institute and Clinic, University of Pittsburgh School of Medicine, Pittsburgh, Pennsylvania

Henny A. Westra, PhD, Department of Psychology, York University, Toronto, Ontario, Canada

Erica M. Woodin, PhD, Department of Psychology, University of Victoria, Victoria, British Columbia, Canada

Rebecca Yeh, BA, Center for the Treatment and Study of Anxiety, University of Pennsylvania, Philadelphia, Pennsylvania

David Yusko, PsyD, Center for the Treatment and Study of Anxiety, University of Pennsylvania, Philadelphia, Pennsylvania

Allan Zuckoff, PhD, Department of Psychology, University of Pittsburgh, Pittsburgh, Pennsylvania

Preface

Motivational interviewing (MI) is an approach for helping people change that was originally developed by William R. Miller and Stephen Rollnick. It has had a substantial impact on research and practice in the fields of substance abuse and health-related problems in the United States and many other countries.

There are several reasons for its appeal. First, it directly addresses a significant problem common to all therapies: client ambivalence about change. The primary goals of MI are to help clients resolve ambivalence and increase their intrinsic motivation for change. Second, it is flexible and can be used as a "stand-alone" therapy, a pretreatment or adjunct to other therapies, a method to motivate people in need of therapy to seek it, or an integrative framework within which other therapies can be conducted. Third, there is a considerable body of research evidence supporting both the efficacy and effectiveness of MI with substance use and health-related problems. Fourth, research has demonstrated that MI achieves significant therapeutic effects in relatively few sessions. Because of these appealing features, MI has much to offer the field of psychotherapy.

In the preface to the first edition, we wrote, ". . . it is surprising that MI has hardly been employed or studied outside of the fields of substance use and health-related concerns." As the chapters in this book illustrate, this situation has changed a great deal. MI is being applied to many more problems. For example, this edition contains chapters on MI and suicidal ideation, intimate partner violence, and the transdiagnostic treatment of emotional disorders. At the time of the first edition, there was little or no research in these areas. Furthermore, there are now more publications using rigorous research designs than there were in the past.

The scope has widened and the number of empirical studies using strong designs has increased. MI is clearly gaining momentum in the field of psychotherapy because of its ability to increase motivation in clients and enhance clinical outcomes. We approached this second edition with the goal of further encouraging this momentum.

These chapters represent advances in research and practice in MI. Each describes a clinical problem and its usual treatments, how MI has been used, any modifications that were necessary to tailor MI to the problem and population, detailed clinical case histories, and a summary of the relevant research.

A recent search of the literature on MI found extensions to clinical problems not covered in the book. We have listed these below. Unfortunately, these works were published too late for us to invite these authors to contribute to this book.

- Phobias: Abramsky (2013)
- Sex offenders: Marshall and O'Brien (2014)
- Sleep problems: Willgerodt, Kieckhefer, Ward, and Lentz (2014)
- Teaching MI to parents of young adults with schizophrenia: Smeerdijk et al. (2014)

There is still a long way to go in developing clinical treatment methods that incorporate MI for a wider array of clinical problems, and to evaluate these treatments with strong research designs. Our goal in this edition is to further encourage work on MI and psychotherapy.

This book represents a truly collaborative effort on the part of the coeditors. William R. Miller and Stephen Rollnick have done a great deal of research and clinical work using MI with substance use disorders and health-related problems. Hal Arkowitz has done research and clinical work extending the use of MI to depression and anxiety.

Clinical practitioners from a number of disciplines will find a wealth of information in this book on applications of MI, along with numerous case histories and vignettes. Clinical researchers will find in it a rich source of hypotheses to be tested regarding the efficacy, effectiveness, and mechanisms of MI. Graduate students in clinical, counseling, and rehabilitation psychology as well as those in social work programs will also find this book of interest. We view MI as a clinical tool that does not compete with or displace, but rather can be integrated with, a variety of other psychotherapeutic interventions. We look forward to what future research and practice will reveal about such integration.

For several years, one of us (H. A.) has taught a clinical research practicum on MI to clinical psychology graduate students at the University of Arizona. It has been very well received, and at the end of the course most students said they expected to incorporate it into their future clinical work, and some into their future research. Later contact with some of these students showed that, for the most part, they have. For two decades in the PhD training program in clinical psychology at the University of New Mexico, another of us (W. R. M.) offered an introductory practicum, teaching MI as foundational interviewing and counseling skills within which other clinical interventions can be provided. We hope other universities will offer courses and practica on MI. If they do, this book can serve as a text or as supplementary reading in seminars and practica on other forms of psychotherapy.

References

Abramsky, L. (2013). *Therapist self-disclosure and motivational interviewing statements on treatment seeking of aviophobics.* Unpublished doctoral dissertation, Hofstra University, Hempstead, New York.

Marshall, W. L., & O'Brien, M. D. (2014). Balancing clients' strengths and deficits in sexual offender treatment: The Rockwood treatment approach. In R. C. Tafrate & D. Mitchell (Eds.), *Forensic CBT: A handbook for clinical practice* (pp. 281–301). Hoboken, NJ: Wiley-Blackwell.

Smeerdijk, M., Keet, R., de Haan, L., Barrowclaw, C., Linszen, D., & Schippers, G. (2014). Feasibility of teaching motivational interviewing to parents of young adults with recent onset schizophrenia and co-occurring caanbis use. *Journal of Substance Abuse Treatment, 46,* 340–345.

Willgerodt, M., Kieckhefer, G. M., Ward, T. M., & Lentz, M. J. (2014). Feasibility of using actigraphy and motivational-based interviewing to improve sleep among school-age children and their parents. *Journal of School Nursing, 30,* 136–148.

Contents

CHAPTER 1

• • • • • •

Learning, Applying, and Extending Motivational Interviewing

William R. Miller
Hal Arkowitz

Since the first clinical description of motivational interviewing (MI; Miller, 1983), research and clinical applications have blossomed like wildflowers. From its original use with problem drinkers, MI is now being implemented in a broad array of other applications including health promotion, social work, psychotherapy, coaching, medicine, dentistry, and education. In this chapter we offer an overview of MI and the ways it has been used in clinical practice, and then we address the evidence base, why MI works, and how clinicians learn it.

Motivation in Clinical Practice and Research

The concept of motivation has played a significant role in the history of psychology (Cofer & Apley, 1964; Myers, 2011; Petri & Govern, 2012), though this scientific knowledge base has seldom been applied in psychotherapy. The concept of motivation is particularly pertinent when clients seem "stuck." A traditional therapeutic view is that such "stuckness" represents resistance to change. Clients are sometimes said to be resistive, oppositional, or "in denial," terms that have a pejorative connotation

1

implying pathology and willful (even if unconscious) obstruction of the therapist's benevolent efforts. Schools of psychotherapy have had differing views on the nature and origins of resistance and how to work with it. Focusing instead on the psychological dynamics of motivation can invoke a more positive emphasis on how and why people *do* change and how therapists can facilitate it (Engle & Arkowitz, 2006; Miller, 1985).

Social psychologist Kurt Lewin (1935) described various motivational conflicts (such as approach–avoidance) whereby people can be immobilized by ambivalence. Rather than being a pathological phenomenon, ambivalence is a normal and common human condition whereby people simultaneously want and do not want something. Clients who seek therapy are often ambivalent about change, and their motivation may ebb and flow during the course of treatment. MI is a method for helping clients to get unstuck and resolve such ambivalence in favor of positive change.

Within the transtheoretical model of change (Prochaska & Norcross, 2013), ambivalence is a normal process on the road to change. In fact, ambivalence (the contemplation stage) is a step forward from the earlier precontemplation stage, where change is not even being considered. Many therapies and therapists are prepared to help clients who have already progressed two steps further to the action stage—but what about those who are not yet ready for change? In addiction treatment, such clients were once told to go away and come back when they were motivated. That's not good enough. Helping people to work through ambivalence and readiness for change is an important therapeutic skill, enabling one to work with a broader range of clients than just those who are already sufficiently "motivated."

Now, consider the interpersonal dynamic when a client who is ambivalent about change sits down to talk with a therapist who wants to promote change. Miller and Rollnick (2013) have described a natural "righting reflex" of professional helpers to educate, persuade, and advise clients about change. Doing so takes up one side of the client's ambivalence, the prochange side. A predictable result is for the person to then respond with the other side of ambivalence, "Yes, but . . . " If the therapist reciprocates with counterargument, he or she has thereby in essence externalized the person's ambivalence, with the clinician advocating for change while the client argues against it. There are both theoretical and empirical reasons to be concerned that this pattern is countertherapeutic, actually *decreasing* clients' commitment to change.

Daryl Bem (1967) posited that, from a conceptual perspective, people learn what they believe in the same way that others do, namely, by hearing what they say. If a noncoercive context (such as counterattitudinal role play) causes them to defend a particular position, they become more committed to that position. Bem's self-perception theory offered an alternative explanation for the large literature on cognitive dissonance (Festinger, 1957). It is also clear that external pressure can undermine the desire to change. Brehm and Brehm (1981) adduced that an aversive state of reactance arises when people perceive a threat to their behavioral freedom. One motivational response is to intensify one's attitudes and behaviors in opposition to the persuasion or coercion.

Empirical evidence can be derived from studies of psycholinguistic processes in MI. In spontaneous speech, clients' ambivalence is represented by the balance of change talk (verbalizations favoring change) and sustain talk (favoring the status quo). The ratio of change talk to sustain talk during treatment sessions predicts the likelihood of subsequent behavior change (Moyers, Martin, Houck, Christopher, & Tonigan, 2009). This finding parallels similar ones from the transtheoretical model that movement from contemplation to action is signaled by an increase in the pros relative to the cons of change (Prochaska, 1994). This relationship might be of only passing interest ("Motivated people are the ones who change") were it not that levels of client change talk and sustain talk or resistance are strongly influenced by therapist responses, as demonstrated in both correlational (Bertholet, Faouzi, Gmel, Gaume, & Daeppen, 2010; Daeppen, Bertholet, Gmel, & Gaume, 2007; Gaume, Bertholet, Faouzi, Gmel, & Daeppen, 2010; Moyers & Martin, 2006; Moyers et al., 2009) and experimental studies (Glynn & Moyers, 2010; Miller, Benefield, & Tonigan, 1993; Patterson & Forgatch, 1985). Thus, if therapists counsel in a way that evokes more sustain talk or "resistance" than change talk, clients are less likely to change. In contrast, change is promoted by differentially evoking from clients their own change talk.

Related findings from social psychology are found in the literature on decisional balance. As mentioned above, a person's balance of pros to cons (a passive *measure* of decisional balance) reflects readiness for and probability of change. As a clinical procedure, however, decisional balance involves actively evoking and exploring *all* the pros and cons of change, thus causing clients to voice both change talk and sustain talk. Clinical studies indicate that doing this with people who are ambivalent consistently *decreases* their commitment to change (Miller & Rose, 2015), perhaps by perpetuating rather than resolving ambivalence.

What Is MI?

MI is a particular way of having a conversation about change so that it is the client rather than the clinician who voices the arguments for change (Miller, 1983; Miller & Rollnick, 2013). It is strongly rooted in the person-centered approach of Carl Rogers (1951, 1959, 1980) in its emphasis on understanding the client's internal frame of reference and concerns. In both MI and client-centered counseling the therapist provides the conditions for growth and change by communicating attitudes of acceptance and accurate empathy.

MI can be thought of as an evolution of client-centered counseling. It differs from a classic "nondirective" approach in that there is clear direction toward one or more specific outcome goals, and the therapist uses systematic strategies to move toward those goals. Usually it is the client who brings the change goal(s), although in certain contexts (such as addiction treatment or probation) the clinician may by role have change goals that the client does not necessarily share, at least at the outset.

Four Processes of MI

MI is now described as comprising four processes. The first of these is *engaging*, developing a therapeutic alliance that facilitates working together. Client-centered counseling skills are prominent here from the very beginning. A second process is *focusing*, clarifying the goals and direction of counseling. With a clear goal in place, the *evoking* process involves eliciting the client's own motivations for change. It is here that the therapist attends in particular to the client's change talk, seeking to evoke, understand, reflect, explore, and summarize it. When there seems to be sufficient readiness for change MI proceeds to the fourth process of *planning*. Though the four processes sound linear, in practice they are quite recursive. One may double back from planning to evoking if motivation seems to wane. It is common for the focus of consultation to change, and at times it is important to strengthen engagement. Somewhat different skills are involved in each process, though the client-centered engaging skills form a foundation throughout MI.

Underlying Spirit of MI

There is also strong overlap between a person-centered approach and what the codevelopers have described as the underlying *spirit* of MI

(Miller & Rollnick, 2013; Rollnick & Miller, 1995). Without this larger mindset and "heartset" in practice, MI can be confused with and reduced to a set of techniques. Accurate empathy has been a key element in MI from the start (Miller, 1983) and is linked to therapeutic efficacy (Moyers & Miller, 2013). Empathy is central to the first of four fundamentals of the spirit of MI: *acceptance*, which also includes honoring clients' autonomy, affirming their strengths, and respecting each person's absolute worth as a human being. A second component of MI spirit is an attitude of *partnership*, a collaboration between the clinician's expertise and clients' own expertise about themselves. The component of *compassion* is the intention to give primacy to the client's own welfare, growth, and best interests. Finally *evocation* is the mindset of calling forth the client's own wisdom, values, ideas, and plans. Evocation is the opposite of a deficit model—that the client is lacking something that the therapist needs to install. Rather than communicating "I have what you need, and I will give it to you," the underlying message in MI is "You have what you need, and together we will find it."

Compatibility with Other Methods

MI was never intended to be a comprehensive psychotherapy. It is a therapeutic tool for addressing the common issue of ambivalence about change. Miller (1983) first conceptualized it as a prelude to or preparation for treatment, and a surprise in early studies was that after MI clients often proceeded to change their drinking on their own without seeking further treatment (Miller et al., 1993; Miller, Sovereign, & Krege, 1988). Thus MI is sometimes practiced as a free-standing treatment, often as a brief opportunistic intervention. More commonly, though, MI is being combined with other treatments such as cognitive-behavioral therapies (Longabaugh, Zweben, LoCastro, & Miller, 2005). A meta-analysis found that MI had the most enduring effects when it was combined with another active treatment (Hettema, Steele, & Miller, 2005).

In one common adaptation known as motivational enhancement therapy (MET), the client is given personal feedback based on individual results from standardized assessment measures (Ball, Todd, et al., 2007; Miller, Zweben, Diclemente, & Rychtarik, 1992; Stephens, Babor, Kadden, & Miller, 2002). This feedback, which concerns the client's level of severity on target symptoms compared to norms, is delivered in an MI style. MET may be particularly useful in working with clients at a "precontemplation" level, who perceive little or no reason to change (Miller & Rollnick, 2013).

Basic Engaging Skills of MI

Four clinical microskills derived from client-centered counseling are used throughout MI, abbreviated by the mnemonic acronym OARS. The O component is to ask *Open* questions that give clients latitude in how to respond. Often intake interviews consist of a long litany of closed, short-answer questions that leave the client in a fairly passive role: "I ask the questions, and you give me the information I want." Carl Rogers's tongue-in-cheek skepticism about assessment was that it's of limited use because the client already knows all this! Beyond the asymmetrical power relationship of question and answer, this approach also implies that once you have enough information then you will have the solution. MI generally avoids this "expert role" where the therapist pretends to know more about clients than they do themselves. If change is to be integrated into people's daily lives, their own expertise about themselves is a vital resource. There are also informal guidelines to limit questioning, such as not to ask three questions in a row (even open questions).

A is for *Affirming.* In MI, clinicians watch for and affirm clients' strengths and abilities. Each step in the right direction, no matter how small, is recognized and affirmed. Clients are often asked to describe their own strengths, a "self-affirmation" process that tends to strengthen therapeutic alliance and reduce defensiveness. Rather than focusing on pathology or criticizing shortcomings, the clinician seeks to "catch people doing something right." This affirming of strengths and efforts is consistent with communicating positive regard. Some simple examples of affirmations are "It took courage to do that" and "That's a really good idea."

Perhaps the most frequently used microskill in MI is *Reflection,* a key method for experiencing and communicating accurate empathy. Simple reflections repeat all or part of what the client said. Though helpful at times, they are quite limited and often feel unnatural. Therapeutic momentum is much better promoted through complex reflections that make a guess about what the person means but has not quite said yet. One way to think about this is "continuing the paragraph"—not repeating what the client has just said but instead saying what *might* be the next phrase or sentence in the paragraph. The goal is to understand clearly how clients are experiencing their reality and to reflect that understanding back to them in a way that encourages continued experiencing.

Many therapists learn about reflective listening as part of their early training in basic interviewing skills. It is easy to underestimate the difficulty of skillful empathic reflection. High-quality reflective listening is a core skill in MI and in the person-centered approach more generally. The majority of responses from a skillful MI practitioner should be reflective guesses about the client's meaning. It can be a challenge for novices as well as experienced professionals to rely primarily on empathic reflection rather than asking questions, offering advice, and relating in other ways that impose an external frame of reference.

Finally, the *S* in OARS is a reminder to *Summarize*. Summaries play an important role in client-centered counseling and have more particular uses in MI. They not only show that you have been listening and value what clients say enough to remember it; good summaries also link material together and can help emphasize certain points.

Beyond the OARS, MI includes a particular way of offering information and advice when appropriate. The most general guideline is to offer information or advice *with permission* and not tell clients what they already know. A client may ask you for suggestions ("What do you think I should do?"), and you can ask directly for permission ("Would it be helpful if I told you some things that other people have done that worked for them?"). Such offerings in MI are often accompanied by autonomy-supporting statements like "You may or may not agree" or "I don't know whether this will concern you or not—it's up to you, really." Rather than downloading an uninterrupted sequence of information, the interviewer offers it in small chunks, checking in regularly for the client's own responses and perceptions, a sequence that Rollnick has termed "elicit–provide–elicit" (Rollnick, Miller, & Butler, 2008).

Focusing

Sometimes the focus for conversations about change is set by the context. A person who walks into a smoking cessation clinic does not wonder what the topic of conversation will be. In more general health and social services it is usually the client who offers presenting concerns to be addressed. Then there is the situation where the clinician has a focus or concern that the client may not share. Brief opportunistic interventions are of this kind. A patient comes to a clinic wanting relief from a cough and sore throat, and the physician wants to talk about smoking. Probation officers and disciplinary administrators regularly enter into conversations about change with less-than-eager participants. Many clients are referred to addiction treatment services by the courts or relatives and offer mostly sustain talk at the beginning. MI can be used in any of these circumstances to move toward an identified goal. The focusing process is to identify mutually acceptable goals. When a change goal is prescribed by the context or a client is ambivalent, a challenge is to find the client's own motivation to move toward that goal. That is the process of evoking.

Evoking

Evoking is the process that is most unique to MI. Having identified a clear focus for the conversation about change, the clinician proceeds to steer the conversation toward finding and exploring the client's own motivations for change. This involves three sets of skills for *recognizing, eliciting,* and *responding* to change talk. This is not to stay that sustain talk is ignored or disrespected. When a client offers sustain talk, as happens naturally in ambivalence, the clinician listens to and often reflects it. It is interesting that sometimes when you reflect sustain talk, the client responds with the other side of ambivalence. Consider this actual exchange:

CLIENT: I really don't think alcohol is a problem for me.

INTERVIEWER: Drinking hasn't really caused you any problems.

CLIENT: Well, it does. Anybody who drinks as much as I do is bound to have some problems.

The MI clinician, however, is particularly interested in finding and exploring change talk and usually does not go looking for sustain talk (as one might do in a decisional balance intervention). This emphasis requires, first, being able to recognize change talk when you hear it and, second, realizing that, of all the things clients say to you, this is particularly important material because it predicts change.

Recognizing Change Talk

So, what is change talk? In the most general sense, it is anything clients say that signals a move toward or openness to change. You already know much about this just by virtue of being a member of society. When you ask someone to do something, you pay particularly close attention to what he or she says in response to your request because the person's words contain clues as to how likely it is to happen:

"I'll do it this afternoon."
"I'll try to do it."

"I might be able to."
"I would if I could."

Each culture has a natural language for transactions about change. The psycholinguist Paul Amrhein was particularly helpful in clarifying and specifying different kinds of change talk in MI (Amrhein, 1992; Amrhein, Miller, Yahne, Palmer, & Fulcher, 2003; Moyers et al., 2007).

Some kinds of change talk are termed *preparatory* in that they signal inclination toward change without committing to it. Four types of preparatory change talk are abbreviated in the acronym DARN: Desire, Ability, Reasons, and Need.

Every language on earth has a way of saying "I want" (Goddard & Wierzbicka, 1994). Desire statements imply an approach motivation: I want, like, wish, prefer, and the like.

"I *want* to feel less anxious."
"I would *like* to lose some weight."
"I *wish* I were more comfortable talking to people."

Ability statements imply the possibility of change:

"I know I *can* be kinder to my wife."
"I am *able* to resist temptation sometimes."
"I *could* just keep my mouth shut."

Reason statements have an if–then quality, expressing a desirable outcome if the change were made or an undesirable outcome without change.

"If I get arrested again I'll lose my job."
"My kids would be happy if I didn't criticize them so much."
"I should take my medication so I can concentrate at work."

Finally, Need statements have an imperative quality of must, have to, need to without necessarily stating a reason why:

"Something has got to change in our relationship."
"I have to get over this performance anxiety."
"I need to have a better relationship with my kids."

Other kinds of statements are called *mobilizing* change talk because they signal movement in the direction of change. An acronym here is CATs: Commitment, Activation, and Taking steps.

Commitment language is how we make promises and agreements. In a way, the strongest committing speech is also the simplest: I will. I do. I promise. There are also endless subtleties to signal greater or lesser degrees of willingness:

"I probably will."
"I promise, I guess."
"I guarantee that I will."

Then there are Activation statements that are not quite commitment but do signal willingness.

"I'll consider it."
"I'm willing to."
"I might."

Taking steps statements refer to something the person has already done to move toward change. This might occur when a client returns for the next session and says:

"I bought a pair of running shoes this week [with the goal of exercising more]."
"I filled the prescription you gave me."
"I did the diary that you asked me to keep."
"I went 2 days without smoking this week."

Change talk matters because it presages change. It literally is clients talking themselves into change (Miller & Rollnick, 2004). Some good news is that it is not the client's level of change talk and sustain talk at the beginning of a session that predicts change (or the lack thereof); rather, it is client speech toward the *end* of an MI session and the pattern over the course of the session (Amrhein et al., 2003). During a successful MI session the balance of change talk to sustain talk gradually shifts. In an experimental design, this balance rises and drops as the counselor shifts back and forth between MI and a more directive method (Glynn & Moyers, 2010).

Sustain talk is simply the opposite of change talk. It consists of statements that reflect an inclination toward the status quo and away from change. If the topic were whether to begin exposure-based treatment for posttraumatic stress disorder [PTSD], a client might say:

"I really don't *want* to do it!" [Desire]
"I *can't* do it." [Ability]
"It would bring up all of those memories for me again." [Reason]
"I don't *need* to do it." [Need]
"I'm not going to do it, period." [Commitment]
"I'm not ready." [Activation]
"I cancelled my appointment." [Taking steps]

With people who are ambivalent, it is normal to hear both change talk and sustain talk together, even in the same sentence and often with a "but" in the middle.

"I want to [change talk], but I don't think I can do it [sustain talk]."
"I'm not very happy about it [sustain talk], but I need to [change talk]."
"It's not what I want to do [sustain talk], it's what I'm going to do [change talk]."

The key to recognizing change talk is to tune your ear to hear it so that it stands out in your perception whenever it occurs.

Eliciting Change Talk

You don't have to wait for change talk to occur (though with ambivalent people you're likely to hear it regardless). There are evoking skills that invite clients to express change talk.

Perhaps the easiest and most common way to elicit change talk is to ask for it with an open question. This involves thinking one step ahead: If I ask this, what is the client likely to answer? Consider the expected answers to these open questions:

"What are some good reasons for you to make this change?" [Change talk]
"Why haven't you done it?" [Sustain talk]
"Knowing what you do about yourself, how might you be able to do it?" [Change talk]
"What do you like about how things are now?" [Sustain talk]

Ask open questions the answer to which is change talk.
Another evoking strategy involves looking ahead, asking clients

what could be the advantages of making the change and what might happen if they continue on their present course. Exploring hopes and values also can be useful.

> "How would you like for your life to be different a year from now?"
> "What is the worst that might happen if you keep on as you have been?"
> "What do you care about most? How would you like to be remembered?"

A simple scaling question is to ask "On a scale from 0 to 10, where 0 is not at all important and 10 is the most important thing in your life right now, how important would you say it is for you to _____?" The client offers a number, perhaps a 4. Which would be the better follow-up question?

> "And why are you at a 4 instead of 0 or 1?"
> "And why are you at a 4 instead of a 6 or 7?"

The answer to the former is likely to be change talk, whereas the answer to the latter would probably be sustain talk.

These are just a few examples of ways to evoke change talk. There are hundreds of ways to do it, and you get immediate feedback from your client as to whether you're doing it well.

Responding to Change Talk

When you hear change talk, don't just sit there. If you respond in particular ways, you are likely to hear more change talk. For those four ways there is yet another acronym: EARS.

Actually EARS is just OARS with the first letter changed to an *E* because it is a specific type of open question—one that asks for *Elaboration* or an *Example*. If a client were to say "I think I would feel better if I exercised more," an *E* response could be:

> "In what ways do you think you would feel better?"
> "When have you felt good after exercising? Give me an example."
> "How do you think exercising more might help you?"

All of these encourage the client to keep exploring the change talk theme that was just offered. Ask such questions with curiosity and a desire to understand better what the person means.

A again is for *Affirm*. You can offer a statement of appreciation or encouragement in response to change talk:

"Good for you!"
"That sounds like a good idea!"
"You really want to stay healthy."

Perhaps the most natural response to change talk is to *Reflect* it. This again encourages the person to keep exploring and elaborating on the change talk.

CLIENT: We just never talk. We don't communicate.

INTERVIEWER: You'd like to be communicating better. [Simple reflection]

CLIENT: Yes! Sometimes we go for hours at home without saying anything.

INTERVIEWER: That sounds kind of lonely. [Complex reflection]

CLIENT: Well, it is. I feel like he takes me for granted.

INTERVIEWER: And you would like to feel closer and cared for. [Complex reflection, continuing the paragraph]

CLIENT: Isn't that what a marriage is all about?

INTERVIEWER: It's really important to you, important enough that you're willing to work on it. [Trying out some additional change talk]

CLIENT: I am.

In general training on empathic listening, there is often little guidance about what to reflect out of all that a client says. In MI, it is particularly important to hear and reflect the client's change talk.

Similarly, although *Summarizing* is often taught as a basic counseling skill, there are usually few guidelines about what to include in a summary. In MI, one is first listening for and evoking change talk and reflecting it when it occurs. As change talk accumulates, the clinician offers summaries that pull it together. Each bit of change talk is like a flower, and the interviewer is assembling a bouquet. After hearing two or three flowers, offer back a small summary:

"So far, you've said that you would like to be communicating better in your relationship and you wish you would spend more time together doing fun things instead of just the routine. How else do you think you might strengthen your relationship?"

The open question invites more flowers, and as they come the bouquet grows larger. When you sense that you have collected all the change talk that is readily available, you can offer a recapitulation summary that pulls it all together. Thus, clients first hear themselves expressing change talk, then hear it again as you reflect it, and then hear it again in summaries alongside their other change talk. This is a path out of ambivalence, and one that is more difficult to do alone, when self-talk tends to vacillate between change talk and sustain talk that negate each other.

Planning

The fourth process in MI is planning, developing a specific plan for how to implement change or at least a first step. Clients often signal you that they are ready to begin the planning process by offering more mobilizing change talk and less sustain talk. You can test the water by offering a recapitulation summary of change talk and then asking a key question the essence of which is "So, what next?"

> "Given what you've said so far, what do you think you ought to do?"
> "So, what are you thinking at this point about how to proceed?"
> "If you do want to move in this direction, what might be a good first step for you?"

Perhaps the main point about planning in MI is that you are still evoking the plan from the client, drawing on the person's expertise. The MI style encourages a change plan that comes primarily from the client rather than the therapist. Switching into a directive mode at this point can undermine the motivational progress that has been made. As stated earlier, it is fine to offer some information or advice with permission, but beware of uninvited advice. What is the person ready, willing, and able to do? You may encourage the client to think about change with questions like "How do you think you can make that happen?" At times, clients may be motivated to change but not know what they need to do in order to accomplish the change (e.g., to reduce panic attacks). At such times, your own expertise is a useful and necessary part of therapy. The issue isn't whether or not advice and suggestions are offered but rather *how and when* they are offered. In MI, this input is given by a therapist who assumes the role of guide or change consultant. A guide doesn't decide when or where you should go but instead helps you get to where you want to go. If the client wishes, you may make suggestions about various possible ways to proceed, with the attitude that the client will choose those options that fit best at present. For example, a therapist might say the following to a client who appears ready to change but doesn't know how to do it: "I have some thoughts about approaches that have been helpful for other people with a similar problem. Would you be interested in hearing them?" In this way, the therapist conveys respect for the clients' ability to choose what's best for them while being ready to provide input to facilitate change.

We should note that people often vacillate in their degree of motivation and ambivalence within and across sessions. As Mahoney (2001) suggested, change is best described as an oscillating process. It is seldom linear or unidimensional. Most people who seek therapy have more than one concern or are weighing change at various levels—for example, depression is often accompanied by relationship problems and substance abuse. There may be different degrees of motivation for change in these different problem areas. In addition, Arkowitz and Burke (2008) and Zuckoff, Swartz, and Grote (Chapter 6, this volume) distinguish between motivation to change the overall problem (e.g., anxiety) and motivation to engage in the actions necessary to accomplish the change. A person highly motivated to decrease distress may nevertheless be unwilling to pursue a particular strategy for doing so. There may be ambivalence about one or both of these.

It is normal for there to be multiple goals. More than half of those with a diagnosis of either an anxiety or depressive disorder meet the criteria for at least one additional anxiety or depressive disorder (Brown, Campbell, Lehman, Grisham, & Mancill, 2001). With substance use disorders as with many others, comorbidity seems to be the rule rather than the exception (Miller, Forcehimes, & Zweben, 2011). Clients may be at different stages of readiness for change in each problem area. A client might be highly motivated to work on his or her anxiety disorder but disinclined to change his or her substance use. Fortunately, therapeutic change in one problem area is often associated with improvement in other problem areas (Newman, Przeworski, Fisher, & Borkovec, 2010).

Resistance

In the first two editions of *Motivational Interviewing* (Miller & Rollnick, 1991, 2002) the concept of resistance was prominent. In fact, during the first decade or two a common motivation for clinicians to seek

MI training was the unanswered question "How can I deal with my most resistant and difficult clients?"

The third edition (Miller & Rollnick, 2013) signaled a significant shift away from the concept of resistance, which as noted earlier has somewhat pejorative overtones that imply it is a client problem. Two findings prompted this movement away from "resistance." The first was abundant evidence that the behavior termed "resistance" is highly responsive to therapist style. It can literally be dialed up or down by changes in therapist response (Glynn & Moyers, 2010; Patterson & Forgatch, 1985). It takes two to "resist." Secondly, it became clear that most of what had been described as resistance was merely *sustain talk*, a normal manifestation of ambivalence.

If one subtracts sustain talk from resistance, what is left? Miller and Rollnick (2013) termed it "discord," behavior that signals dissonance in the therapeutic relationship. Unlike sustain talk, which is about the change target, discord statements often contain the word "you":

"You don't understand how hard it is for me."
"You can't tell me what to do."
"I'm not sure if you can really help me."
"You're not listening to me."

Both sustain talk and discord are highly responsive to therapist style, and high levels of either predict a lack of change.

Both sustain talk and discord are important and warrant your notice and response. Our clinical experience, however, is that if you start with an MI style from the beginning you are unlikely to encounter much discord along the way. Sustain talk will still be there, of course, because it is normal with ambivalence, but as MI proceeds sustain talk tends to wane while change talk increases. Neither is sustain talk or discord necessarily a product of client pathology; both are clearly responsive to interpersonal dynamics.

Relationship of MI to Other Psychotherapies

MI is more of a "way of being" with people than it is another "school" of therapy (Rogers, 1980). Yet, as in other types of psychotherapy, the goal is to facilitate therapeutic change. In this section, we will compare and contrast MI with other psychotherapies and briefly discuss how MI can be used in conjunction with these other therapies.

While MI is strongly rooted in Carl Rogers's client-centered therapy, it also shares similarities with other therapeutic approaches. MI and psychoanalytic therapies view ambivalence or resistance as providing meaningful information that can be used productively in therapy. However, they differ sharply in the types of information that they consider important and how they respond to it. In psychoanalytic theories, resistance is usually thought of as conflict, mostly unconscious, between the client and therapist. A central construct in psychodynamic theories and therapies is transference, the unconscious tendency for the client to assign to the therapist feelings and attitudes associated with the client's early significant and problematic relationships, especially with parents, early in life. In this context, resistance provides clues to repressed conflicts that are carried over from the past, and re-enactment in therapy allows the therapist to help the client resolve the resistance and the early conflicts associated with it. By contrast, MI is almost entirely focused on the here and now, without *a priori* views about why ambivalence occurs. Ambivalence and discord are not seen as reflecting pathology. In MI, what is important is to understand the client's perspective and evoke his or her own motivations for change.

In cognitive-behavioral therapy (CBT) ambivalence is seldom discussed and is not given any special status, though some behavior therapists (e.g., Patterson & Forgatch, 1985) and cognitive-behavioral therapists (e.g., Leahy, 2002) have addressed resistance. A behavioral perspective attributes "resistance" to the therapist's inadequate conceptualization of the conditions that control the behaviors. Cognitive therapists (e.g., Beck, Rush, Shaw, & Emery, 1979) regard resistance as providing information about a client's distorted thinking and beliefs. For example, when a depressed client in cognitive therapy doesn't comply with homework assignments, cognitive therapists search for the beliefs and schemas that may be causing the resistance, such as pessimism about change.

In contrast to MI, CBT is a fairly didactic approach that emphasizes teaching clients new behaviors and ways to correct dysfunctional beliefs. CBT operates largely from a deficit model, implying that the client's problems emanate from something that is missing (e.g., skills, rational thinking, appropriate contingencies) that the therapist can teach. The use of the phrase "homework assignments" in CBT highlights the role of the therapist as more of a teacher in the change enterprise. The CBT therapist is regarded as an expert who can provide direction for the client in facilitating change. By contrast, MI involves more of an equal partnership than an expert–patient relationship.

MI has the potential for enhancing the effectiveness of CBT and other therapies. MI can provide a context for integrative therapy and the use of cognitive-behavioral methods (Arkowitz, 2002; Engle & Arkowitz, 2006; Miller, 1988). Strategies of both cognitive-behavioral and psychoanalytic therapies (such as structuring between-session activities in the former and giving interpretations in the latter) can be conducted in the context of a relationship that is more congruent with MI rather than in a manner that is more expert-driven. With the benefits of accurate empathy and evoking clients' own motivations for change, MI has the potential to enhance the efficacy of other active treatments.

How Effective Is MI?

How well does MI work, for what, and for whom? Across four decades a large body of research has accumulated to answer these questions. We summarize this literature here in three sections: (1) the efficacy of MI in clinical trials, (2) the relative efficacy of MI when compared with other approaches, and (3) studies of clinical effectiveness—how well the method holds up in community practice, outside the controlled conditions of clinical research. The MI website includes a cumulative bibliography of this literature (see *www.motivationalinterviewing.org*).

Efficacy Trials

Randomized clinical trials are often considered to be the gold standard in demonstrating treatment efficacy. In these studies participants agree to be randomly assigned to receive different treatments (such as MI or a comparison condition). Those in the comparison condition may receive no treatment, be placed on a waiting list, or receive treatment as usual or a different type of treatment. As we completed this chapter, more than 200 randomized clinical trials had been published for interventions identified with MI, along with many reviews and meta-analyses summarizing research findings (Britt, Hudson, & Blampied, 2004; Heckman, Egleston, & Hofmann, 2010; Hettema et al., 2005; Lundahl et al., 2013; Lundahl, Kunz, Brownell, Tollefson, & Burke, 2010; Rubak, Sandbaek, Lauritzen, & Christensen, 2005).

Several general conclusions may be drawn from this literature. There is strong evidence that MI can be effective in triggering behavior change, with average effect size generally in the small to medium range across a wide variety of target problems. Another clear pattern is high variability in the efficacy of MI across studies, therapists, and sites within multisite trials, related in part to the quality or fidelity of MI that is delivered (Miller & Rollnick, 2014). The outcome literature ranges from null findings to large effect sizes, suggesting that other unidentified factors may mediate or moderate the efficacy of MI. As with many psychotherapies, the specific effect of MI tends to diminish with the length of follow-up. An interesting exception is that MI has continued to show a sizable effect (0.6) that holds up over time when MI is added to another active treatment (Hettema et al., 2005). MI and other treatment methods seem to have a synergistic effect. MI may increase the efficacy of other methods by enhancing adherence, and the efficacy of MI benefits from the additive effect of adhering to another active treatment. In many such studies MI was used as a pretreatment to another therapy. Some studies have found that the effectiveness of MI is greater with clients who have more severe problems (e.g., Handmaker, Miller, & Manicke, 1999; Westra, Arkowitz, & Dozois, 2009).

Relative Efficacy of MI

What happens when MI is compared directly with other treatment methods? Here, MI is not added to another approach, but instead clients are assigned at random to receive MI or a different treatment. Across studies, people receiving MI tend to show more change relative to those given advice or treated with educational, didactic, or persuasive interventions. When MI is compared with other active treatment approaches (such as CBT), outcomes tend to be similar, though the MI treatment usually involves fewer sessions (Babor & Del Boca, 2003; Hodgins, Currie, & el-Guebaly, 2001; Marijuana Treatment Project Research Group, 2004; UKATT Research Team, 2005).

Clinical Effectiveness

Published studies tend to show significant positive effects of MI on behavior change under the highly controlled conditions of a randomized clinical trial, though there are also noteworthy examples of null findings (e.g., Miller, Yahne, & Tonigan, 2003). Efficacy trials, however, do not guarantee effectiveness when MI is applied by frontline clinicians under ordinary conditions of community practice with diverse populations (Ball, Martino, et al., 2007). Nevertheless, many studies have demonstrated significant clinical benefits of MI when delivered by frontline providers for problems such as alcohol (e.g., Senft, Polen, Freeborn,

& Hollis, 1997) and drug abuse (e.g., Bernstein et al., 2005; Marijuana Treatment Project Research Group, 2004), hypertension (e.g., Woollard et al., 1995), smoking (e.g., Heckman et al., 2010), and health promotion (e.g., Resnicow et al., 2001; Thevos, Quick, & Yanduli, 2000).

Several aspects of the clinical trial literature are also encouraging in regard to generalizability. MI has shown efficacy across a wide range of target problems, populations, providers, and nations. U.S. studies of MI with ethnic minority populations have shown, on average, substantially *larger* effects than those with primarily white Anglo-American populations (Hettema et al., 2005). MI may offer advantages in cross-cultural counseling, particularly because of the therapist's focus on understanding the client's unique context and perspective. Furthermore, studies in which clinicians delivered manual-guided MI showed *smaller* effects than those observed when MI did not follow the constrained guidelines of a manual (Hettema et al., 2005). This finding is consistent with an emphasis on the overall approach or spirit of MI rather than on specific techniques, and overly prescriptive manuals run the risk of decreasing therapist flexibility in a way that disadvantages effective use of the method. In any event, across multiple trials these findings indicate that MI is applicable to a range of populations and problems and does not require the structure of a procedural manual and adherence monitoring. Nevertheless, adequate training is needed for clinicians to be able to deliver MI with sufficient fidelity to impact client outcomes (Miller & Rollnick, 2014).

Why Does MI Work?

When the effectiveness of a therapy varies across providers and programs, it suggests the need to understand the critical elements that contribute to its effects. One component of MI regarded by its codevelopers (Miller, 1983; Miller & Rollnick, 1991) as central to its efficacy is the therapist quality of *accurate empathy* (Rogers, 1959; Truax & Carkhuff, 1967). Sometimes misunderstood as having had similar life experiences, accurate empathy actually refers to a learnable clinical skill for identifying and reflecting the client's own experiencing. In research preceding the introduction of MI, therapist interpersonal skill in this domain predicted subsequent client change (Miller, Taylor, & West, 1980; Truax & Carkhuff, 1967; Valle, 1981).

As practiced within MI, accurate empathy blends with other interpersonal skill components to constitute an underlying MI spirit, assessed by global ratings of clinician–client interactions (Baer et al., 2004; Miller & Mount, 2001; Moyers, Martin, Catley, Harris, & Ahluwalia, 2003; Moyers, Martin, Manuel, Hendrickson, & Miller, 2005). Observers' ratings of clinicians on this global scale predict more favorable client responses during an MI session (Moyers, Miller, & Hendrickson, 2005). Thus, one important component of the impact of MI appears to be the quality of the therapeutic relationship, reflected particularly in the skill of accurate empathy (Moyers & Miller, 2013).

Miller (1983) further hypothesized that MI would work by causing clients to verbalize their own arguments for change. Client ambivalence is resolved in the direction of change as clients express aloud the disadvantages of the status quo, the advantages of change, and their ability and intentions to change (Miller & Rollnick, 1991). Such client statements are now called change talk, and the strategic eliciting of client change talk differentiates MI from more general client-centered counseling (Miller & Rollnick, 2013). A wide range of studies has now confirmed a relationship between change talk expressed by clients during MI sessions and subsequent behavior change (Amrhein et al., 2003; Bertholet et al., 2010; Gaume et al., 2010; Hendrickson et al., 2004; Moyers et al., 2007, 2009).

In contrast, client speech that defends the status quo (sustain talk) predicts a lack of subsequent change (Amrhein et al., 2003; Miller, Benefield, & Tonigan, 1993). The more a client argues against change, the less likely it is to happen. This is not particularly surprising in itself ("Resistant clients don't change"). The implications for practice come from findings that client resistance is strongly influenced by the clinician's counseling style (Miller, Benefield, & Tonigan, 1993; Patterson & Forgatch, 1985). An important part of the impact of MI training may be to decrease counselors' countertherapeutic responses that evoke sustain talk and discord associated with poorer outcomes (White & Miller, 2007)

Much remains to be learned about the mechanisms underlying the efficacy of MI. Our current understanding of how MI works is this. If the clinician counsels in a way that elicits client defensiveness and sustain talk, change is unlikely to follow. If, on the other hand, the clinician provides accurate empathy and counsels in a way that evokes clients' own motivations for and commitment to change, then behavior change often follows.

A more complex question would be "Why or under what conditions does change talk lead to change?" Is change talk itself causal, or does it simply reflect some underlying process that leads to change? Simply reading, writing, or chanting change talk seems unlikely to effect change. Neural activation patterns during spontaneous change talk are quite different from those with artificially induced change talk (Feldstein Ewing, Filbey, Sabbineni, Chandler, & Hutchinson, 2011).

Are there clients for whom MI is particularly indicated or contraindicated? Here the evidence base is thin, but a trend is apparent. The more resistant (oppositional, angry) a client, the greater seems to be the advantage of MI relative to more prescriptive approaches (Karno & Longabaugh, 2004, 2005; Project MATCH Research Group, 1997). MI was specifically developed for clients who are ambivalent and less ready to proceed with change. Conversely, MI has been found to be unhelpful for people who have already decided to change. Within the new four-process model of MI (Miller & Rollnick, 2013), it is the evoking process that is unnecessary if a client is already prepared for change, and the appropriate method (with adequate engaging) would be to proceed to planning. Continuing to use evoking with clients who are already highly motivated may damage therapeutic rapport or even lead to dropout because therapist and client are not on the same page.

How Do Clinicians Learn MI?

Understanding how and why a treatment method works is helpful in knowing how to help clinicians learn it. This section focuses on what is known about how counselors learn the method of MI.

Eight Skills in Learning MI

Miller and Moyers (2006) have described eight skills by which clinicians acquire proficiency in MI. The first of these involves at least openness to the underlying assumptions and spirit of the method: a collaborative rather than prescriptive approach, eliciting motivation from the client rather than trying to install it, and honoring client autonomy rather than taking a more authoritarian or confrontational stance. Internalization of this overall spirit increases with practice, but one is unlikely to learn MI (or want to) without first being willing to entertain the feasibility of this approach. Learning MI is, in our experience, particularly difficult for those with a directive-expert perspective on the helping process. At the University of Arizona, Arkowitz has taught a semester-long MI practicum for students primarily trained in the directive style of cognitive-behavioral therapy. At first, MI seems to students like not doing anything useful. As their skill in MI progresses, however, the evidence of client changes usually convinces them that they are indeed "doing" something therapeutic with MI.

A next task, and a challenging one in itself, is to develop proficiency in the interpersonal skills of client-centered counseling, particularly accurate empathy. A skillful clinician makes reflective listening look easy, but it is a proficiency that is developed and honed over years of practice. To take the next steps in MI, the clinician needs skill and comfort in forming accurate reflections that move the client forward, encouraging continued exploration.

MI differs from client-centered counseling in the focus of MI on ambivalence and in particular on change talk. A third skill in learning MI, then, is for the counselor to learn to recognize change talk when hearing it, and to distinguish it from other forms of client speech. Being able to recognize change talk, the clinician next learns how to elicit and reinforce it. In other words, the counselor employs specific strategies to evoke change talk and responds differentially in order to increase and strengthen it. This is linked to a fifth skill, learning how to respond to sustain talk and discord so as not to increase it.

The exploration of client ambivalence can continue almost indefinitely, and there is another skill in knowing when the client is ready to proceed to planning. Helping clients to formulate change plans represents a sixth skill in learning MI. Prematurely pursuing a change plan, however, can elicit pushback, increasing client commitment to the status quo. In MI, the change planning process continues to be one of collaborative negotiation. With a change plan developed, it remains to engage client commitment to the plan—a seventh task in acquiring MI skillfulness.

Finally, there is the skill of flexibly blending MI with other therapeutic methods. MI was never intended to be a comprehensive treatment, displacing all others. In fact, some of its most consistent beneficial effects are in combination with other forms of treatment. Some counselors with a high level of skill in MI sometimes have difficulty switching back and forth flexibly with other styles when needed (Miller, Moyers, Arciniega, Ernst, & Forcehimes, 2005). Others find a way to blend the clinical style of MI with other therapeutic approaches without a feeling of switching back and forth (Longabaugh et al., 2005).

Initial Training

From the above-described set of skills, it is apparent that there is only so much a practitioner could learn from a one-time workshop on MI. Even a 2- to 3-day initial workshop led by a proficient MI trainer is likely to provide primarily an introduction to the basic style and spirit of MI, first steps toward learning reflective listening, and an ability to recognize change talk. A workshop is not the means but rather the *beginning* of learning MI. Some ambitious learning goals for an introductory workshop are:

1. To understand the underlying spirit and approach of MI.
2. To recognize reflective listening responses and differentiate them from other counseling responses.
3. To be able to provide at least 50% reflective listening responses during a conversation.
4. To recognize change talk and be able to differentiate commitment language from other types of change talk.
5. To list and demonstrate several different strategies for eliciting client change talk.

A workshop without follow-up, however, is unlikely to make a significant difference in practice. In an initial evaluation of Miller's own 2-day workshop, clinicians were able to demonstrate some skills on demand, but the changes in ongoing practice were minimal (Miller & Mount, 2001). More tellingly, there was no change in how clients responded to their therapists (e.g., change talk) after the workshop, suggesting no likely improvement in client outcomes.

What does seem to help in initially learning MI is a combination of ongoing feedback and coaching. This is sensible in that these two components—personal feedback and performance coaching—are helpful in learning most any complex skill. To yield a significant gain in clinical skill in MI, an introductory workshop should be followed by some ongoing individual feedback and coaching based on observation of actual practice with clients (Miller, Yahne, Moyers, Martinez, & Pirritano, 2004). Graduate training affords an opportunity for such ongoing shaping of clinical skillfulness. As mentioned earlier, the University of Arizona clinical psychology graduate program has offered a practicum on MI that involves lectures and discussion, demonstrations, roleplaying exercises, and ongoing supervision of clinical cases referred from the community. In a randomized trial of MI training strategies, therapists' clients showed increased change talk only when both feedback and coaching were provided after initial training (Amrhein, Miller, Yahne, Knupsky, & Hochstein, 2004).

Continuing to Learn

Excellent introductory training in MI, even with a few months of coaching support, still constitutes only an introduction to the clinical method.

(Imagine a 2-day workshop to learn psychoanalysis, tennis, piano, or chess.) The real learning is in doing, and that requires ongoing practice with feedback.

As it turns out, the needed feedback is built into the process of MI and depends upon knowing what to watch for. In response to a good reflective listening statement, the person keeps talking, reveals a bit more, explores a little further. The very process of reflective listening helps the counselor improve because clients continually provide immediate corrective feedback. In response to a reflection, a client basically says "Yes" or "No," "Yes, that's right," or "No, that's not quite what I meant," and in either case tends to continue the story and elaborate. This is the kind of feedback that permits learning, just as reliable as seeing where the golf ball goes after a swing.

Similarly, once one knows the sequence of client language in successful MI, there is immediate feedback as to how sessions are going. Counselor responses that lead to change talk are the "right stuff." In essence, client change talk becomes a reinforcer for counselor behavior. Counselors also learn what responses evoke sustain talk and discord. In essence, sustain talk or discord serves as an immediate signal not to repeat that response but to try another approach. In this way, clients become your teachers, offering ongoing information much as archers receive immediate feedback after each arrow shot in target practice.

There are other possible aids to continued learning of MI beyond the feedback provided by clients themselves. Computerized simulated encounters have been developed to which clinicians can generate responses and receive feedback (e.g., Baer et al., 2012). Recording and listening to one's own sessions can be helpful, particularly when using a structured coding system to focus on particular processes within MI sessions (Lane et al., 2005; Madson & Campbell, 2006; Pierson et al., 2007). Such session recordings can also be reviewed by a supervisor or coach whose task it is to help clinicians develop skill in MI. Some clinicians form peer learning groups to review session recordings together and discuss ongoing challenges in applying MI.

Conclusions

In its relatively brief life, MI has already had a significant impact on both research and practice for helping people change. A large evidence base has accumulated supporting the efficacy of MI in addressing a number of problematic health and lifestyle behaviors. Much has been learned about how to help practitioners develop proficiency in MI. A puzzling phenomenon is the high variability in efficacy across studies, sites, and therapists, suggesting a need to understand better what factors influence the effectiveness or ineffectiveness of MI (Miller & Rollnick, 2014).

MI took root first in addiction treatment and medical health care. Applications of MI within mainstream mental health services, as reflected in this volume, is a newer enterprise. Studies continue to explore its utility with common clinical problems such as anxiety, depression, eating disorders, suicidality, and other issues that bring people to seek psychotherapy. MI has potential not only as a "stand-alone" treatment but perhaps more importantly as an approach that can be combined or integrated with other effective therapeutic methods. A meta-analysis of treatments (primarily CBT) for depression and some anxiety disorders by Westen and Morrison (2001) has revealed considerable efficacy, but with one-half to two-thirds of clients showing significant improvement. However, there is considerable room for improvement in treatment retention, reduction of problem severity, and prevention of recurrences. Using MI as a pretreatment for CBT (e.g., Westra, Arkowitz, & Dozois, 2009) or delivering other evidence-based treatments such as CBT in the "MI spirit" (Arkowitz & Burke, 2008; Miller, 2004) both have the potential to improve upon these results.

Some promising starts have been made to understand how and why MI facilitates change. Therapist empathy, client change talk, and diminished "resistance" all seem to play a role in the efficacy of MI, but still we are just getting started in understanding the specific and relational elements that yield change (Miller & Rose, 2009). Research on the critical elements and processes within MI will continue to inform practice, quality assurance, and training of MI. Look how far we've come! How can we still have so far to go?

References

Amrhein, P. C. (1992). The comprehension of quasi-performance verbs in verbal commitments: New evidence for componential theories of lexical meaning. *Journal of Memory and Language, 31*, 756–784.

Amrhein, P. C., Miller, W. R., Yahne, C., Knupsky, A., & Hochstein, D. (2004). Strength of client commitment language improves with therapist training in motivational interviewing. *Alcoholism: Clinical and Experimental Research, 28*(5), 74A.

Amrhein, P. C., Miller, W. R., Yahne, C. E., Palmer, M., & Fulcher, L. (2003). Client commitment language during motivational interviewing predicts drug use outcomes. *Journal of Consulting and Clinical Psychology, 71*, 862–878.

Arkowitz, H. (2002). An integrative approach to psychotherapy based on common processes of change. In J. Lebow (Ed.), *Comprehensive handbook of psychotherapy: Vol, 4. Integrative and eclectic therapies* (pp. 317–337). New York: Wiley.

Arkowitz, H., & Burke, B. (2008). Motivational interviewing as an integrative framework for the treatment of depression. In H. Arkowitz, H. A. Westra, W. R. Miller, & S. Rollnick, (Eds.), *Motivational interviewing in the treatment of psychological problems* (pp. 145–173). New York: Guilford Press.

Babor, T. F., & Del Boca, F. K. (Eds.). (2003). *Treatment matching in alcoholism*. Cambridge, UK: Cambridge University Press.

Baer, J. S., Carpenter, K. M., Beadnell, B., Stoner, S. A., Ingalsbe, M. H., Hartzler, B., et al. (2012). Computer assessment of simulated patient interviews (CASPI): Psychometric properties of a web-based system for the assessment of motivational interviewing skills. *Journal of Studies on Alcohol and Drugs, 73*(1), 154–164.

Baer, J. S., Rosengren, D. B., Dunn, C. W., Wells, W. A., Ogle, R. L., & Hartzler, B. (2004). An evaluation of workshop training in motivational interviewing for addiction and mental health clinicians. *Drug and Alcohol Dependence, 73*(1), 99–106.

Ball, S. A., Martino, S., Nich, C., Frankforter, T. L., van Horn, D., Crits-Christoph, P., et al. (2007). Site matters: Multisite randomized trial of motivational enhancement therapy in community drug abuse clinics. *Journal of Consulting and Clinical Psychology, 75*, 556–567.

Ball, S. A., Todd, M., Tennen, H., Armeli, S., Mohr, C., Affleck, G., et al. (2007). Brief motivational enhancement and coping skills interventions for heavy drinking. *Addictive Behaviors, 32*, 1105–1118.

Beck, A. T., Rush, A. J., Shaw, B. E., & Emery, G. (1979). *Cognitive therapy of depression*. New York: Guilford Press.

Bem, D. J. (1967). Self-perception: An alternative interpretation of cognitive dissonance phenomena. *Psychological Review, 74*, 183–200.

Bernstein, J., Bernstein, E., Tassiopoulos, K., Heeren, T., Levenson, S., & Hingson, R. (2005). Brief motivational intervention at a clinic visit reduces cocaine and heroin use. *Drug and Alcohol Dependence, 77*, 49–59.

Bertholet, N., Faouzi, M., Gmel, G., Gaume, J., & Daeppen, J. B. (2010). Change talk sequence during brief motivational intervention, towards or away from drinking. *Addiction, 105*, 2106–2112.

Brehm, S. S., & Brehm, J. W. (1981). *Psychological reactance: A theory of freedom and control*. New York: Academic Press.

Britt, E., Hudson, S. M., & Blampied, N. M. (2004). Motivational Interviewing in health settings: A review. *Patient Education and Counseling, 53*(2), 147–155.

Brown, T. A., Campbell, L. A., Lehman, C. L., Grisham, J. R., & Mancill, R. B. (2001). Current and lifetime comorbidity of the *DSM-IV* anxiety and mood disorders in a large clinical sample. *Journal of Abnormal Psychology, 110*, 585–599.

Cofer, C. N., & Apley, M. H. (1964). *Motivation*. New York: Wiley.

Daeppen, J-B., Bertholet, N., Gmel, G., & Gaume, J. (2007). Communication during brief intervention, intention to change, and outcome. *Substance Abuse, 28*(3), 43–51.

Engle, D., & Arkowitz, H. (2006). *Ambivalence in psychotherapy: Facilitating readiness to change.* New York: Guilford Press.

Feldstein Ewing, S. W., Filbey, F. M., Sabbineni, A., Chandler, L. D., & Hutchinson, K. E. (2011). How psychological alcohol interventions work: A preliminary look at what fMRI can tell us. *Alcoholism: Clinical and Experimental Research, 35*(4), 643–651.

Festinger, L. (1957). *A theory of cognitive dissonance.* Stanford, CA: Stanford University Press.

Gaume, J., Bertholet, N., Faouzi, M., Gmel, G., & Daeppen, J. B. (2010). Counselor motivational interviewing skills and young adult change talk articulation during brief motivational interventions. *Journal of Substance Abuse Treatment, 39,* 272–281.

Glynn, L. H., & Moyers, T. B. (2010). Chasing change talk: The clinician's role in evoking client language about change. *Journal of Substance Abuse Treatment, 39,* 65–70.

Goddard, C., & Wierzbicka, A. (1994). *Semantic and lexical universals.* Amsterdam: John Benjamins.

Handmaker, N. S., Miller, W. R., & Manicke, M. (1999). Findings of a pilot study of motivational interviewing with pregnant drinkers. *Journal of Studies on Alcohol, 60,* 285–287.

Heckman, C. J., Egleston, B. L., & Hofmann, M. T. (2010). Efficacy of motivational interviewing for smokng cessation: A systematic review and meta-analysis. *Tobacco Control, 19*(5), 410–416.

Hendrickson, S. M. L., Martin, T., Manuel, J. K., Christopher, P. J., Thiedeman, T., & Moyers, T. B. (2004). Assessing reliability of the Motivational Interviewing Treatment Integrity Behavioral Coding System under limited range. *Alcoholism: Clinical and Experimental Research, 28*(5), 74A.

Hettema, J., Steele, J., & Miller, W. R. (2005). Motivational interviewing. *Annual Review of Clinical Psychology, 1,* 91–111.

Hodgins, D. C., Currie, S. R., & el-Guebaly, N. (2001). Motivational enhancement and self-help treatments for problem gambling. *Journal of Consulting and Clinical Psychology, 69,* 50–57.

Karno, M. P., & Longabaugh, R. (2004). What do we know?: Process analysis and the search for a better understanding of Project MATCH's anger-by-treatment matching effect. *Journal of Studies on Alcohol, 65,* 501–512.

Karno, M. P., & Longabaugh, R. (2005). An examination of how therapist directiveness interacts with patient anger and reactance to predict alcohol use. *Journal of Studies on Alcohol, 66,* 825–832.

Lane, C., Huws-Thomas, M., Hood, K., Rollnick, S., Edwards, K., & Robling, M. (2005). Measuring adaptations of motivational interviewing: The development and validation of the behavior change counseling index (BECCI). *Patient Education and Counseling, 56,* 166–173.

Leahy, R. L. (2002). *Overcoming resistance in cognitive therapy.* New York: Guilford Press.

Lewin, K. (1935). *A dynamic theory of personality.* New York: McGraw-Hill.

Longabaugh, R., Zweben, A., LoCastro, J. S., & Miller, W. R. (2005). Origins, issues and options in the development of the Combined Behavioral Intervention. *Journal of Studies on Alcohol, 66*(4), S179–S187.

Lundahl, B., Moleni, T., Burke, B. L., Butters, R., Tollefson, D., Butler, C., et al. (2013). Motivational interviewing in medical care settings: A systematic review and meta-analysis of randomized controlled trials. *Patient Education and Counseling, 93*(2), 157–168.

Lundahl, B. W., Kunz, C., Brownell, C., Tollefson, D., & Burke, B. L. (2010). A meta-analysis of motivational interviewing: Twenty-five years of empirical studies. *Research on Social Work Practice, 20*(2), 137–160.

Madson, M. B., & Campbell, T. C. (2006). Measures of fidelity in motivational enhancement: A systematic review. *Journal of Substance Abuse Treatment, 31*, 67–73.

Mahoney, M. J. (2001). *Human change processes.* New York: Basic Books.

Marijuana Treatment Project Research Group. (2004). Brief treatments for cannabis dependence: Findings from a randomized multisite trial. *Journal of Consulting and Clinical Psychology, 72*, 455–466.

Miller, W. R. (1983). Motivational interviewing with problem drinkers. *Behavioural Psychotherapy, 11*, 147–172.

Miller, W. R. (1985). Motivation for treatment: A review with special emphasis on alcoholism. *Psychological Bulletin, 98*, 84–107.

Miller, W. R. (1988). Including clients' spiritual perspectives in cognitive behavior therapy. In W. R. Miller & J. E. Martin (Eds.), *Behavior therapy and religion: Integrating spiritual and behavioral approaches to change* (43–55). Newbury Park, CA: Sage.

Miller, W. R. (Ed.) (2004). *Combined Behavioral Intervention manual: A clinical research guide for therapists treating people with alcohol abuse and dependence* (COMBINE Monograph Series, Vol. 1). Bethesda, MD: National Institute on Alcohol Abuse and Alcoholism.

Miller, W. R., Benefield, R. G., & Tonigan, J. S. (1993). Enhancing motivation for change in problem drinking: A controlled comparison of two therapist styles. *Journal of Consulting and Clinical Psychology, 61*, 455–461.

Miller, W. R., Forcehimes, A. A., & Zweben, A. (2011). *Treating addiction: Guidelines for professionals.* New York: Guilford Press.

Miller, W. R., & Mount, K. A. (2001). A small study of training in motivational interviewing: Does one workshop change clinician and client behavior? *Behavioural and Cognitive Psychotherapy, 29*, 457–471.

Miller, W. R., & Moyers, T. B. (2006). Eight stages in learning motivational interviewing. *Journal of Teaching in the Addictions, 5*, 3–17.

Miller, W. R., Moyers, T. B., Arciniega, L. T., Ernst, D., & Forcehimes, A. (2005). Training, supervision and quality monitoring of the COMBINE study behavioral interventions. *Journal of Studies on Alcohol* (Suppl. 15), S188–S195.

Miller, W. R., & Rollnick, S. (1991). *Motivational interviewing: Preparing people to change addictive behavior.* New York: Guilford Press.

Miller, W. R., & Rollnick, S. (2002). *Motivational interviewing: Preparing people for change* (2nd ed.). New York: Guilford Press.

Miller, W. R., & Rollnick, S. (2004). Talking oneself into change: Motivational interviewing, stages of change, and the therapeutic process. *Journal of Cognitive Psychotherapy, 18,* 299–308.

Miller, W. R., & Rollnick, S. (2013). *Motivational interviewing: Helping people change* (3rd ed.). New York: Guilford Press.

Miller, W. R., & Rollnick, S. (2014). The effectiveness and ineffectiveness of complex behavioral interventions: Impact of treatment fidelity. *Contemporary Clinical Trials, 37*(2), 234–241.

Miller, W. R., & Rose, G. S. (2009). Toward a theory of motivational interviewing. *American Psychologist, 64,* 527–537.

Miller, W. R., & Rose, G. S. (2015). Motivational interviewing and decisional balance: Contrasting procedures to client ambivalence. *Behavioural and Cognitive Psychotherapy, 43*(2), 129–141.

Miller, W. R., Sovereign, R. G., & Krege, B. (1988). Motivational interviewing with problem drinkers: II. The Drinker's Check-up as a preventive intervention. *Behavioural Psychotherapy, 16,* 251–268.

Miller, W. R., Taylor, C. A., & West, J. C. (1980). Focused versus broad spectrum behavior therapy for problem drinkers. *Journal of Consulting and Clinical Psychology, 48,* 590–601.

Miller, W. R., Yahne, C. E., Moyers, T. B., Martinez, J., & Pirritano, M. (2004). A randomized trial of methods to help clinicians learn motivational interviewing. *Journal of Consulting and Clinical Psychology, 72,* 1050–1062.

Miller, W. R., Yahne, C. E., & Tonigan, J. S. (2003). Motivational interviewing in drug abuse services: A randomized trial. *Journal of Consulting and Clinical Psychology, 71,* 754–763.

Miller, W. R., Zweben, A., Diclemente, C. C., & Rychtarik, R. G. (1992). *Motivational enhancement therapy manual: A clinical research guide for therapists treating individuals with alcohol abuse and dependence* (Vol. 2). Rockville, MD: National Institute on Alcohol Abuse and Alcoholism.

Moyers, T. B., & Martin, T. (2006). Therapist influence on client language during motivational interviewing sessions. *Journal of Substance Abuse Treatment, 30,* 245–252.

Moyers, T. B., Martin, T., Catley, D., Harris, K. J., & Ahluwalia, J. S. (2003). Assessing the integrity of motivational interventions: Reliability of the Motivational Interviewing Skills Code. *Behavioural and Cognitive Psychotherapy, 31,* 177–184.

Moyers, T. B., Martin, T., Christopher, P. J., Houck, J. M., Tonigan, J. S., & Amrhein, P. C. (2007). Client language as a mediator of motivational interviewing efficacy: Where is the evidence? *Alcoholism: Clinical and Experimental Research, 31*(Suppl.), 40S–47S.

Moyers, T. B., Martin, T., Houck, J. M., Christopher, P. J., & Tonigan, J. S. (2009). From in-session behaviors to drinking outcomes: A causal chain for motivational interviewing. *Journal of Consulting and Clinical Psychology, 77*(6), 1113–1124.

Moyers, T. B., Martin, T., Manuel, J. K., Hendrickson, S. M. L., & Miller, W. R. (2005). Assessing competence in the use of motivational interviewing. *Journal of Substance Abuse Treatment, 28,* 19–26.

Moyers, T. B., & Miller, W. R. (2013). Is low therapist empathy toxic? *Psychology of Addictive Behaviors, 27*(3), 878–884.

Moyers, T. B., Miller, W. R., & Hendrickson, S. M. L. (2005). How does motivational interviewing work? Therapist interpersonal skill predicts involvement within motivational interviewing sessions. *Journal of Consulting and Clinical Psychology, 73,* 590–598.

Myers, D. G. (2011). *Psychology* (10th ed.). New York: Worth Publishers.

Newman, M. G., Przeworski, A., Fisher, A. J., & Borkovec, T. D. (2010). Diagnostic comorbidity in adults with generalized anxiety disorder: Impact of comorbidity on psychotherapy outcome and impact of psychotherapy on comorbid diagnoses. *Behavior Therapy, 41,* 59–72.

Patterson, G., & Chamberlain, P. (1994). A functional analysis of resistance during parent training. *Clinical Psychology: Research and Practice, 1,* 53–70.

Patterson, G. R., & Forgatch, M. S. (1985). Therapist behavior as a determinant for client noncompliance: A paradox for the behavior modifier. *Journal of Consulting and Clinical Psychology, 53,* 846–851.

Pierson, H. M., Hayes, S. C., Gifford, E. V., Roget, N., Padilla, M., Bissett, R., et al. (2007). An examination of the Motivational Interviewing Treatment Integrity code. *Journal of Substance Abuse Treatment, 32,* 11–17.

Petri, H. L., & Govern, J. M. (2012). *Motivation: Theory, research and application.* Belmont, CA: Wadsworth.

Prochaska, J. O. (1994). Strong and weak principles for progressing from precontemplation to action on the basis of twelve problem behaviors. *Health Psychology, 13,* 47–51.

Prochaska, J., & Norcross, J. (2013). *Systems of psychotherapy: A transtheoretical analysis* (8th ed.). Stamford, CT: Cenage Learning.

Project MATCH Research Group (1997). Project MATCH secondary a priori hypotheses. *Addiction, 92,* 1671–1698.

Resnicow, K., Jackson, A., Wang, T., De, A. K., McCarty, F., Dudley, W. N., et al. (2001). A motivational interviewing intervention to increase fruit and vegetable intake through Black churches: Results of the Eat for Life trial. *American Journal of Public Health, 91*(10), 1686–1693.

Rogers, C. R. (1951). *Client-centered therapy.* Boston: Houghton Mifflin.

Rogers, C. R. (1959). A theory of therapy, personality, and interpersonal relationships as developed in the client-centered framework. In S. Koch (Ed.), *Psychology: The study of a science: Vol. 3. Formulations of the person and the social contexts* (pp. 184–256). New York: McGraw-Hill.

Rogers, C. R. (1980). *A way of being.* Boston: Houghton Mifflin.

Rollnick, S., & Miller, W. R. (1995). What is motivational interviewing? *Behavioural and Cognitive Psychotherapy, 23,* 325–334.

Rollnick, S., Miller, W. R., & Butler, C. (2008). *Motivational interviewing in health care.* New York: Guilford Press.

Rubak, S., Sandbaek, A., Lauritzen, T., & Christensen, B. (2005). Motivational interviewing: A systematic review and meta-analysis. *British Journal of General Practice, 55,* 305–312.

Senft, R. A., Polen, M. R., Freeborn, D. K., & Hollis, J. F. (1997). Brief intervention in a primary care setting for hazardous drinkers. *American Journal of Preventive Medicine, 13*, 464–470.

Stephens, R. S., Babor, T. F., Kadden, R., & Miller, M. (2002). The Marijuana Treatment Project: Rationale, design and participant characteristics. *Addiction, 97*, 109–124.

Thevos, A. K., Quick, R. E., & Yanduli, V. (2000). Application of motivational interviewing to the adoption of water disinfection practices in Zambia. *Health Promotion International, 15*, 207–214.

Truax, C. B., & Carkhuff, R. R. (1967). *Toward effective counseling and psychotherapy*. Chicago: Aldine.

UKATT Research Team. (2005). Effectiveness of treatment for alcohol problems: Findings of the randomized UK Alcohol Treatment Trial (UKATT). *British Medical Journal, 331*, 541–544.

Valle, S. K. (1981). Interpersonal functioning of alcoholism counselors and treatment outcome. *Journal of Studies on Alcohol, 42*, 783–790.

Westen, D., & Morrison, K. (2001). A multi-dimensional meta-analysis of treatments for depression, panic, and generalized anxiety disorder: An empirical examination of the status of empirically supported therapies. *Journal of Consulting and Clinical Psychology, 69*, 875–899.

Westra, H. A., Arkowitz, H., & Dozois, D. J. A. (2009). Adding a motivational interviewing pretreatment to cognitive behavioral therapy for generalized anxiety disorder: A randomized controlled trial. *Journal of the Anxiety Disorders, 23*, 1106–1117.

White, W. L., & Miller, W. R. (2007). The use of confrontation in addiction treatment: History, science, and time for a change. *The Counselor, 8*(4), 12–30.

Woollard, J., Beilin, L., Lord, T., Puddey, I., MacAdam, D., & Rouse, I. (1995). A controlled trial of nurse counselling on lifestyle change for hypertensives treated in general practice: Preliminary results. *Clinical and Experimental Pharmacology and Physiology, 22*, 466–468.

CHAPTER 2

• • • • • •

Motivation Facilitation in the Unified Protocol for Transdiagnostic Treatment of Emotional Disorders

James F. Boswell
Kate H. Bentley
David H. Barlow

Cognitive-behavioral therapies (CBT) have demonstrated efficacy for a wide variety of problem areas (Butler, Chapman, Forman, & Beck, 2006), and this is particularly the case for the treatment of emotional disorders, such as anxiety and mood disorders (Hollon & Beck, 2013). Nevertheless, a significant percentage of clients fail to respond to "gold standard" CBT (as well as other evidence-based approaches; Lambert, 2013), with many of these individuals failing to engage sufficiently in treatment and/or terminating prematurely (Boswell, Llera, Newman, & Castonguay, 2011; Swift & Greenberg, 2012). Clinicians and researchers have increasingly recognized the potential for enhancing the effectiveness of CBT through the integration of specific strategies aimed at facilitating client engagement and retention (e.g., Arkowitz & Westra, 2004; Constantino, Castonguay, Zack, & DeGeorge, 2010). Motivational interviewing principles and strategies hold considerable promise for achieving these aims (Constantino, DeGeorge, Dadlani, & Overtree, 2009).

Clinical Problems and Usual Treatments

Decades of research have led to the identification of numerous evidence-based psychological treatments for specific problems (Lambert, 2013; Nathan & Gorman, 2007). Although the impact on behavioral health has been considerable, the treatment research *Zeitgeist* has led to the proliferation of treatment manuals that prescribe narrowly defined techniques aimed at narrowly defined problems (Boswell & Goldfried, 2010; Norcross, 2005). The ever narrowing slicing of problem areas to be studied and treated has no doubt been influenced by recent iterations of the *Diagnostic and Statistical Manual of Mental Disorders* (e.g., DSM-IV-TR, DSM-5; American Psychiatric Association, 2000, 2013). However, the field has recognized the conceptual, empirical, and practical limitations of this approach to the study and treatment of common mental health problems (Barlow, Allen, & Choate, 2004), leading to the development of principle-driven integrative, *transdiagnostic* treatments.

Basic and applied psychological research has questioned the utility of DSM disorder constructs in the assessment and treatment of psychological problems (Brown & Barlow, 2009). For example, research has demonstrated a considerable degree of overlap among various anxiety and mood disorders where high rates of current and lifetime comorbidity have consistently been observed (Brown, Campbell, Lehman, Grisham, & Mancill, 2001; Kessler et al., 2005; Zimmerman, Chelminski, & McDermut, 2002). The high degree of comorbidity may be explained by the presence of common underlying factors that contribute to the etiology and maintenance of diverse emotional problems (Andrews, 1996; Tyrer, 1989; Wolfe, 2011), with manifest differences (e.g., fear of social evaluation vs. contamination) representing relatively superficial variations of the same process. In fact, research in the areas of neuroscience (e.g., Etkin & Wager, 2007), emotion science (e.g., Fellous & LeDoux, 2005; LeDoux, 1996), and psychopathology (Brown, 2007) has elucidated common higher-order dimensions of temperament that underlie emotional difficulties, most significantly negative/positive affect and behavioral inhibition/activation (Brown, 2007; Brown, Chorpita, & Barlow, 1998; Carver & White, 1994; Watson & Clark, 1984). These dimensions have been linked to other observed shared factors, such as cognitive–emotional processing biases (Beck & Clark, 1997; Dalgleish & Watts, 1990; McLaughlin, Borkovec, & Sibrava, 2007; Mobini & Grant, 2007) and increased emotional reactivity and cognitive-behavioral avoidance (Brown & Barlow, 2009; Campbell-Sills, Barlow, Brown, & Hofmann, 2006).

Although the aim of developing manualized protocols has been to facilitate training and implementation of evidence-based psychosocial interventions, from the perspective of clinical practice the abundance of increasingly specific treatment manuals (many of which include minor and somewhat trivial variations in treatment procedures) has actually led to an increased burden on practicing clinicians and trainees as well as significant strain on transportability and dissemination (McHugh & Barlow, 2010). This reality has led to the development of transdiagnostic CBT treatments that integrate common evidence-based change strategies (Fairburn, Cooper, & Shafran, 2003; Norton & Philipp, 2008). Driven by the accumulating empirical psychopathology and emotion science literature, the *Unified Protocol for Transdiagnostic Treatment of Emotional Disorders* (UP; Barlow et al., 2011a, 2011b) is a unique example of this transdiagnostic focus. Along with the integration of evidence-based CBT change strategies, the UP seeks to target directly core mechanisms implicated in the development and maintenance of anxiety, mood, and related disorders.

The Unified Protocol

The UP is a transdiagnostic emotion-focused CBT treatment designed to be applicable to mental health conditions that involve a prominent emotional component (e.g., mood, anxiety, and somatic symptom disorders). The UP is composed of a series of treatment modules: Motivation Enhancement for Treatment Engagement (Module 1); Recognition and Tracking of Emotional Experiences (Module 2); Emotion Awareness Training (Module 3); Cognitive Appraisal and Reappraisal (Module 4); Emotion Avoidance and Emotion-Driven Behaviors (Module 5); Awareness and Tolerance of Physical Sensations (Module 6); Interoceptive and Situational Emotion Exposures (Module 7); and Relapse Prevention (Module 8; Payne, Ellard, Farchione, Fairholme, & Barlow, 2014). Each module includes one or more core intervention strategies that are embedded within an evidence-based principle of change (Boswell, 2013). A modular framework was chosen to enhance-flexibility of application; for example, more time and attention to emotion driven behaviors (e.g., social withdrawal) may be needed with depressed clients. Material from previously covered modules can be reintegrated at later points in treatment as needed. As we will discuss, this is particularly relevant for the Motivation Enhancement for Treatment Engagement module, as many clients are likely to require motivation facilitation strategies throughout treatment.

Rationale for Integrating
Motivation Facilitation Strategies

Motivation Enhancement for Treatment Engagement is the entry-level module of the UP. The decision to assimilate motivational interviewing (MI) strategies was relatively straightforward, given the ultimate goal of integrating evidence-based treatment principles and intervention strategies that cut across problem areas and approaches (Boswell, 2013). Decades of research, much of which is summarized in this volume (as well as in Miller & Rollnick, 2013), has demonstrated the effectiveness of MI in diverse problem areas, thereby confirming its transdiagnostic relevance. Clinical and research evidence has demonstrated that clients begin psychotherapy with variable degrees of motivation for change (Engle & Arkowitz, 2006), and ambivalence regarding change is a relatively common phenomenon that is not unique to a given client population or problem area (Constantino, Boswell, Bernecker, & Castonguay, 2013).

The integration of MI-derived strategies in the UP was based heavily on the work of Westra, Arkowitz, and colleagues (e.g., Arkowitz & Westra, 2004; Westra, 2004; Westra, Arkowitz, & Dozois, 2009), who have demonstrated the benefits of augmenting CBT for anxiety disorders with MI. In a recent UP study involving principally anxious and depressed clients, the majority of clients began treatment in the *contemplation* stage of change (Boswell, Sauer-Zavala, Gallagher, Delgado, & Barlow, 2012). Within Prochaska and colleagues' transtheoretical model (TTM; Prochaska & DiClemente, 1984; Prochaska & Norcross, 2002), clients in the contemplation stage are aware that a problem exists and are interested in information about the problem, yet they are still ambivalent and have not made a commitment to take action. We tested the hypothesis that overall readiness to change at pretreatment would function as a moderator of the relationship between initial problem severity and the magnitude of change experienced during treatment. Consistent with previous research (see Clarkin & Levy, 2004; Newman, Crits-Christoph, Connolly Gibbons, & Erickson, 2006), higher initial severity was negatively correlated with overall change; however, this relationship was essentially reversed when the interaction with readiness was examined. Clients who presented with high initial severity and high readiness demonstrated the greatest degree of change in the trial. Consistent with Westra et al. (2009), these results highlighted not only the relevance of change readiness for individuals with primary anxiety and depression but also the particular relevance of motivation enhancement strategies for clients entering treatment with high levels of severity and low levels of readiness to change.

Theory and the scope of treatment research in this area, therefore, support the transdiagnostic relevance of motivation and motivation enhancement strategies. Within the framework of the UP's transdiagnostic focus on emotion, emotional experience itself is often the source of ambivalence. Research has shown that many clients are ambivalent about having *any* emotional experience, whether positive or negative (Campbell-Sills et al., 2006; Mennin, Heimberg, Turk, & Fresco, 2005). This predisposition to experience heightened levels of negative affect and to perceive such experiences as threatening (i.e., neuroticism) can lead to attempts (both cognitive and behavioral) to control, suppress, and avoid emotions (Campbell-Sills, Ellard, & Barlow, 2014). Such responses typically result in short-term reductions in negative arousal (Borkovec, Lyonfields, Wiser, & Diehl, 1993). Emotion avoidance strategies are, therefore, maintained through negative reinforcement as well as the lost opportunity for corrective learning (Borkovec, Alcaine, & Behar, 2004; Boswell, 2013; Hayes, Beck, & Yasinksi, 2012). For example, it is extremely difficult to disconfirm a strongly held expectation that one will be socially rejected if one avoids all interpersonal contact.

Unfortunately, emotion avoidance strategies often increase and generalize to new situations and experiences. Furthermore, the paradoxical effects of suppression and avoidance on subsequent subjective distress have been well documented (Abramowitz, Tolin, & Street, 2001; Gross & John, 2003; Wegner, Schneider, Carter, & White, 1987). These consequences and behaviors can lead to an increasingly restricted life. Many clients who enter psychotherapy have some awareness of the negative consequences of their avoidance; however, this may not be their primary reason for seeking help. Many clients believe that the emotions *are* the problem and that reduction (or complete elimination) of the emotions themselves is the appropriate target of treatment. This belief is the driving force behind their sustain talk. When offered a different perspective in the UP, clients are often forced to ask themselves, "Can I give up learned behaviors if it means facing what I fear most—my own emotions?" MI-derived stances and strategies can be highly useful in facilitating awareness of such ambivalence, evoking change talk, and increasing the client's commitment to treatment tasks and goals.

The decision to label the UP module "motivation enhancement" rather than motivational interviewing is worthy of note. While CBT therapists are taught to assume the role of expert and often adopt a directive style, MI requires a less directive, *guiding* style. Although this distinction represents an important theoretical difference, in practice there are likely wide variations in the level of directiveness among CBT therapists and within a given course of treatment. Regardless, motivation facilitation in the UP can be considered a CBT adaptation of core MI strategies. Specifically, the UP takes an assimilative integration (Boswell, Nelson, Nordberg, McAleavey, & Castonguay, 2010; Messer, 2001) approach to the transdiagnostic application of MI. In assimilative integration, case formulations and treatment plans are anchored within a specific theoretical framework (e.g., CBT) while simultaneously incorporating techniques and from other approaches (as needed for a particular client) that might address underemphasized factors in the primary approach (e.g., assimilating MI strategies into CBT). Assimilation in the UP occurs in two ways, beginning with the Motivation Enhancement for Treatment Engagement Module (Module 1), during which the topics of motivation and ambivalence are brought up explicitly by the therapist. The following points are specifically addressed: (1) motivation exists on a continuum and is likely to ebb and flow over the course of treatment; (2) motivation will be relevant to the process and outcome of the treatment; and (3) the identification of concrete value-driven goals will be important for both the process and outcome of the treatment (Gollwitzer, 1999). The second method of assimilation is the flexible application of MI-consistent strategies throughout the course of treatment, based on relevant markers such as ambivalence and the increased use of sustain talk (Constantino et al., 2013).

General Considerations

The level of attention devoted to specific motivation enhancement strategies depends on the individual client. Regardless of duration or intensity, the primary goals of the motivation enhancement module are to use evidence-based motivational strategies to increase clients' (1) overall readiness for behavior change, (2) positive engagement, (3) openness/receptivity to an emotion-focused transdiagnostic problem conceptualization, and (4) change efficacy (e.g., goal selection and hope regarding the likelihood of goal attainment). These goals effectively span the four MI processes of *engaging*, *focusing*, *evoking*, and *planning*. Motivation is addressed at the beginning of treatment, prior to the introduction of specific CBT skills, because change readiness and self-efficacy are viewed as prerequisites for treatment engagement, which in turn will greatly influence the likelihood of achieving positive lasting change.

Furthermore, low levels of readiness, receptivity, and mutual goal specification are indicators of a poor-quality working alliance, which itself is a transdiagnostic, pantheoretical prognostic indicator of subsequent treatment process and outcome (Castonguay, Constantino, Boswell, & Kraus, 2010). Collaborative engagement is the mortar that holds together the bricks in CBT (Castonguay, Constantino, McAleavey, & Goldfried, 2010), and one of the primary functions of integrating MI-derived strategies in the UP is to increase engagement and facilitate the development and maintenance of a positive working alliance. The conceptualization of the working alliance in this transdiagnostic treatment is consistent with Bordin's (1979) three-component model—(1) affective bond, (2) agreement on treatment goals, and (3) agreement on tasks (in order to reach identified goals)—although more emphasis is admittedly placed on tasks and goals. For example, Webb et al. (2011) found that agreement on tasks and goals explained more of the outcome variance in CBT for depression than the quality of the affective bond.

Clinical Applications

Motivation Facilitation in Early Treatment

Along with engaging, other core MI processes are facilitated by an early functional assessment of the client's emotions (Barlow et al., 2011b). Due to its transdiagnostic framework, the UP generally eschews a focus on diagnostic labels or specific symptoms. Rather, the focus is on the client's emotional experience, in particular (1) the types, frequencies, intensities, and contexts for strong emotions; (2) how the client responds to this experience (e.g., efforts to control or suppress distressing affects); and (3) the impact on functioning, quality of life, and the achievement of short- and long-term life goals. In our experience, clients respond more openly to this form of assessment because it is closer to their subjective experience and values. This assessment also facilitates discussion of functional treatment goals, which can otherwise be experienced as disembodied when the primary focus is on the presence or absence of a diagnosis or symptom frequencies.

With sufficient engagement, the functional assessment process flows naturally into focusing, evoking, and subsequent planning. A key element of focusing during Module 1 is achieving a shared conceptualization of the problem and treatment plan. It should be emphasized that a shared agreement is not tantamount to convincing the client to see things the therapist's way. The therapist's goal is to maintain a guiding stance. For example, an important element of the engagement and focusing process in the UP is a discussion of the nature and function of emotions along with the long-term costs of emotion avoidance. This discussion may trigger ambivalence within clients because the therapist will ultimately convey that "getting rid of" or eliminating painful emotions *is* the primary problem and, therefore, will not be a viable goal for treatment. Ambivalence may be a marker of progress at this early stage because it indicates that the client (or at least a part of him or her) recognizes the costs of emotion avoidance.

Therefore, the early guiding style of the functional assessment serves multiple aims, such as increasing openness/receptivity to an emotion-focused transdiagnostic problem conceptualization and promoting change efficacy. Both of these aims serve the complementary function of developing discrepancy, and well-described evoking questions are commonly used (see Miller & Rollnick, 2013). For example, clients who describe a restricted life owing to increased reliance on avoidance strategies can be asked, "How would you like to live a less restricted life?" or, alternatively, "What could be some advantages to getting out of your head and taking some action?" With patience, this discussion can shift into increasingly concrete planning.

Treatment cannot progress to a subsequent UP module until planning has begun, underscoring the importance of evoking and reinforcing change talk and change efficacy. Nevertheless, as previously noted, motivation is not a "finish line" to be crossed and never thought of again. The therapist must be responsive to the individual client and judge whether or not to move forward with particular treatment tasks. Therefore, clients who are still in the *precontemplation* stage of change (Prochaska & DiClemente, 1984) are not ready to proceed to subsequent modules; such cases are examples of when ambivalence may be a sign of progress. In these instances, decisional balance exercises are conducted where the client is guided to weigh the pros and cons of both changing and staying the same (e.g., the cost of continuing to work so hard to control or avoid emotions). The goal in such cases is to foster and clarify ambivalence, which can then be explored through focusing and evoking strategies.

For clients exhibiting a higher level of readiness, the transition into the planning process begins with the identification of "higher-order" values and goals articulated in the focusing and evoking process. A common client higher-order goal statement is "I feel like I don't have a life. I'm afraid of everything. I want to actually start living." Within Module 1, the next step is making this general goal-directed stance more concrete. A common therapist follow-up question is "What would you be doing, let's say 6 months from now, if you were living your life? How would you know?" The client may choose to focus on developing meaningful relationships, or seeking out new experiences, or obtaining employment. If a client wishes to focus on social concerns and relationship issues, for example, then the therapist guides the discussion toward collaborative agreement on increasingly concrete goals (e.g., improving interactions with coworkers or finding a romantic partner) and the necessary steps to achieve those goals.

Motivation throughout Treatment

Although we advocate addressing motivation with every client, and Module 1 serves as a prerequisite for subsequent UP modules, the degree of attention devoted to motivation and engagement maintenance and enhancement throughout the course of treatment will vary considerably among individual clients. Because of the importance of between-session activities (i.e., homework), collaborative engagement is paramount; therefore, the therapist must be sensitively attuned to fluctuations in motivation and engagement. Consistent with the growing alliance rupture–repair literature (Safran, Muran, & Eubanks-Carter, 2011), markers of disengagement can be either subtle or overt. A common form of subtle disengagement is when a pliant client acquiesces to a directing therapist in the absence of a shared understanding of the value and purpose of the task or goal. Compared to more overt markers of disengagement (e.g., a comment that explicitly devalues the therapy or therapist) or ambivalence ("I'm not sure that I can do this"), subtle markers are more difficult to detect and, therefore, address. MI-derived strategies are integrated into the UP so that therapists can be mindful of maintaining a guiding style and fostering collaboration on both within- and between-session tasks and activities. Furthermore, therapists are prepared to identify markers of disengagement and ambivalence, such as sustain talk. When the "going gets tough," the therapist may need to shift to the engaging and evoking strategies of MI. This discussion may include revisiting the client's initially articulated values and goals as well as metacommunicating about the therapy process.

It is important to note that acknowledging and working with ambivalence may itself be a primary focus of UP treatment for some clients. We have found that some clients have difficulty tolerating *ambivalence* because of the strong emotions that are attached and the natural anxiety it triggers. This represents a particularly interesting complementary relationship between MI and UP processes where not only is ambivalence normalized but also clients may be asked simply to sit with and fully experience their ambivalence and uncertainty as a form of exposure (Boswell, Thompson-Hollands, Farchione, & Barlow, 2012). The primary goal in this instance, at least initially, is learning to tolerate the presence of ambivalence and associated affect. Premature foreclosure on a resolution of ambivalence may function as an emotion avoidance strategy that leads to short-term relief but yet will likely prove to be problematic in the long term, as with other forms of emotion avoidance (e.g., behavioral, cognitive) that clients may be using.

Clinical Illustration

Given the transdiagnostic focus of the UP, we describe a clinical case that involved complex mood and anxiety disorder comorbidity. Satoko[1] was a 36-year-old single Japanese woman. She moved to the United States to attend college when she was 22 years old. She was referred to the Center for Anxiety and Related Disorders by her psychiatrist. Satoko initially completed a clinical assessment that involved self-report measures and administration of the Anxiety Disorders Interview Schedule for DSM-IV (Lifetime Version, ADIS-IV-L; DiNardo, Brown, & Barlow, 1994). Based on this assessment, she was given a principal diagnosis (most severe and interfering) of recurrent major depression (clinical severity rating [CSR] = 6, on a scale from 0 to 8, with 8 being most severe and interfering) and secondary diagnoses of social phobia (CSR = 5), posttraumatic stress disorder (CSR = 4), and marijuana dependence (CSR = 4).

Satoko reported feeling "overwhelmed" and "stuck." She described pervasive feelings of worthlessness, shame, and guilt, which she often connected to her inability to complete college (largely owing to financial limitations), find steady employment, and "have a successful life." She reported being interested in art and interior design; however, after leaving college, she could only find a job at a local restaurant. She reported having no friends until she began to socialize with some of her co-workers. These individuals were heavy users of drugs and alcohol, and she began to use these substances as well, which she attributed to perceived social pressure. However, Satoko also found the effects of marijuana and

---

[1]This client participated in a university Institutional Review Board approved (#3126E) case series study. She provided informed consent to have her sessions' audio recorded and clinical information used for research and publication purposes. The client's name and certain characteristics (e.g., precise age) have been altered to ensure confidentiality.

alcohol to be highly reinforcing through the subsequent, albeit short-term, reductions of her negative affect, worry, and rumination. On one occasion when she was intoxicated, she was sexually assaulted by one of her coworkers. She did not report the assault; instead, she quit her job and withdrew further. She eventually found a job at a different restaurant and, through an acquaintance, was introduced to an individual who owned a home decor and interior design shop. To Satoko's amazement, this person offered her a position in his shop as a consultant/sales associate. Although this was her "dream job," Satoko reported intense anticipatory social anxiety and worry-precipitated panic attacks. She experienced intense anxiety and intrusive worry/rumination when interacting with clients as well as intense shame ("The clients were always white . . . wealthy and successful. I would be shaking talking to them. My English is not good, and I don't have a college education. I had no business being there. They must be thinking I am so stupid . . . that I don't belong"). Eventually, Satoko stopped showing up for work, and it became increasingly rare for her to leave her apartment. At the time that she began psychotherapy at our center, she was extremely socially isolated and smoking marijuana most days of the week.

Satoko was visibly upset and in tears throughout most of her first appointment. At the beginning of treatment, she received total scores of 18 and 16 (out of a possible 20) on the Overall Depression Severity and Impairment (ODSIS; Bentley, Gallagher, Carl, & Barlow, 2014) and Overall Anxiety Severity and Impairment (OASIS; Norman, Hami-Cissell, Means-Christensen, & Stein, 2006) scales, respectively. She also received a total score of 41 on the Beck Depression Inventory–II (BDI-II; Beck, Steer, & Brown, 1996) and a total score of 28 on the Beck Anxiety Inventory (BAI; Beck, Epstein, Brown, & Steer, 1988). In addition, she received a percent maximum score of 23 on the Quality of Life Enjoyment and Satisfaction Questionnaire (Q-LES-Q; Endicott, Nee, Harrison, & Blumenthal, 1993) and a total score of 16 (out of a possible 48) on the State Hope Scale (SHS; Snyder et al., 1996). Her initial expectancy rating on the Credibility and Expectancy Questionnaire (CEQ; Borkovec & Nau, 1972) was 50%, and her highest URICA (University of Rhode Island Change Assessment) subscale score was for the contemplation stage.

Motivation Enhancement Module

The first session with Satoko focused on conducting a functional analysis of her emotions and behaviors (i.e., the identification of antecedent and reinforcing factors that influence the occurrence of specific thoughts, feelings, and behaviors), providing basic information (e.g., regarding the overall treatment model), and gauging expectations and motivation for CBT-oriented treatment. Satoko described a life largely characterized by extreme cognitive and behavioral avoidance. Although her recognition of the costs of these strategies led her to seek nonpharmacological treatment for the first time and she frequently referred to herself as "desperate," she was openly skeptical of her ability to change and comply with any treatment approach that would ask her to begin facing her emotions and reducing her reliance on avoidance strategies. This apparent ambivalence regarding the tasks of treatment and the likelihood of improvement was consistent with her quantitative indicators of outcome expectations and readiness.

More formal motivation facilitation strategies were introduced in the second session. The therapist began by asking Satoko about her experience of the first session. Satoko reported finding the session "OK" and beginning to experience more hope (because "this therapy could be helpful"). The therapist summarized the concerns that Satoko had communicated in the first session and discussed the dynamic nature of motivation and ambivalence. He asked if there was anything in particular that led Satoko to feel "desperate." Satoko described feeling as if her "life is ticking by." This feeling had been amplified by a sense that she "ruined" her opportunity at the home decor store. Concomitantly, she reported experiencing a sense of dread at the prospect of reentering a context that consistently triggered feelings of intense shame and worthlessness. The therapist chose to explore this feeling of shame in more depth and provide some psychoeducation regarding the nature and function of both basic and "moral" emotions. He empathized with Satoko's urges to avoid situations and people who trigger such strong negative emotion; yet, he also noted the costs when quitting a job owing to anxiety becomes the most recent piece of evidence to support one's negative view of self, which, in turn, leads to greater distress and subsequent avoidance (e.g., resorting to substance use). The therapist wondered what it would mean to Satoko to no longer be ashamed or driven by negative emotion. Satoko was able to describe general indicators, such as having a meaningful job and friends whom she can trust and spend time with. The therapist encouraged Satoko to complete two tasks prior to the next session: a values analysis that involved rating the relative importance of different life domains and a review of the motivation enhancement and goal-setting chapter in the UP workbook.

Prior to the third session, Satoko completed the Working Alliance

Inventory—Short Form (Tracey & Kokotovic, 1989). Her mean item rating was 5.42, indicating her perception of a moderately strong bond as well as moderate agreement on treatment tasks and goals. Consistent with this rating, she had completed the suggested values activity and reading. The results of her values analysis indicated that Satoko highly valued work and social domains. In addition, she communicated an increased willingness to engage in treatment tasks that involved confronting feared emotions and situations if it meant that she "could have a better life." The therapist noted this change talk and encouraged Satoko to expand on her emerging sense of hope and trust in the psychotherapy process. This evoking process led directly into concrete planning. Satoko identified the following goals: (1) find employment in her area of interest; (2) build social connections with people in her age range who share similar interests; and (3) develop a more balanced and accepting sense of self. Each goal was discussed in more detail, and Satoko was encouraged to write down any further goal-related considerations over the following week in addition to reviewing the next chapter in the workbook.

This marked the beginning of a shift from the motivation enhancement module into the first formal UP skills module. Prior to the subsequent session, Satoko once again completed the URICA, CEQ, and WAI-S. Her expectancy rating was 90% (a 40% increase from her baseline rating) and her SHS total score was 25 (compared to 16 at baseline). Her highest URICA subscale score was for the action stage, and her mean WAI-S item score was 6.75.

Motivation and Engagement in Subsequent Sessions

Motivation and engagement are rarely linear or uniformly high throughout treatment. Satoko's frequent and intense experience of shame and anxiety not only triggered subjective distress but also contributed to the generalization of avoidance behaviors that maintained and exacerbated her difficulties. These very emotions colored her ambivalence regarding treatment, including both the task of therapy and its likelihood of success. The decision to move ahead with subsequent treatment modules was based on the therapist's judgment that Satoko was sufficiently motivated and oriented toward engaging in new learning experiences.

The therapist had witnessed sufficient change talk and instillation of hope to facilitate the identification of value-driven treatment goals. Nevertheless, difficulties arose throughout the course of treatment that required the therapist to reintegrate motivation facilitation strategies. For instance, when discussing potential between-session activities related to initiating social contact, Satoko suggested visiting a coworker at the home decor store where she had previously been an employee. This particular individual designed pieces for the shop, and Satoko admired this person's talent and knowledge. In addition, this coworker had disclosed to Satoko that she was a "recovering alcoholic," which she identified with to some extent. However, after offering this example, Satoko quickly dismissed its viability. The therapist attempted to clarify Satoko's experience at that moment, and she described experiencing a mix of sadness, shame, and anxiety. In Satoko's mind, this activity would surely trigger intense negative emotion and cognitive appraisals (e.g., "Why would she waste her time with me? She is brilliant, and I have nothing to offer. I would be boring or irritating, and I won't be able to speak clearly"). The therapist took this opportunity not only to evoke and strengthen Satoko's arguments for change (including revisiting previously identified values and long-term goals) but also to practice increasing cognitive flexibility prior to and during the between-session task. At the beginning of the subsequent session, Satoko reported visiting her former coworker despite experiencing significant anticipatory anxiety. She described being "shocked" by her coworker's level of excitement to see Satoko. They spoke for over an hour, and at one point the coworker told Satoko that she had always admired her creativity. This represented a major corrective experience for Satoko (see Castonguay & Hill, 2012) that had important implications for the remainder of treatment.

Because Satoko was able to (1) engage in value-driven behaviors despite experiencing negative emotion and (2) hear and "take in" her coworker's feedback, this experience marked a transition toward genuine self-acceptance for her. Similar instances of doubt and occasional sustain talk emerged over the course of treatment (e.g., in anticipation of exposure tasks and further efforts to reduce emotion avoidance); however, the therapist maintained a guiding style and integrated motivation facilitation strategies as needed. Over time, Satoko developed a friendship with this former coworker, and she was eventually invited back to work in the store. Satoko did return to the store. She chose not to start full-time on the retail floor, yet she gradually increased her contact with clients. At the end of 20 sessions, Satoko had ODSIS and OASIS total scores of 8. Her total BDI-II score was 11, and her total BAI score was 18. She received a percent maximum score of 48 on the Q-LES-Q.

Relevant Research

Research to date has examined the overall efficacy of the UP with all eight modules delivered sequentially (although the number of sessions devoted to each module has varied). Studies have included intensive case analyses (Boswell, Anderson, & Barlow, 2014), open trials (Ellard, Deckersbach, Sylvia, Nierenberg, & Barlow, 2012; Ellard, Fairholme, Boisseau, Farchione, & Barlow, 2010), and randomized controlled trials (RCTs; Farchione et al., 2012) with clients presenting with diverse principal anxiety and secondary/comorbid conditions (e.g., anxiety, mood, or somatic symptom disorders). Moderate to large pre- to posttreatment effect sizes, in terms of symptom reduction and functional improvement within and between groups (i.e., UP compared to a wait-list control; Farchione et al., 2012), have been observed across principal and comorbid problem areas. Results have shown that these changes are typically maintained or enhanced at 6-month follow-up (Ellard et al., 2010; Farchione et al., 2012).

Research on the application of motivation facilitation in transdiagnostic psychotherapy such as the UP is also still in its infancy. As noted above, Boswell et al. (2012) found that the level of pretreatment readiness for change functioned as a moderator of the relationship between initial severity and magnitude of change in UP treatment. In addition, Thompson-Hollands, Bentley, Gallagher, Boswell, and Barlow (2014) found that clients reported an average percentage of expected improvement of 70% following the introduction of the UP motivational enhancement module at Session 2. However, the wait-list/delayed treatment control group in this RCT (Farchione et al., 2012) did not provide expectancy ratings. Consequently, the specific impacts of the Motivation Enhancement for Treatment Engagement Module or the integration of MI-derived strategies throughout UP treatment have yet to be examined empirically.

Our research group is currently conducting a large RCT comparing the UP to single-diagnosis protocols (SDPs) for diverse principal anxiety disorders (as well as a wait-list/delayed treatment condition). All clients receive 16 sessions of weekly psychotherapy with the exception of individuals with principal panic disorder, who receive only 12 weekly sessions to be consistent with existing empirically supported CBT protocols (e.g., Craske & Barlow, 2007). The motivation enhancement strategies described above are introduced with all clients who are randomized to the UP condition. The trial is still in the active treatment phase; however, we will present some preliminary results that are relevant to the motivational enhancement module here.

We are examining readiness to change with the University of Rhode Island Change Assessment (URICA; McConnaughy, DiClemente, Prochasta, & Velicer, 1983; McConnaughy Prochasta, & Velicer, 1989). Participating clients are asked to complete the URICA at pretreatment and after Session 4. Using the sample to date ($n = 115$), we conducted two MANOVAs testing between condition differences (UP [$n = 58$], compared to SDPs [$n = 57$]) in URICA stage of change scores. The first MANOVA examined stages of change at baseline. Interestingly, no clients have thus far entered the trial at the precontemplation stage of change. As expected (given randomization), the between-condition effect on subscale scores at baseline was not significant, Wilks' λ (4, 110) = .99, p = .88, partial η^2 = .01. A significant between-condition effect was observed, however, at Session 4, Wilks' λ (4, 89) = .89, p < .05, partial η^2 = .11. Univariate tests indicated a significant difference in action stage scores, $F(1, 92)$ = 4.65, p < .05. Clients in the UP condition exhibited higher action scores (M = 4.32, SD = .46) as compared to SDP participants (M = 4.11, SD = .47, Hedges' g = .44). For those clients in the UP condition, 42% would be categorized as being in the action stage, compared to 18% of clients in the SDP condition. Some 54% of the UP participants would be categorized as being in the contemplation stage, compared to 82% of the SDP participants. These results are quite preliminary, however, given that the trial recruitment phase is only at its midpoint. Further, it is important to note that these results cannot conclusively be attributed to the motivational enhancement module, as psychoeducation and emotion monitoring strategies are also introduced by Session 4 of the treatment.

Problems and Suggested Solutions

Although few significant difficulties in applying motivation facilitation strategies arose in the case of Satoko (perhaps owing to her willingness to identify and disclose treatment-related concerns and ambivalence), conceptual and practical difficulties can certainly arise when utilizing MI-derived strategies in CBT-oriented transdiagnostic treatments such as the UP. As noted above, one conceptual difficulty is the role and style of the psychotherapist. Traditionally, CBT therapists assume the expert role and maintain a directive style. Conversely, MI deemphasizes the therapist as expert and encourages a guiding style. These differences, of course, have practical implications for the nature of the working relationship and the tasks and goals of treatment. Clearly, we do not believe that these approaches are irreconcilable. There will be times when it is necessary for a therapist to adopt a more directive style; however, we are in favor of adopting a guiding style early in treatment as well as shifting to it in a flexible manner throughout the course of treatment. With the establishment of a positive working alliance, the therapist will have more "degrees of freedom" to adopt a directive stance when needed. It is also good practice to frequently check in with clients ("Does this fit with your goals?").

The modular structure of the UP presents another potential difficulty. Although the modular approach is aimed at increasing flexibility and personalization, there is the risk that therapists will approach the motivation enhancement module as a box that is simply checked after one or two sessions. This approach may result in either moving ahead prematurely with other treatment elements or failing to address motivation and engagement issues as they arise over the course of treatment. The likelihood of the former result is diminished with sufficient patience and attunement. To avoid the latter, therapists will do well to attend to process markers (Constantino et al., 2013), such as increased sustain talk and subtle alliance ruptures. Just as one would not ignore an opportunity to practice cognitive reappraisal after it was formally introduced several sessions earlier, one should not abandon potentially useful motivation enhancement strategies because "they were already covered." Nevertheless, flexibility should operate in both directions. Formal implementation of the motivation enhancement module may ultimately be unnecessary for some clients. In such instances, motivation enhancement strategies are best integrated on an as-needed basis in response to specific markers. Empirical evidence is lacking in this area, unfortunately, which makes it difficult to advocate for any particular set of guidelines.

Another potential difficulty is highlighted by the transdiagnostic conceptualization. In many ways, the aim of the UP is to address underlying neurotic temperament (Barlow, Sauer-Zavala, Carl, Bullis, & Ellard, 2014). Negative self-views are part and parcel of the so-called neurotic spectrum, as illustrated in the case described above. Indeed, a major focus of treatment is the modification of this negative self-view, and one of the goals of the motivation enhancement module is the instillation of hope (or an activation of positive self-striving). Basic social psychological theory and research has shown that people possess both self-enhancement and self-consistency strivings (Swann, 1996). For individuals with a neurotic temperament, these may be in conflict. In these instances, patients may employ strategies to protect the self from inconsistent feedback (see Pinel & Constantino, 2003). Therefore, therapists will need to be sensitive to patients' self-strivings by balancing their need for self-verification with movement toward change-oriented strategies. Moving too quickly toward changing this self-view (e.g., by attempting to provide corrective feedback—"This isn't the *real* you") may actually hinder engagement and disrupt the development of the working alliance (Constantino et al., 2010).

Conclusions

Considerable research has led to the identification of evidence-based treatments (Lambert, 2013), intervention principles (Castonguay & Beutler, 2006), and relationship factors (Norcross, 2011). Despite significant advances in these areas, a routine challenge is whether or not, and the degree to which, these elements generalize and can be effectively assimilated into ostensibly different treatment approaches and problem areas. Accumulating research and the chapters in this volume provide strong evidence that we are taking strides toward meeting this challenge. In this chapter, we have described how a specific transdiagnostic treatment approach (Unified Protocol for Transdiagnostic Treatment of Emotional Disorders) integrates MI-derived motivation enhancement strategies and principles. The cognitive-affective basis of motivation and ambivalence makes these factors particularly well suited for an emotion-focused treatment such as the UP. Moreover, the focus on shared underlying factors— which we believe are at the core of emotional difficulties—requires a level of conceptualization that goes beyond the more superficial variations in symptom constellations that have traditionally been the focus of CBT. This approach offers a pathway for the transdiagnostic application of MI strategies.

Research on the transdiagnostic application of MI principles and strategies is firmly in the action stage, and thus continued empirical attention is warranted. We believe that future work in this area should focus on the following questions:

1. What are the specific effects of motivational enhancement strategies on the process and outcome of transdiagnostic psychotherapy?
2. What are the client characteristics that moderate the relationship between motivational enhancement and treatment outcome, and for whom is it indicated (or contraindicated)?
3. What are the evidence-based within-treatment markers for responsively integrating motivational enhancement strategies?
4. How do we train clinicians to apply these strategies and principles in a flexible manner, particularly with complex clients?

Results from the current UP RCT will be an excellent resource for beginning to address the first three questions in transdiagnostic CBT. Addressing the fourth question will require additional research on the dissemination and implementation of intervention principles in routine treatment settings.

References

Abramowitz, J., Tolin, D., & Street, G. (2001). Paradoxical effects of thought suppression: a meta-analysis of controlled studies. *Clinical Psychology Review, 21*, 683–703.

American Psychiatric Association. (2000). *Diagnostic and statistical manual of mental disorders* (4th ed., text rev.). Washington, DC: Author.

American Psychiatric Association. (2013). *Diagnostic and statistical manual of mental disorders* (5th ed.). Arlington, VA: Author.

Andrews, G. (1996). Comorbidity in neurotic disorders: The similarities are more important than the differences. In R. M. Rapee (Ed.), *Current controversies in the anxiety disorders* (pp. 3–20). New York: Guilford Press.

Arkowitz, H., & Westra, H. A. (2004). Integrating motivational and cognitive behavioral therapy in the treatment of depression and anxiety. *Journal of Cognitive Psychotherapy, 18*, 337–350.

Barlow, D. H., Allen, L. B., & Choate, M. L. (2004). Toward a unified treatment for emotional disorders. *Behavior Therapy, 35*, 205–230.

Barlow, D. H., Ellard, K. K., Fairholme, C. P., Farchione, T. J., Boisseau, C. L., Allen, L. B., et al. (2011a). *Unified Protocol for Transdiagnostic Treatment of Emotional Disorders: Client workbook.* New York: Oxford University Press.

Barlow, D. H., Farchione, T. J., Fairholme, C. P., Ellard, K. K., Boisseau, C. L., Allen, L. B., et al. (2011b). *Unified Protocol for Transdiagnostic Treatment of Emotional Disorders: Therapist guide.* New York: Oxford University Press.

Barlow, D. H., Sauer-Zavala, S., Carl, J. R., Bullis, J. R., & Ellard, K. K. (2014). The nature, diagnosis, and treatment of neuroticism: Back to the future. *Clinical Psychological Science, 21*, 344–365.

Beck, A. T., & Clark, D. A. (1997). An information processing model of anxiety: Automatic and strategic processes. *Behaviour Research and Therapy, 35*, 49–58.

Beck, A. T., Epstein, N., Brown, G., & Steer, R. A. (1988). An inventory for measuring clinical anxiety: Psychometric properties. *Journal of Consulting and Clinical Psychology, 56*(6), 893–897.

Beck, A. T., Steer, R. A., & Brown, G. K. (1996). *Manual for the Beck Depression Inventory–II.* San Antonio, TX: Psychological Corp.

Bentley, K. H., Gallagher, M. W., Carl, J. R., & Barlow, D. H. (2014). Development and validation of the Overall Depression Severity and Impairment Scale. *Psychological Assessment, 26*, 815–830.

Bordin, E. S. (1979). The generalizability of the psychoanalytic concept of the working alliance. *Psychotherapy: Theory, Research and Practice, 16*, 252–260.

Borkovec, T. D., Alcaine, O. M., & Behar, E. (2004). Avoidance theory of worry and generalized anxiety disorder. In R. G. Heimberg, C. L. Turk, & D. S. Mennin (Eds.), *Generalized anxiety disorder: Advances in research and practice* (pp. 320–350). New York: Guilford Press.

Borkovec, T. D., Lyonfields, J. D., Wiser, S. L., & Diehl, L. (1993). The role of worrisome thinking in the suppression of cardiovascular response to phobic imagery. *Behaviour Research and Therapy, 31*, 321–324.

Borkovec, T. D., & Nau, S. D. (1972). Credibility of analogue therapy rationales. *Journal of Behavior Therapy and Experimental Psychiatry, 3*, 257–260.

Boswell, J. F. (2013). Intervention strategies and clinical process in transdiagnostic cognitive-behavioral therapy. *Psychotherapy, 50*, 381–386.

Boswell, J. F., Anderson, L. M., & Barlow, D. H. (2014). An idiographic analysis of change processes in the unified transdiagnostic treatment of depression. *Journal of Consulting and Clinical Psychology, 82*, 1060–1071.

Boswell, J. F., & Goldfried, M. R. (2010). Psychotherapy integration. In I. B. Weiner & W. E. Craighead (Eds.), *The Corsini encyclopedia of psychology* (4th ed, pp. 1–3). New York: Wiley.

Boswell, J. F., Llera, S. J., Newman, M. G., & Castonguay, L. G. (2011). A case of premature termination in a treatment for generalized anxiety disorder. *Cognitive and Behavioral Practice, 18*, 326–337.

Boswell, J. F., Nelson, D. L., Nordberg, S. S., McAleavey, A. A., & Castonguay, L. G. (2010). Competency in integrative psychotherapy: Perspectives on training and supervision. *Psychotherapy Theory, Research, Practice, Training, 47*, 3–11.

Boswell, J. F., Sauer-Zavala, S. E., Gallagher, M. W., Delgado, N., & Barlow, D. H. (2012). Readiness to change as a moderator of outcome in transdiagnostic treatment. *Psychotherapy Research, 22*, 570–578.

Boswell, J. F., Thompson-Hollands, J., Farchione, T. J., & Barlow, D. H. (2013). Intolerance of uncertainty: A common factor in the treatment of emotional disorders. *Journal of Clinical Psychology, 69*, 630–645.

Brown, T. A. (2007). Temporal course and structural relationships among dimensions of temperament and DSM-IV anxiety and mood disorders. *Journal of Abnormal Psychology, 116*, 313–328.

Brown, T. A., & Barlow, D. H. (2009). A proposal for a dimensional classification system based on the shared features of the DSM-IV anxiety and mood disorders: Implications for assessment and treatment. *Psychological Assessment, 21*, 256–271.

Brown, T. A., Campbell, L. A., Lehman, C. L., Grisham, J. R., & Mancill, R. B. (2001). Current and lifetime comorbidity of the DSM-IV anxiety and mood disorders in a large clinical sample. *Journal of Abnormal Psychology, 110*, 49–58.

Brown, T. A., Chorpita, B. F., & Barlow, D. H. (1998). Structural relationships among dimensions of the DSM-IV anxiety and mood disorders and dimensions of negative affect, positive affect, and autonomic arousal. *Journal of Abnormal Psychology, 107*, 179–192.

Butler, A. C., Chapman, J. E., Forman, E. M., & Beck, A. T. (2006). The empirical status of cognitive-behavioral therapy: A review of meta-analyses. *Clinical Psychology Review, 26*, 17–31.

Campbell-Sills, L., Barlow, D. H., Brown, T. A., & Hofmann, S. G. (2006). Acceptability and suppression of negative emotion in anxiety and mood disorders. *Emotion, 6*, 587–595.

Campbell-Sills, L., Ellard, K. K., & Barlow, D. H. (2014). Emotion regulation in anxiety disorders. In J. J. Gross (Ed.), *Handbook of emotion regulation* (2nd ed., pp. 393–412). New York: Guilford Press.

Carver, C. S., & White, T. L. (1994). Behavioral inhibition, behavioral activation, and affective responses to impending reward and punishment: The BIS/BAS scales. *Journal of Personality and Social Psychology, 67*, 319–333.

Castonguay, L. G., & Beutler, L. E. (2006). Principles of therapeutic change: A task force on participants, relationships, and technique factors. *Journal of Clinical Psychology, 62*, 631–638.

Castonguay, L. G., Constantino, M. J., Boswell, J. F., & Kraus, D. (2010). The therapeutic alliance: Research and theory. In L. Horowitz & S. Strack (Eds.), *Handbook of interpersonal psychology: Theory, research, assessment, and therapeutic interventions* (pp. 509–518). New York: Wiley.

Castonguay, L. G., Constantino, M. J., McAleavey, A. A., & Goldfried, M. R. (2010). The alliance in cognitive-behavioral therapy. In J. C. Muran & J. P. Barber (Eds.), *The therapeutic alliance: An evidence-based guide to practice* (pp. 150–171). New York: Guilford Press.

Castonguay, L. G., & Hill, C. E. (Eds.). (2012). *Transformation in psychotherapy: Corrective experiences across cognitive behavioral, humanistic, and psychodynamic approaches*. Washington, DC: American Psychological Association Press.

Clarkin, J., & Levy, K. N. (2004). Client variables. In M. J. Lambert (Ed.), *Bergin and Garfield's handbook of psychotherapy and behavior change*. New York: Oxford University Press.

Constantino, M. J., Boswell, J. F., Bernecker, S., & Castonguay, L. G. (2013). Context-responsive psychotherapy integration as a framework for a unified clinical science: Conceptual and empirical considerations. *Journal of Unified Psychotherapy and Clinical Science, 2*, 1–20.

Constantino, M. J., Castonguay, L. G., Zack, S. E., & DeGeorge, J. (2010). Engagement in psychotherapy: Factors contributing to the facilitation, demise, and restoration of the therapeutic alliance. In D. Castro-Blanco & M. S. Karver (Eds.), *Elusive alliance: Treatment engagement strategies with high-risk adolescents* (pp. 21–57). Washington, DC: American Psychological Association.

Constantino, M. J., DeGeorge, J., Dadlani, M. B., & Overtree, C. E. (2009). Motivational interviewing: A bellwether for context-response integration. *Journal of Clinical Psychology: In Session, 65*, 1246–1253.

Craske, M. G., & Barlow, D. H. (2007). *Mastery of your anxiety and panic: Therapist guide*. New York: Oxford University Press.

Dalgleish, T., & Watts, F. N. (1990). Biases of attention and memory in disorders of anxiety and depression. *Clinical Psychology Review, 10*, 589–604.

DiNardo, P. A., Brown, T. A., & Barlow, D. H. (1994). *Anxiety Disorders Interview Schedule for DSM-IV: Lifetime Version (ADIS-IV-L)*. San Antonio, TX: Psychological Corp.

Ellard, K. K., Deckersbach, T., Sylvia, L. G., Nierenberg, A. A., & Barlow, D. H. (2012). Transdiagnostic treatment of bipolar disorder and comorbid anxiety with the Unified Protocol: A clinical replication series. *Behavior Modification, 36*, 482–508.

Ellard, K. K., Fairholme, C. P., Boisseau, C. L., Farchione, T., & Barlow, D. H. (2010). Unified protocol for the transdiagnostic treatment of emotional disorders: Protocol development and initial outcome data. *Cognitive and Behavioral Practice, 17*, 88–101.

Endicott, J., Nee, J., Harrison, W., & Blumenthal, R. (1993). Quality of Life Enjoyment and Satisfaction Questionnaire: A new measure. *Psychopharmacology Bulletin, 29*, 321–326.

Engle, D. E., & Arkowitz, H. (2006). *Ambivalence in psychotherapy: Facilitating readiness to change*. New York: Guilford Press.

Etkin, A., & Wager, T. D. (2007). Functional neuroimaging of anxiety: A meta-analysis of emotional processing in PTSD, social anxiety disorder, and specific phobia. *American Journal of Psychiatry, 164*, 1476–1488.

Fairburn, C. G., Cooper, Z., & Shafran, R. (2003). Cognitive behavior therapy for eating disorders: A "transdiagnostic" theory and treatment. *Behaviour Research and Therapy, 41*, 509–528.

Farchione, T. J., Fairholme, C. P., Ellard, K. K., Boisseau, C. L., Thompson-Hollands, J., Carl, J. R., et al. (2012). Unified Protocol for Transdiagnostic Treatment of Emotional Disorders: A randomized controlled trial. *Behavior Therapy, 43*, 666–678.

Fellous, J., & LeDoux, J. E. (2005). Toward basic principles for emotional processing: What the fearful brain tells the robot. In J. Fellous & M. A. Arbib (Eds.), *Who needs emotions?: The brain meets the robot* (pp. 79–115). New York: Oxford University Press.

Gollwitzer, P. M. (1999). Implementation intentions: Simple effects of simple plans. *American Psychologist, 54*, 493–503.

Gross, J. J., & John, O. (2003). Individual differences in two emotion regulation processes: Implications for affect, relationships, and well-being. *Journal of Personality and Social Psychology, 85*, 348–362.

Hayes, A. M., Beck, G., & Yasinski, C. (2012). A cognitive behavioral perspective on corrective experiences. In L. G. Castonguay & C. E. Hill (Eds.), *Transformation in psychotherapy: Corrective experiences across cognitive behavioral, humanistic, and psychodynamic approaches* (pp. 69–83). Washington, DC: American Psychological Association Press.

Hollon, S. D., & Beck, A. T. (2013). Cognitive and cognitive-behavioral therapies. In M. J. Lambert (Ed.), *Bergin and Garfield's handbook of psychotherapy and behavior change* (6th ed., pp. 393–442). New York: Wiley.

Kessler, R. C., Berglund, P., Demler, O., Jin, R., Merikangas, K. R., & Walters, E. E. (2005). Lifetime prevalence and age-of-onset distributions of DSM-IV disorders in the National Comorbidity Survey Replication. *Archives of General Psychiatry, 62,* 593–602.

Lambert, M. J. (Ed.). (2013). *Bergin and Garfield's handbook of psychotherapy and behavior change* (6th ed.). New York: Wiley.

LeDoux, J. E. (1996). *The emotional brain: The mysterious underpinnings of emotional life.* New York: Simon & Schuster.

McConnaughy, E. A., DiClemente, C. C., Prochaska, J. O., & Velicer, W. F. (1989). Stages of change in psychotherapy: A follow-up report. *Psychotherapy, 26,* 494–503.

McConnaughy, E. A., Prochaska, J. O., & Velicer, W. F. (1983). Stage of change in psychotherapy: Measurement and sample profiles. *Psychotherapy, 20,* 368–375.

McHugh, R. K., & Barlow, D. H. (2010). Dissemination and implementation of evidence-based psychological interventions: A review of current efforts. *American Psychologist, 65,* 73–84.

McLaughlin, K. A., Borkovec, T. D., & Sibrava, N. J. (2007). The effects of worry and rumination on affect states and cognitive activity. *Behavior Therapy, 38,* 23–38.

Mennin, D., Heimberg, R., Turk, C., & Fresco, D. (2005). Preliminary evidence for an emotional dysregulation model of generalized anxiety disorder. *Behaviour Research and Therapy, 43,* 1281–1310.

Messer, S. B. (2001). Introduction to the special issue on assimilative integration. *Journal of Psychotherapy Integration, 11,* 1–4.

Miller, W. R., & Rollnick, S. (2013). *Motivational interviewing: Helping people change* (3rd ed.). New York: Guilford Press.

Mobini, S., & Grant, A. (2007). Clinical implications of attentional bias in anxiety disorders: An integrative literature review. *Psychotherapy: Theory, Research, Practice, Training, 44,* 450–462.

Nathan, P., & Gorman, J. (Eds.). (2007). *A guide to treatments that work* (3rd ed.). New York: Oxford University Press.

Newman, M. G., Crits-Christoph, P., Connolly Gibbons, M. B., & Erickson, T. E. (2006). Participant factors in the treatment of anxiety disorders. In L. G. Castonguay and L. E. Beutler (Eds.), *Principles of therapeutic change that work* (pp. 121–154). New York: Oxford Press.

Norcross, J. C. (2005). A primer on psychotherapy integration. In J. C. Norcross & M. R. Goldfried (Eds.), *Handbook of psychotherapy integration* (2nd ed., pp. 3–23). New York: Oxford University Press.

Norcross, J. C. (Ed.). (2011). *Psychotherapy relationships that work: Evidence-based responsiveness* (2nd ed.) New York: Oxford University Press.

Norman, S. B., Hami-Cissell, S., Means-Christensen, A. J., & Stein, M. B. (2006). Development and validation of an Overall Anxiety Severity and Impairment Scale (OASIS). *Depression and Anxiety, 23,* 245–249.

Norton, P. J., & Philipp, L. M. (2008). Transdiagnostic approaches to the treatment of anxiety disorders: A meta-analytic review. *Psychotherapy: Theory, Research, Practice, Training, 45,* 214–226.

Payne, L. A., Ellard, K. K., Farchione, T. J., Fairholme, C. P., & Barlow, D. H. (2014). Emotional disorders: A unified transdiagnostic protocol. In D. H. Barlow (Ed.), *Clinical handbook of psychological disorders: A step-by-step treatment manual* (5th ed., pp. 237–274). New York: Guilford Press.

Pinel, E. C., & Constantino, M. J. (2003). Putting self psychology to good use: When social psychologists and clinical psychologists unite. *Journal of Psychotherapy Integration, 13,* 9–32.

Prochaska, J. O., & DiClemente, C. C. (1984). *The transtheoretical approach: Crossing the traditional boundaries of therapy.* Homewood, IL: Dow-Jones/Irwin.

Prochaska, J. O., & Norcross, J. C. (2002). *Systems of psychotherapy: A transtheoretical analysis* (5th ed.). Pacific Grove, CA: Brooks-Cole.

Safran, J. D., Muran, J. C., & Eubanks-Carter, C. (2011). Repairing alliance ruptures. *Psychotherapy, 48,* 80–87.

Snyder, C. R., Sympson, S. C., Ybasco, F. C., Borders, T. F., Babyak, M. A., & Higgins, R. L. (1996). Development and validation of the State Hope Scale. *Journal of Personality and Social Psychology, 2,* 321–335.

Swann, W. B., Jr. (1996). *Self-traps: The elusive quest for higher self-esteem.* New York: Freeman.

Swift, J. K., & Greenberg, R. P. (2012). Premature discontinuation in adult psychotherapy: A meta-analysis. *Journal of Consulting and Clinical Psychology, 80,* 547–559.

Thompson-Hollands, J., Bentley, K. H., Gallagher, M. W., Boswell, J. F., & Barlow, D. H. (2014). Credibility and outcome expectancy in the Unified Protocol: Relationship to outcomes. *Journal of Experimental Psychopathology, 5,* 72–82.

Tracey, T. J., & Kokotovic, A. M. (1989). Factor structure of the Working Alliance Inventory. *Psychological Assessment, 1,* 207–210.

Tyrer, P. J. (1989). *Classification of neurosis.* Chichester, UK: Wiley.

Watson, D., & Clark, L. A. (1984). Negative affectivity: The disposition to experience aversive emotional states. *Psychological Bulletin, 96,* 465–490.

Webb, C. A., DeRubeis, R. J., Amsterdam, J. D., Shelton, R. C., Hollon, S. D., & Dimidjian, S. (2011). Two aspects of the therapeutic alliance: Differential relations with depressive symptom change. *Journal of Consulting and Clinical Psychology, 79,* 279–283.

Wegner, D. M., Schneider, D. J., Carter, S., & White, T. (1987). Paradoxical effects of thought suppression. *Journal of Personality and Social Psychology, 53,* 5–13.

Westra, H. A. (2004). Managing resistance in cognitive behavioural therapy: Application of motivational interviewing in mixed anxiety depression. *Cognitive Behaviour Therapy, 33,* 161–175.

Westra, H. A., Arkowitz, H., & Dozois, D. J. A. (2009). Adding motivational interviewing pretreatment to cognitive behavioral therapy for generalized anxiety disorder: A preliminary controlled trial. *Journal of Anxiety Disorders, 23,* 1106–1117.

Wolfe, B. E. (2011). Anxiety disorders. In J. C. Norcross, G. R. VandenBos, & D. K. Freedheim (Eds.), *History of psychotherapy: Continuity and change* (2nd ed., pp. 561–573). Washington, DC: American Psychological Association.

Zimmerman, M., Chelminski, I., & McDermut, W. (2002). Major depressive disorder and axis I diagnostic comorbidity. *Journal of Clinical Psychiatry, 63,* 187–193.

CHAPTER 3

• • • • • •

Enhancing the Effectiveness of Exposure and Response Prevention in the Treatment of Obsessive–Compulsive Disorder

Exploring a Role for Motivational Interviewing

Allan Zuckoff
Iván C. Balán
Helen Blair Simpson

With a lifetime prevalence of 2–3%, obsessive–compulsive disorder (OCD) is an important cause of illness-related disability. This disproportionate impact reflects the fact that OCD typically starts in childhood or adolescence, persists throughout a person's life, and produces substantial impairment in functioning because of the severe and chronic nature of the illness.

The hallmarks of OCD are obsessions (i.e., recurrent intrusive thoughts, images, or urges that cause anxiety or distress) and compulsions (i.e., repetitive mental or behavioral acts). Compulsions are typically performed in response to an obsession (e.g., fears of contamination leading to washing rituals) to reduce the distress triggered by obsessions or to prevent a feared event (e.g., becoming ill). However, these compulsions are either not realistic (e.g., repeatedly calling up a positive image to prevent harm befalling a loved one) or are clearly excessive (e.g., showering for many hours each day).

Although all people with OCD have obsessions and/or compulsions, the specific content of the obsessions and compulsions differs among individuals with the disorder. Certain themes are common, including forbidden or taboo thoughts (e.g., aggressive, sexual, and religious obsessions and related compulsions), cleaning (with fears of contamination associated with related cleaning rituals), harm (with fears of harm to oneself or others resulting in checking compulsions), and symmetry (with symmetry obsessions resulting in repeating, ordering, and counting compulsions). Historically, hoarding concerns (the obsessive collecting and maintaining of worthless objects) have also been included with OCD, although the *Diagnostic and Statistical Manual of Mental Disorders* now recognizes a separate diagnosis of hoarding disorder. People with OCD also differ significantly in their recognition of the irrationality of their obsessions and compulsions ("insight"), and the level of insight can fluctuate over the course of the illness and thereby complicate treatment.

Usual Treatments

Practice guidelines for OCD recommend pharmacotherapy with serotonin reuptake inhibitors (i.e., clomipramine and the selective serotonin reuptake inhibitors [SSRIs] like fluoxetine) and cognitive-behavioral therapy (CBT) alone or in combination as first-line treatments (Koran, Hanna, Hollander, Nestadt, & Simpson, 2007). The form of CBT employed is called exposure and response prevention (EX/RP). Randomized controlled trials have shown that 70–80% of clients who enter EX/RP treatment will respond to it, and up to 50% will achieve minimal symptoms after acute treatment (Foa et al., 2005; Simpson, Foa, et al., 2008, 2013). Not only does EX/RP lead to acute improvement in OCD symptoms, but many clients can also maintain their gains over time. In some randomized controlled trials, CBT with or without medication has been shown to be more effective than medication alone (Foa et al., 2005; Simpson et al., 2013).

EX/RP teaches people new strategies to cope with obsessions and compulsions (Kozak & Foa, 1997). Specifically, clients are taught to confront what they fear ("exposure") and to refrain from performing compulsions (also known as "ritualizing") when doing so ("response prevention"). Exposures involve live confrontations with feared situations (e.g., touching objects in public bathrooms for a client with contamination fears) and imaginal confrontations with feared consequences (e.g., imagining killing someone for a client with aggressive concerns). When clients face their fears for a prolonged period without ritualizing, their belief that the consequences they fear will inevitably follows is typically disconfirmed; the usual result is a reduction in their anxiety and in the perceived need to ritualize.

When clients adhere to these procedures, EX/RP is highly efficacious. For example, in a recent trial of EX/RP, client adherence to EX/RP procedures significantly predicted posttreatment OCD severity (Simpson et al., 2011; Simpson, Marcus, Zuckoff, Franklin, & Foa, 2012). Moreover, the degree of client adherence was significantly associated with the degree of improvement and the odds of response.

However, some clients refuse EX/RP, and others choose not to adhere by dropping out of treatment or by not fully implementing the procedures as recommended (Abramowitz, Franklin, Zoellner, & DiBernardo, 2002; Foa et al., 1983; Simpson et al., 2006). It is estimated that at least 50% of OCD clients who try EX/RP do not respond optimally, even when combined with pharmacotherapy (Simpson, Huppert, Petkova, Foa, & Liebowitz, 2006; Simpson, Foa, et al., 2008; Simpson et al., 2013; Sookman & Steketee, 2007). If the link between client adherence and EX/RP outcome is causal, then increasing treatment entry, reducing dropout, and improving client adherence to EX/RP procedures should improve treatment outcomes. We and others have explored whether motivational interviewing (MI) can be used to improve client adherence to EX/RP.

Rationale for Employing MI in the Treatment of OCD

MI has demonstrated efficacy in increasing adherence to a variety of treatments for substance use, mental health, and chronic medical conditions (Lundahl, Kunz, Brownell, Tollefson, & Burke, 2010; Zuckoff & Hettema, 2007). In particular, MI has been used to foster participation in cognitive-behavioral therapies for persons with anxiety disorders (see Westra & Aviram, Chapter 4, and Yusko, Drapkin, & Yeh, Chapter 5, this volume for discussions of the use of MI in the treatment of generalized anxiety disorder and posttraumatic stress disorder). MI appears to be especially effective when employed as a prelude or adjunct designed to enhance the effects of lengthier or more intensive treatments, including cognitive-behavioral therapy (Hettema, Steele, & Miller, 2005).

MI has motivated people with alcohol dependence to adhere to alcohol treatment (Connors, Walitzer, & Dermen, 2002), people with uncontrolled pain to attend a pain reduction workshop (Habib, Morrissey, & Helmes, 2005), overweight women with diabetes to adhere to behavioral weight control treatment (West, DiLillo, Bursac, Gore, & Greene, 2007), and depressed Hispanics to remain in antidepressant treatment (Lewis-Fernandez et al., 2013). In all these cases, MI can be conceived of as increasing motivation to do something challenging or unpleasant in the short term (i.e., resist urges to drink and make a variety of behavioral, emotional, and lifestyle changes; engage in difficult physical rehabilitation activities; self-monitor dietary intake and blood-sugar levels; take medications as prescribed) for long-term gains. Analogously, MI might also be able to help motivate OCD clients to resist or ignore urges to ritualize (even if rituals relieve short-term distress) and to confront fears (even if exposures produce short-term distress) in order to improve their OCD symptoms, functioning, and general well-being.

Zuckoff and colleagues (Zuckoff & Daley, 2001; Zweben & Zuckoff, 2002) argued that the likelihood that a person will enter, participate in, and complete treatment may be impacted by ambivalence not only about change but also about the treatment itself as a pathway toward change. For clients with OCD, the benefits of reducing the time spent obsessing and engaging in rituals, and the negative impact of these symptomatic behaviors on their lives, may be balanced or outweighed by the benefits of symptomatic behaviors (e.g., perceived safety, short-term anxiety reduction). Additionally, their confidence in their ability to change their symptomatic ways of thinking and acting may be low. If MI were successful in helping OCD clients resolve their ambivalence about change, they might commit more fully to EX/RP treatment. However, the aversiveness of the EX/RP procedures may be an especially potent obstacle. In EX/RP, OCD clients are asked to expose themselves repeatedly and at length to feared stimuli without ritualizing or avoiding. Successful outcomes in EX/RP thus require the willingness to tolerate the considerable anxiety and discomfort such exposures evoke and to commit substantial time and energy to a highly structured and demanding treatment. If ambivalence about taking these actions were resolved, clients might participate more fully in EX/RP.

Important aspects of MI include building engagement and developing a collaborative focus. Clients with OCD express a wide variety of reasons for being uncertain about change and for reluctance to initiate EX/RP, attend consistently, participate actively, and continue until the therapy is complete. The receptive, exploratory nature of the MI style and its highly individualizing approach would therefore seem a good fit. EX/RP relies primarily on psychoeducation and encouragement to motivate clients to participate in treatment; EX/RP therapist manuals do not provide an explicit framework for recognizing when the therapist has "gotten ahead" of clients' readiness to change and for responding accordingly. MI's emphasis on recognizing, evoking, and responding to change talk before collaborating on action toward change could also bring added value.

Whether the clinical style of MI represents a good match with the approach of EX/RP is more ambiguous. On the one hand, MI does not promote behaviors that could undermine the effectiveness of EX/RP, such as "neutralizing" (i.e., compulsively canceling out unwanted thoughts with positive alternatives), and it does promote factors upon which standard EX/RP relies for its effectiveness: a strong therapeutic alliance, a collaborative relationship, and a client's sense of self-efficacy.

On the other hand, although EX/RP relies on a strong therapeutic alliance for its effects, there is a directive component as well that conflicts with the interactional style of MI. The foci of treatment are identification of and treatment of OCD symptoms. It is assumed that the client has come to treatment to learn a new set of skills and that the therapist's role is to teach these skills and direct the treatment; client adherence to the procedures the therapist recommends is crucial. Possible ramifications of tension between this expert-driven approach and the client-centered style of MI will be discussed later in this chapter.

Clinical Applications

Research by Others on Enhancing the Effects of CBT for OCD

To date, few studies have been conducted to assess how MI might enhance the effects of CBT for clients with OCD. Maltby and Tolin (2005) developed a four-session readiness intervention that was intended to decrease EX/RP refusal among clients with OCD. The readiness intervention consisted of 4 individual visits with a therapist over 1 month and included (1) psychoeducation focused on OCD and the empirical data supporting the efficacy of EX/RP; (2) explicit use of MI procedures in two of the four sessions; (3) presentation of a videotape about EX/RP; (4) construction of a sample exposure hierarchy; and (5) speaking with a client who had completed EX/RP. Twelve clients who had previously refused EX/RP (for other than logistical reasons) were randomly assigned to receive this readiness intervention ($n = 7$) or to remain on a waiting list (n = 5) for 1 month. After 1 month, they were offered 15 EX/RP sessions. Of the participants who received the readiness intervention, 86% agreed to begin EX/RP treatment as compared to 20% of those who received the waiting-list condition. When EX/RP treatment followed the readiness intervention (but not when it followed the waiting-list condition), clients experienced a decrease in OCD symptoms comparable to that observed in OCD clients who did not refuse EX/RP. However, the dropout rate for EX/RP following the readiness intervention was 50%, a rate higher than the typical EX/RP dropout rate. These data provide preliminary support for the hypothesis that a multimodal intervention that includes some MI elements can increase the rates of acceptance of EX/RP, but the data also suggest that this intervention is insufficient to prevent later dropout. However, the small sample size precludes strong conclusions. Moreover, the fact that the readiness intervention was multimodal makes it impossible to ascertain the importance of the addition of the MI procedures per se.

Meyer and colleagues (2010) provided two individual sessions of MI and thought mapping (TM) prior to group CBT. TM is a structured approach based on the transtheoretical model (Prochaska & DiClemente, 1984) that aims to help clients understand the relationship between thoughts and actions (Leukefeld, Brown, Clark, Godlaski, & Hays, 2000; Leukefeld et al., 2005; Inciardi et al., 2006). The group CBT sessions were conducted over a period of 12 weeks, with eight participants per cohort. These sessions included psychoeducation, EX/RP techniques, cognitive techniques to change dysfunctional beliefs, and general group therapy techniques. Results from the study (n = 93) showed that the group receiving the MI+TM pretreatment showed a greater reduction in OCD symptoms as compared to those with CBT alone. They also noted that there was further symptom reduction at the 3-month follow-up for the MI+TM group. However, because once again MI was combined with another intervention, it is not possible to determine its specific contribution to outcome.

Focusing on children and adolescents (n = 16) with OCD, Merlo and colleagues (2010) compared clients who received a three-session pretreatment to those who received psychoeducation (PE), both followed by group CBT. The CBT intervention consisted of providing information about OCD and the treatment rationale, EX/RP exercises, and later in the treatment cognitive interventions for obsessive thinking. The MI or PE sessions were conducted before the first session of the CBT, immediately following Session 4, and before Session 8. Results showed that by Week 5 of treatment, OCD symptoms were significantly lower for the CBT+MI group than for the CBT+PE group. The difference found between groups at week 5 was not sustained posttreatment. However, clients in the CBT+MI group achieved their treatment gains in fewer sessions than those in the CBT+PE groups (10.75 vs. 13.75 sessions, respectively).

Research by Our Group

We have explored two ways of using MI to enhance OCD treatment engagement and adherence. First, in what we called the "MI stuck" procedure, we employed MI to motivate clients to seek evidence-based treatment for OCD (i.e., medication or EX/RP or both). Second, in the CBT+MI procedure, we added MI to EX/RP with the goal of enhancing treatment adherence and improving client outcomes. We describe each of these interventions and summarize the results of our research in the two sections that follow.

"MI Stuck"

The "MI stuck" intervention focused on clients who had declined referral for OCD treatment despite experiencing significant symptoms and wishing for relief from those symptoms. We thus conceptualized them as "stuck" in ambivalence about change and/or treatment. Clients received four weekly MI sessions that each lasted 1 hour, with the goal of motivating them to pursue an evidence-based treatment for OCD (i.e., either EX/RP or pharmacotherapy or both) (Simpson & Zuckoff, 2011).

The intervention was structured as follows. In Session 1, the therapist began by asking what clients identified as their main problem (without assuming *a priori* that it was OCD or that the client would call it OCD). After developing a shared perspective about the problem, the therapist then elicited how this problem affected clients' lives. The aim was to use MI to increase motivation for change by developing and highlighting discrepancy between how their life was and how they would like it to be. The therapist also assessed how important clients felt it was to make a change in their OCD symptoms and worked to increase the importance of change as needed.

Assuming that the client expressed that change was important, Session 2 focused on assessing and building confidence for change. This included reviewing clients' prior attempts at change, specifically eliciting clients' perspective on any negative aspects of prior treatments as well as why the treatments failed (Grote, Zuckoff, Swartz, Bledsoe, &

Geibel, 2007; Swartz et al., 2008). The therapist's goal was to build confidence in change by reflecting what had worked in the past, providing a different perspective on past failures where appropriate (e.g., attributing disappointing outcomes to factors other than the efficacy of the treatments or clients' inability to succeed), and offering key information about evidence-based treatments in an MI-congruent way. Inevitably, ambivalence not only about treatment but also about change emerged, and the therapist shifted between building importance for change and building confidence in being able to make the needed changes.

If the client expressed that change was necessary and possible, Session 3 focused on what options for change, if any, clients were considering now. The goal was to help those clients who appeared ready for change (as indicated by their level of change talk in Sessions 1 and 2) to express a commitment to change by engaging in evidence-based treatments (EX/RP and/or medication).

If the client made a commitment to change using one or both of these treatments, Session 4 was used to help the client develop a specific change plan. This entailed evoking the specific changes the clients wanted to make, the reasons for making them, steps they planned to take to achieve their goals (i.e., what treatments), and hurdles they anticipated and potential solutions to address these obstacles. Appropriate referrals were offered if requested. If a client continued to express ambivalence about change or treatment in Session 3, Session 4 was used to continue to evoke change talk with the goal of moving the client closer to commitment.

Six clients received this intervention. One month after Session 4, the therapist called the clients to assess their current perspective about their OCD and their need for change as well as to learn whether they had sought (or planned to seek) OCD treatment. Three would have met the new DSM-5 diagnostic criteria for hoarding disorder. Of these, all had previously tried and failed SSRI treatment, and none wanted EX/RP, primarily because they did not want to discard their clutter. Two expressed the intention to take smaller steps (e.g., to stop acquiring and start organizing their possessions) but were unable to construct a concrete change plan, given the enormity of the task (e.g., apartments full of clutter such that entire rooms were inaccessible) and their inability to decide where and how to start. Despite expressing strong wishes for their lives to be different, all three continued to highly value the perceived benefits of hoarding (e.g., ensuring that objects with potential use did not go to waste, increasing a sense of security that they would not be without material resources, maintaining ties to the past). At follow-up, none of the three had engaged in EX/RP or pharmacotherapy or made significant progress in self-directed activities to address their hoarding. At the same time, all expressed a desire to change their behavior and wished to continue to work with the MI therapist. As one client said: "You are the first person whom I feel really understands my dilemma. I feel hopeful when I speak with you, and I can see that keeping all this stuff is ruining my life. My mind is clear in your office. The problem is when I go home I seem to forget everything I learn here."

In contrast, the other three clients, who would have met DSM-5 criteria for OCD but not for hoarding disorder, did shift in their willingness to pursue evidence-based treatment. One committed to EX/RP treatment in the fourth session and was receiving EX/RP at 1-month follow-up. Another did not commit to evidence-based treatment at the fourth session and was not pursuing treatment at 1-month follow-up; however, 2 weeks later, she spontaneously called the therapist to say that she had sought and received medication for OCD. At the fourth session, the remaining client committed to continuing his SSRI medication and implementing EX/RP procedures on his own. At follow-up, he continued on his SSRI and reported progress in his self-directed efforts. Although we do not have controlled empirical data as yet on the "MI Stuck" approach, these results show promise, at least for clients who do not meet the criteria for hoarding disorder.

Adding MI to EX/RP (EX/RP+MI)

In this intervention, MI was combined with standard EX/RP treatment to help clients who either drop out or only partially adhere to the EX/RP procedures. The goal was to determine whether MI could enhance EX/RP retention and adherence and thereby improve client outcomes.

The two standard introductory sessions of EX/RP were expanded into three, and MI was integrated into the sessions. Although the goals of the introductory sessions included accomplishing the same tasks as in standard EX/RP (assessment, psychoeducation, and treatment planning), therapists conducted the sessions using an MI-congruent stance—empathic, affirming, and autonomy-supportive—and with the intention of developing a collaborative relationship by finding the place where the therapist's aspirations for the client intertwined with the client's aspirations for him- or herself. Consistent with this stance, therapists were taught to use the elicit–provide–elicit framework for exchanging information and offering feedback. They were also taught to listen for, respond effectively to, and evoke client talk in the direction of motivation for and commitment to change and treatment adherence, using the full range of MI strategies and in particular drawing out clients' values and goals and highlighting how change through EX/RP could help achieve them.

During the 15 exposure sessions that followed, standard EX/RP procedures were employed (therapist-supervised exposures, assignment of between-session EX/RP practice, and review of between-session EX/RP practice). If clients balked at completing in-session exposures, reported not doing between-session exposures, or otherwise expressed reluctance to proceed with the treatment, therapists initially used standard EX/RP methods (e.g., psychoeducation, encouragement) for responding to them in these situations. However, if these strategies were insufficient to achieve adherence with the key procedures of EX/RP, therapists were to shift into use of a short (15- to 30-minute) MI module. The objective of this module was to assess and enhance commitment to the time-limited and intensive EX/RP used in the treatment protocol and to reengage the client before proceeding. Therapists were trained to recognize "resistance" (what we would now call discord) using the Miller and Rollnick (2002) adaptation of the rubric developed by Chamberlain and colleagues (1984) and to respond in MI-consistent ways designed to reduce it. They were also taught to view clients as rich resources for solving problems that arise in treatment and to respect clients' determination to chart their own course through the treatment process. Once the client's commitment to continuing with the EX/RP procedures was reestablished, the therapist shifted back into the standard directive EX/RP stance.

Six clients received this EX/RP–MI intervention in an open prospective pilot trial (Simpson, Zuckoff, Page, Franklin, & Foa, 2008), and all but one completed treatment. Five showed a decrease in the severity of their OCD symptoms and an increase in their quality of life, and three had either no or minimal symptoms at the end of treatment. The outcome in these six clients was at least as good as it is with standard EX/RP (Foa et al., 2005; Simpson, Foa, et al., 2008).

We then conducted a pilot randomized controlled trial comparing EX/RP with and without the addition of MI (Simpson, Zuckoff, et al., 2010). Specifically, 30 adults with OCD were randomized to 18 sessions of EX/RP or EX/RP+MI. Therapists rated client adherence at each exposure session. Independent evaluators assessed the change in OCD and depressive symptoms, and clients completed self-report measures of readiness for change, readiness for treatment, and quality of life. There were no significant between-groups differences either in improvement in OCD symptoms or in client adherence as rated with the Patient EX/RP Adherence Scale.

The failure of MI to enhance adherence or outcomes in this study could be attributable to one or more factors. Perhaps MI cannot resolve ambivalence about change in at least some clients with OCD, or perhaps poor EX/RP adherence is unrelated to ambivalence. On the other hand, clients in both treatment conditions were high in measured readiness for treatment from the start; given that, on average, client adherence was good in both treatment groups, the absence of differences could reflect a ceiling effect. It might also be that the intervention protocol we used did not provide sufficient quantity or quality of MI to yield significant effects, or that the therapist's shifting between MI and CBT stances was confusing for clients. We discuss these considerations in more detail later in this chapter.

Clinical Illustrations

MI Stuck

At the start of Session 1, the client stated that he had tried all evidence-based treatments for OCD, and none had worked. At the same time, he described his obsessions about harm and checking compulsions as an "addiction" that crippled his social and work functioning. Rating the importance of change as a 10 (on a scale from 0 to 10), he rated his confidence that he could change as 3 of 10. As the session progressed, it became clear that the primary issue for this client was not motivation for change but motivation for treatment: he was deeply discouraged about the prospect that treatment could work for him and thus unwilling to initiate either of the two evidence-based treatments available.

In Session 2, the client revealed that he had never fully stopped his rituals during prior EX/RP trials nor done his homework exposures as instructed. The therapist elicited several reasons: the client doubted the procedures would work for him, he didn't like the anxiety he experienced, and he felt his vigilance about harm helped make him an ethical person. The therapist then reframed the client's EX/RP experience not as a treatment failure (as the client had perceived it) but as a question that remained to be answered, namely: What would happen if the client were to complete a course of EX/RP with full engagement? The discussion that followed included information exchange about EX/RP's effectiveness and the necessity of full participation to obtain the desired effects. The therapist was careful not to imply that the client was to blame for the failure of the previous treatment, attributing it instead to a lack of clarity in the dialogue between the client and his previous therapist. Following this discussion, the client expressed a wish that his previous therapist had been clearer. Building on this, the therapist validated the client's anxiety at the prospect of taking on EX/RP again, empathizing with how pointless it would seem to embark on a difficult treatment without any reason to think that it would lead to positive changes—something the client had not had the chance to discover the last time. The session ended with the client expressing less pessimism and the therapist feeling increased hope for the client.

In Session 3, after validating the client's sense that his OCD kept him and others safe, the therapist elicited from the client the view that his checking was "exaggerated" and unrelated to any real threat. As they explored this change talk, the client spoke with increasing conviction about how the checking, instead of generating safety, was simply ruining his life. This seemed to lead the client to reconsider treatment. However, he did not want the sexual side effects of SSRIs and expressed continued doubts about EX/RP, saying that exposures merely "replicated" the anxiety he already felt. Here, the therapist elicited the client's understanding of how EX/RP works, uncovering several misperceptions that appeared to contribute to his prior nonadherence and the failure of the treatment to reduce his symptoms.

A key moment appeared to be when the client mentioned that there were areas of his life in which he did not feel compelled to minimize risk. When the therapist asked for an example, the client recalled military training in how to leap from an airplane with a parachute and accepting that he might need to do so. The therapist reflected that he was the sort of person who did what needed to be done when there were no other options. Shortly thereafter, the client expressed the view that EX/RP was his "only option," and he began to wonder whether it might work this time. The therapist asked what would make a difference, and the client was clear: an EX/RP therapist who gave him explicit directions and a "clear path" so that there was effectively no option to fail. The therapist's perception was that affirming the client by expressing interest in his story and admiring his resolve resulted in a shift in how the client saw himself—that is, as a man of action—and an enhancement of the client's confidence in his ability to take on EX/RP.

In Session 4, the client asked for a referral to an EX/RP therapist of the kind they had discussed previously, one who would communicate clearly and firmly guide the client through the treatment as it was intended to be done. The therapist and client collaboratively completed a change plan that included adherence to between-session exposures and in-session completion of exposures at the top of his hierarchy. The session ended with the client committing to that plan.

Upon follow-up, the client had entered into and completed a

standard treatment course (2 introductory sessions and 15 exposure sessions) of EX/RP, adhered to the homework, and conducted exposures at the top of his hierarchy. Before and after the four MI sessions, his OCD severity scores, based on the Yale–Brown Obsessive Compulsive Scale (Y-BOCS; Goodman, Price, et al., 1989a; Goodman et al., 1989b), were 23 and 22, respectively, indicating moderate severity. After EX/RP treatment, his OCD symptoms decreased dramatically such that his symptoms were no more than mild (Y-BOCS = 8).

EX/RP+MI

At the initial assessment, Client A presented with severe OCD symptoms (Y-BOCS = 30) within two domains: contamination and harm. Her contamination fears were widespread, and she had extensive washing rituals. She also feared harm befalling her or her family, and these fears involved magical thinking (e.g., verbalizing bad thoughts would harm her family). Thus, she initially did not allow sessions to be recorded. Rituals included repeating mantras.

During the introductory sessions, the client expressed clear reasons for change and a commitment to conduct contamination exposures in response to the therapist's evocative questions and empathic reflections. However, she expressed great reluctance about conducting harm exposures. In standard EX/RP, a therapist might try to use the psychoeducational component to convince the client that harm exposures were necessary and ask for the client's commitment to try them. Instead, once reluctance about the exposures surfaced and did not resolve despite empathic reflections or information provided in an MI-congruent way (elicit–provide–elicit), the therapist shifted focus, supporting the client's personal choice and control regarding the focus of exposures to be conducted. The result was that toward the end of the session the client agreed to engage in contamination exposures and to reevaluate the possibility of engaging in harm exposures as treatment progressed.

During the exposure sessions, the client progressed quickly through her hierarchy of contamination exposures, surpassing her worst fears and engaging in previously unimaginable exposures by mid-treatment (e.g., bringing "contaminated" objects into her mother's apartment). However, the client rejected exposures that tested her magical thoughts about harm. At a pivotal moment halfway through treatment, she expressed anger when the therapist suggested such an exposure. In standard EX/RP the therapist might have offered more psychoeducation, called for courage, and emphasized that avoiding the exposure could jeopardize the therapy. Instead, the therapist responded by shifting to the MI module.

This included coming alongside ("This seems like a risk that is too dangerous to take"), looking forward ("What will your life be like if your fears and rituals about doing harm don't change?"), and increasing confidence by eliciting discussion of past successes and strengths ("This seems impossible right now. Tell me about times when you've done things that seemed impossible"). The therapist also developed discrepancy through a discussion of the client's values in which she described how deeply she valued her family's well-being and her realization of how her OCD symptoms caused her family "anxiety and pain" rather than keeping them safe. After this conversation, the client renewed her commitment to EX/RP, thereafter helping the therapist construct exposures that tested her magical thoughts and allowing sessions to be recorded. After EX/RP+MI treatment, she had minimal symptoms (Y-BOCS = 5).

Client B also had severe OCD (Y-BOCS = 29). She had near constant intrusive thoughts of things needing to be perfect or exact and spent hours every day performing compulsions to ensure exactness (e.g., organizing and arranging, reviewing decisions and conversations, rereading and rewriting). Although she had recently received 1 year of weekly CBT, the client had refused to participate in exposures or ritual prevention.

During the introductory sessions, the client expressed great uncertainty about treatment, vacillating between rage at her OCD ("I have no choice—I have to fight this!") and fear of "losing" her OCD ("It's the only thing that makes me a good person"). Similarly, she vacillated between embracing and then rejecting EX/RP, lacking confidence that she could stop ritualizing. In standard EX/RP, this client would likely have received extensive psychoeduction and attempts at persuasion. Instead, she was given key information about EX/RP in MI style after the therapist elicited what she knew, resulting in far less didactic instruction than would typically have been provided. Instead of trying to directly persuade her to embark on the exposures, the therapist focused on accepting and exploring her ambivalence about change and EX/RP, employing amplified reflection ("You are absolutely terrified right now about the thought of doing this impossible thing"; "Without the OCD, you would be totally immoral") and double-sided reflection ("In some ways your rituals feel like a good thing, and at the same time they are stopping you from living the life you want to live"). In exploring the ambivalence, the therapist sought to normalize it and support the client's autonomy while developing discrepancy between her current life and her values (thereby enhancing the importance of change) and evoking change talk without triggering discord (allowing the client to talk herself into change).

Given the client's strong ambivalence, it was unclear whether she would proceed to EX/RP treatment, but at the third introductory session she agreed to try it. However, at the fourth session, she refused to engage in the planned exposure. The therapist responded by reassessing the client's attributed importance and confidence for change through EX/RP while emphasizing her personal choice and control. A pivotal moment came when the therapist, working to enhance confidence, asked if she had ever done something that she thought was impossible. The client vividly recalled her initial terror of riding a rollercoaster and how this terror was transformed into thrill once she did it; the therapist then expressed the idea that EX/RP was like this rollercoaster, a challenge to be overcome. This rollercoaster metaphor was subsequently referred to frequently throughout the remaining treatment sessions whenever the client's confidence in her ability to tolerate the exposures flagged.

Although the next few exposure sessions went well, the client's confidence continued to fluctuate, requiring a shift into the MI module in each session. The therapist employed strategies including exploration of the pros and cons of change and enhancement of self-efficacy by evoking prior situations in which the client demonstrated strength and resolve. The client engaged in increasingly difficult exposures, but she had trouble stopping some rituals. In response, the therapist offered amplified reflections of the client's statements about the relief she experienced from ritualizing ("They feel so good"), agreed with a twist to her description of being controlled by rituals ("You feel completely controlled by the sense of relief you get from doing your rituals"), and reframed the task at hand ("You're not sure that you can eliminate rituals, but you feel that you can and need to try"). By the end of treatment, the client was much improved (Y-BOCS = 16). Although she had not eliminated all rituals, she expressed a sense of accomplishment at having engaged in and completed treatment.

Unanswered Questions about Using MI to Enhance Treatment of OCD

Does the Nature of OCD Limit the Benefits of MI?

One issue worth considering is whether the nature of OCD might limit MI's effectiveness. Miller and Rollnick (2013) have noted that, unless there is something more precious to the client than the behavior in which he or she is currently engaging, MI has no basis for success. MI works by helping clients tap into their most important values and goals, recognize how their current behavior is preventing them from realizing those values and goals, and see how they can move toward change. However, some OCD clients have poor insight into the senselessness of their symptoms and truly believe, at least some of the time, in the power of their thoughts and actions to cause or prevent terrible events. As a result, it is rational for them to continue to avoid feared situations or to ritualize, as they may value protecting themselves on behalf of those they care for more than anything else. In the DSM-IV Field Trial (Foa & Kozak, 1995), only 13% of OCD clients were certain that their feared consequence *would not* occur: 27% were mostly certain; 30% were uncertain; but 26% were mostly certain and 4% were completely certain that it *would* occur. An added complication is that insight can fluctuate over time and in different contexts; for example, some clients can sometimes see the senselessness of their symptoms in the therapist's office and yet lose that perspective when faced with an OCD stimulus. It is an open question as to how effective MI can be in clients who lose reality testing like this.

Another issue relates to the age of onset of the OCD. Half of OCD cases start by age 19 and 25% by age 14 (Kessler et al., 2005). Thus, many adults with OCD can't remember a time when they didn't experience OCD; their OCD has been incorporated not only into their activities of daily living but also into their sense of self. When such clients hesitate about changing their life to be less about OCD, it is not clear whether this is best conceptualized as ambivalence (and thus more amenable to an intervention like MI) or better conceptualized as disrupted development (requiring an intervention that could ameliorate the effects of the missing developmental process).

Finally, our clinical experience was that OCD clients with prominent symmetry and exactness concerns and who had to do things until they felt "just right" did not always respond well to typical MI strategies (e.g., open-ended questions, reflections, the elicit–provide–elicit style of providing information). Instead of experiencing the therapist as empathic, some of these clients found the therapist's MI style at best vague and at worst irritating; it appeared that they would have preferred the more directive therapist-driven style of standard EX/RP.

Which Format Should Be Used to Enhance Treatment of OCD?

The Additive Model

The most common format for using MI to improve adherence to and outcomes of a longer or more intensive treatment is the "additive" model in which one or more MI sessions are offered separately from the primary treatment, usually as a pretreatment. Often these sessions are provided by a different clinician from those who provide the primary treatment, which may involve a therapeutic approach that has little in common with the spirit and practice of MI. One meta-analysis found that, in contrast to other formats, when MI was added to another treatment, the effects of MI were maintained at the 1-year follow-up (Hettema et al., 2005).

Typically, MI sessions are added as a prelude to the primary treatment. Studies by Westra and colleagues (Aviram & Westra, 2011; Westra, Arkowitz, & Dozois, 2009; Westra & Dozois, 2006) provide evidence that offering MI as a prelude to CBT for anxiety disorders can enhance both adherence and outcomes (see Westra & Aviram, Chapter 4, this volume for details). As noted earlier, the prelude model showed promise for enhancing treatment adherence and outcomes in OCD in preliminary studies by Maltby and Tolin (2005) and Meyer and colleagues (2010), but because these researchers blended MI with other approaches, it is difficult to draw meaningful conclusions about the role of MI in treatment outcomes. Our use of the prelude model in the "MI stuck" study returned mixed results, as clients with prominent hoarding symptoms were not helped to change or engage in treatment, but those with classic OCD symptoms seemed to benefit.

A clear advantage of the prelude model lies in the greater likelihood that MI can be provided in a relatively "pure" way. Evidence that a mixture of MI-consistent and MI-inconsistent practice is ineffective (Miller & Mount, 2001) supports the value of avoiding the intermixing of other clinical practices with MI, especially such a structured and directive treatment as EX/RP. Dedicated MI clinicians can more easily be trained, coached, and monitored for MI fidelity, and they benefit from well-recognized practice effects in the presence of objective and supportive feedback on performance. On the other hand, clients' reluctance to adhere to treatment procedures can arise at any point during treatment, and thus confining MI to pretreatment misses the opportunity to reengage ambivalent clients whose commitment to the treatment flags. This is especially salient in EX/RP, where the aversiveness of treatment participation increases as clients approach the top of their exposure hierarchy, before decreasing again as symptoms abate and the functional impairment caused by OCD is reduced.

One alternative is to add MI sessions during active treatment as well as using it before treatment starts. For example, West and colleagues (2007) found that adding five individual MI sessions at intervals throughout the first 12 months of an 18-month-long group behavioral weight control treatment improved treatment adherence and outcomes in overweight women with type 2 diabetes as compared with five individual health education sessions provided at the same intervals. Merlo and colleagues (2010) utilized a similar approach in their pilot study with children and adolescents with OCD, inserting individual MI sessions into the primary CBT intervention. This approach might maintain the advantages of the additive model while also ensuring that all clients receive MI in the midst of exposure sessions. If separate MI and CBT practitioners were required to provide treatment to each client, the real-world applicability of this model would be uncertain, especially for primary treatments that are also delivered individually. However, it may be possible to teach practitioners to provide each intervention with fidelity and to reduce client confusion over shifts in style by transparently informing clients about the reasons behind the shifts.

The Integrative Model

The main alternative to the additive model is to integrate MI into the primary treatment. In this model MI is provided during treatment sessions with the primary clinician, who must thus be trained in both MI and the primary treatment.

The extent to which MI is integrated into the treatment can vary. One approach is to begin treatment sessions with a brief MI intervention designed to improve motivation for change and adherence to the treatment. Nock and Kazdin (2005) had clinicians begin the first, fifth, and seventh of eight sessions of behavioral parent management training (PMT) for children with behavior problems with 5–15 minutes of MI and exploration of barriers and solutions, targeting parents' attendance at treatment sessions and adherence to between-session activities. Compared with parents receiving standard PMT, those receiving the "participation enhancement intervention" scored higher on a parent motivation index, attended more treatment sessions, and adhered more fully to treatment procedures. (Treatment outcomes were not reported.)

Further along the continuum of integration is the approach that we took in our "EX/RP+MI" study: blend MI with the preparatory tasks of the primary treatment during the initial sessions and then provide an MI module that the therapist can deploy as needed during the active treatment sessions, when issues of treatment adherence may arise.

Although it has the advantages of real-world applicability (a single practitioner provides the treatment) and availability of MI to enhance motivation for change and adherence throughout the treatment process, integrating MI into standard EX/RP as we did might have an important drawback. In our protocol, therapists had to shift back and forth between MI and EX/RP during exposure sessions if clients became reluctant to adhere in-session or were inconsistent in between-session adherence. We found that, although the signs of nonadherence were sometimes clear (e.g., clients expressed the desire to drop out of treatment), in many cases the signs were more subtle (e.g., partial adherence to between-session practice) and varied from session to session. With such clients, therapists had to judge at each session whether MI was warranted, and unless the signs were obvious, their tendency was not to shift and to rely instead upon familiar CBT strategies. This perhaps was to be expected, given that the therapists had expertise in EX/RP but were relatively new to MI; moreover, the protocol explicitly stated that the MI module was only to be used during exposure sessions if standard CBT procedures were ineffective. Notably, results of intervention fidelity checks using the Motivational Interviewing Treatment Integrity global codes (MITI 3.0; Moyers, Martin, Manuel, Miller, & Ernst, 2005) suggested that little MI was provided during the exposure sessions

It is possible that therapists who had more experience in MI might make the shift from EX/RP to MI more readily and with greater fidelity— but allegiance to a powerful and effective treatment approach like EX/RP can be strong, and the development of an equal allegiance to two distinct approaches might be unlikely. As a result, the MI might be diluted to the point of being rendered ineffective. If expertise in both treatments is necessary to conduct such an integrated protocol, the applicability of this model to routine treatment settings may be limited.

What, then, of the employment of a *more* integrated approach where exposure and ritual prevention procedures would be conducted in a manner consistent with the MI spirit and where MI elements would be fully integrated into sessions? It is possible that this approach could increase the quality and quantity of MI received. Such an approach would target not only ambivalence about entering treatment but also ambivalence about engaging in the individual exposures and other components of between-session exercises. In such an approach, the clinician would evoke from clients how achieving an individual exposure might make them feel or what it might mean in terms of their progress toward overcoming OCD. Similarly, successes with exposures might more strategically be used to evoke change talk and build commitment and confidence to continuing with treatment and overcoming OCD.

The risk of this approach mirrors that of the one previously discussed, namely, potentially diluting the effectiveness of EX/RP by intermixing it with MI. The skilled practice of MI requires that the therapist take up an egalitarian and empathically expressive stance, whereas the skilled practice of EX/RP requires him or her to direct the client with authority through the complex and demanding set of treatment procedures needed to reduce OCD symptoms. Thus, MI might have the potential to decrease rather than increase the impact of the EX/RP procedures if integrated into the treatment. This risk could strengthen the preference for the additive model in the context of OCD treatment. Many of the studies with positive findings for MI as an adjunct employed prelude interventions prior to other treatments (e.g., traditional inpatient rehabilitation) whose style and procedures likewise presented strong contrasts to those of MI.

Conclusions

Considerations for Future Research

MI should be considered a promising but still unproven approach for enhancing treatment seeking and outcomes in EX/RP for OCD. More research is needed not only to identify whether one format for combining MI and CBT is superior to others in improving outcomes but more generally to determine the degree to which MI is effective among this client population, given certain characteristics of OCD.

Addressing these issues requires reliable and valid measures for assessing the impact of MI (as well as other interventions) on adherence to treatment. A brief therapist-administered measure (Simpson, Maher, et al., 2010) has demonstrated good reliability and predictive validity for assessing adherence to between-session assignments in EX/RP.

Adherence can be also be measured in terms of rates of treatment entry. However, an MI intervention could be considered successful not only if it increases the likelihood that people with OCD will enter treatment but also if people who are very unlikely to adhere to treatment procedures decide *not* to enter treatment. When clients adhere only partially to EX/RP for OCD, treatment is likely to be ineffective. Clients who engage half-heartedly risk demoralization and decreased willingness to access treatment later, even if motivation for change is high. Therefore, when MI is used as a prelude to treatment, perhaps it is not starting treatment that is the most accurate metric of MI's effectiveness but rather the extent to which clients complete MI either fully committed to treatment or resolved not to enter treatment until ready to adhere.

Theoretically, MI should be most useful to those who are ambivalent about treatment by helping them resolve this ambivalence as well as enhancing readiness for change. However, testing this hypothesis requires valid and reliable measures of these constructs. We found that a Readiness Ruler targeting readiness to engage in the components of EX/RP, rather than general readiness to change, predicted adherence, which in turn predicted treatment outcome (Maher et al., 2012; Simpson et al., 2012).

It is not clear how feasible it is to train therapists experienced in providing standard EX/RP for OCD to deliver MI in an integrated protocol. Developing proficiency in MI requires careful training, especially if clinicians have been trained in highly structured treatments (Cook, Schnurr, Biyanova, & Coyne, 2009). It remains to be determined whether the potential benefits to clients make the required commitment of time and effort for EX/RP therapists to learn and use MI worthwhile.

Clinical Observations

In our experience, MI was successful when it helped address two distinct but related decisional conflicts that can lead to treatment ambivalence. The first is whether the advantages of changes in OCD symptoms outweigh those of sustaining the status quo to the client. Here, what seemed particularly helpful was eliciting the values the OCD behaviors reflected (e.g., material security and antiwastefulness or carefulness about the well-being of others) and contrasting these with the values that could be expressed if the OCD behaviors were reduced (e.g., improved intimate relationships, mastery of their own destiny, belief in a benevolent world). The recognition that giving up the OCD behaviors was not just compatible with, but also facilitative of, living out cherished values appeared to fuel the desire for change.

The second conflict we observed centered on whether the aversiveness of treatment itself (i.e., the intense anxiety inherent in EX/RP, the side effects inherent in pharmacotherapy) was outweighed by the potential relief from debilitating symptoms. Here a key appeared to be the therapist's ability to empathize with clients' fears while also evoking and affirming their strengths, especially their courage in the face of daunting obstacles and their willingness to persist despite the difficulty of doing so. Providing a nonjudgmental space for clients to think out loud about the available pathways for achieving change also seemed to play an important role. In those cases where clients sought or participated more fully in evidence-based treatment for OCD after an MI intervention, the clients appeared to come to an acceptance of the reality and limitations of the current treatment options and to feel willing and able to commit to short-term pain for long-term gain because change was so essential.

Motivational interviewing has demonstrated effectiveness in enhancing commitment to treatment for a variety of problems. In light of the distress and impairment caused by OCD, and the availability of empirically supported treatments that nonetheless do not reach many of those who could benefit, we and others have begun to explore the potential of MI to engage OCD sufferers into treatment and enhance their adherence once engaged. The nature of OCD, as well the character of the primary treatments themselves, appears to create special challenges in using MI for these purposes. It's clear that much more research will be needed before we can draw any firm conclusions regarding the value of adding or integrating MI into these treatments. Nonetheless, our initial explorations leave us sufficiently encouraged to warrant continuing those efforts.

References

Abramowitz, J. S., Franklin, M. E., Zoellner, L. A., & DiBernardo, C. L. (2002). Treatment compliance and outcome in obsessive–compulsive disorder. *Behavior Modification, 26*(4), 447–463.

Aviram, A., & Westra, H. A. (2011). The impact of motivational interviewing on resistance in cognitive behavioural therapy for generalized anxiety disorder. *Psychotherapy Research, 21,* 698–708.

Chamberlain, P., Patterson, G., Reid, J., Kavanagh, K., & Forgatch, M. (1984). Observation of client resistance. *Behavior Therapy, 15,* 144–155.

Connors, G. J., Walitzer, K. S., & Dermen, K. H. (2002). Preparing clients for alcoholism treatment: Effects on treatment participation and outcomes. *Journal of Consulting and Clinical Psychology, 70*(5), 1161–1169.

Cook, J. M. Schnurr, P. P., Biyanova, T., & Coyne, J. C. (2009). Apples don't fall far from the tree: Influences on psychotherapists' adoption and sustained use of new therapies. *Psychiatric Services, 60,* 671–676.

Foa, E. B., Grayson, J. B., Steketee, G. S., Doppelt, H. G., Turner, R. M., & Latimer, P. R. (1983). Success and failure in the behavioral treatment of obsessive–compulsives. *Journal of Consulting and Clinical Psychology, 51*(2), 287–297.

Foa, E. B., & Kozak, M. J. (1995). DSM-IV field trial: Obsessive–compulsive disorder. *American Journal of Psychiatry, 152,* 90–96.

Foa, E. B., Liebowitz, M. R., Kozak, M. J., Davies, S., Campeas, R., Franklin, M. E., et al. (2005). Randomized, placebo-controlled trial of exposure and ritual prevention, clomipramine, and their combination in the treatment of obsessive–compulsive disorder. *American Journal of Psychiatry, 162,* 151–161.

Goodman, W. K., Price, L. H., Rasmussen, S. A., Mazure, C., Delgado, P., Henninger, G. R., et al. (1989). The Yale–Brown Obsessive Compulsive Scale: II. Validity. *Archives of General Psychiatry, 46,* 1012–1016.

Goodman, W. K., Price, L. H., Rasmussen, S. A., Mazure, C., Fleischmann, R. L., Hill, C. L., et al. (1989). The Yale–Brown Obsessive Compulsive Scale: I. Development, use, and reliability. *Archives of General Psychiatry, 46,* 1006–1011.

Grote, N. K., Zuckoff, A., Swartz, H. A., Bledsoe, S. E., & Geibel, S. (2007). Engaging women who are depressed and economically disadvantaged in mental health treatment. *Social Work, 52,* 295–308.

Habib, S., Morrissey, S., & Helmes, E. (2005). Preparing for pain management: A pilot study to enhance engagement. *Journal of Pain, 6*(1), 48–54.

Hettema, J., Steele, J., & Miller, W. R. (2005). Motivational interviewing. *Annual Review of Clinical Psychology, 1,* 91–111.

Inciardi, J. A., Surratt, H. L., Pechansky, F., Kessler, F., Von Dimen, L., Meyer da Silva, E., et al. (2006). Changing patterns of cocaine use and HIV risks in the south of Brazil. *Journal of Psychoactive Drugs, 38,* 305–310.

Kessler, R. C., Berglund, P., Demler, O., Jin, R., Merikangas, K. R., & Walters, E. E. (2005). Lifetime prevalence and age-of-onset distributions of DSM-IV disorders in the National Comorbidity Survey Replication. *Archives of General Psychiatry, 62,* 593–602.

Koran, L. M., Henna, G. L., Hollander, E., Nestadt, G., & Simpson, H. B. (2007). Practice guideline for the treatment of patients with obsessive–compulsive disorder. *American Journal of Psychiatry, 164*(Suppl. 7), 5–53.

Kozak, M. J., & Foa, E. B. (1997). *Mastery of obsessive–compulsive disorder: A cognitive-behavioral approach.* San Antonio, TX: Psychological Corp.

Leukefeld, C., Brown, C., Clark, J., Godlaski, T., & Hays, R. (2000). *Behavioral therapy for rural substance abusers.* Lexington: University of Kentucky Press.

Leukefeld, C. G., Pechansky, F., Martin, S. S., Surratt, H. L., Inciardi, J. A., Kessler, F. H. P., et al. (2005). Tailoring an HIV-prevention intervention for cocaine injectors and crack users in Porto Alegre, Brazil. *AIDS Care, 17,* 77–87.

Lewis-Fernandez, R., Balan, I. C., Patel, S. R., Sanchez-Lacay, J. A., Alfonso, C., Gorritz, M., et al. (2013). Impact of motivational pharmacotherapy on treatment retention among depressed Latinos. *Psychiatry, 76,* 210–222.

Lundahl, B. W., Kunz, C., Brownell, C., Tollefson, D., & Burke, B. L. (2010). A meta-analysis of motivational interviewing: Twenty-five years of empirical studies. *Research on Social Work Practice, 20*(2), 137–160.

Maher, M. J., Wang, Y., Zuckoff, A., Wall, M. W., Franklin, M., Foa, E. B., et al. (2012). Predictors of patient adherence to cognitive behavioral therapy for obsessive–compulsive disorder. *Psychotherapy and Psychosomatics, 81,* 124–126.

Maltby, N., & Tolin, D. F. (2005). A brief motivational intervention for treatment-refusing OCD patients. *Cognitive Behavioral Therapy, 34*(3), 176–184.

Merlo, L. J., Storch, E. A., Lehmkuhl, H. D., Jacob, M. L., Murphy, T. K.,

Goodman, W. K., et al. (2010). Cognitive behavioral therapy plus motivational interviewing improves outcome for pediatric obsessive–compulsive disorder: A preliminary study. *Cognitive Behavioral Therapy, 39,* 24–27.

Meyer, E., Souza, F., Heldt, E., Knapp, P., Cordioli, A., Shavitt, R. G., et al. (2010). A randomized clinical trial to examine enhancing cognitive-behavioral group therapy for obsessive–compulsive disorder with motivational interviewing and thought mapping. *Behavioural and Cognitive Psychotherapy, 38,* 319–336.

Miller, W. R., & Mount, K. A. (2001). A small study of training in motivational interviewing: Does one workshop change clinician and client behavior? *Behavioural and Cognitive Psychotherapy, 29,* 457–471.

Miller, W. R., & Rollnick, S. (2002). *Motivational interviewing: Preparing people for change* (2nd ed.). New York: Guilford Press.

Miller, W. R., & Rollnick, S. (2013). *Motivational interviewing: Helping people change* (3rd ed.). New York: Guilford Press.

Moyers, T., Martin, T., Manuel, J. K., Miller, W. R., & Ernst, D. (2005). *Motivational Interviewing Treatment Integrity 3.0: Increasing participation in parent management training.* Available at *http://casaa.unm.edu/download/miti3.pdf.*

Nock, M. K., & Kazdin, A. E. (2005). Randomized controlled trial of a brief intervention for increasing participation in parent management training. *Journal of Consulting and Clinical Psychology, 73,* 872–879.

Prochaska, J. O., & DiClemente, C. C. (1984). *The transtheoretical approach: Crossing traditional boundaries of therapy.* Homewood, IL: Dow-Jones/Irwin.

Simpson, H. B., Foa, E. B., Liebowitz, M. R., Huppert, J. D., Cahill, S., Maher, M. J., (2013). Cognitive-behavioral therapy vs risperidone for augmenting serotonin reuptake inhibitors in obsessive–compulsive disorder: A randomized clinical trial. *JAMA Psychiatry, 70,* 1190–1199.

Simpson, H. B., Foa, E. B., Liebowitz, M. R., Ledley, D. R., Huppert, J. D., Cahill, S., et al. (2008). A randomized, controlled trial of cognitive-behavioral therapy for augmenting pharmacotherapy in obsessive–compulsive disorder. *American Journal of Psychiatry, 165,* 621–630.

Simpson, H. B., Huppert, J. D., Petkova, E., Foa, E. B., & Liebowitz, M. R. (2006). Response versus remission in obsessive–compulsive disorder. *Journal of Clinical Psychiatry, 67*(2), 269–276.

Simpson, H. B., Maher, M., Page, J. R., Gibbons, C. J., Franklin, M. E., & Foa, E. B. (2010). Development of a patient adherence scale for exposure and response prevention therapy. *Behavior Therapy, 41,* 30–37.

Simpson, H. B., Maher, M. J., Wang, Y., Bao, Y., Foa, E. B., & Franklin, M. (2011). Patient adherence predicts outcome from cognitive behavioral therapy in obsessive–compulsive disorder. *Journal of Consulting and Clinical Psychology, 79,* 247–252.

Simpson, H. B., Marcus, S. M., Zuckoff, A., Franklin, M., & Foa, E. B. (2012). Patient adherence to cognitive-behavioral therapy predicts long-term outcome in obsessive–compulsive disorder. *Journal of Clinical Psychiatry, 73,* 1265–1266.

Simpson, H. B., & Zuckoff, A. (2011). Using motivational interviewing to enhance treatment outcome in people with obsessive–compulsive disorder. *Cognitive and Behavioral Practice, 18*, 28–37.

Simpson, H. B., Zuckoff, A., Maher, M. J., Page, J., Franklin, M., Foa, F. B., et al. (2010). Challenges using motivational interviewing as an adjunct to exposure therapy for obsessive–compulsive disorder. *Behavior Research and Therapy, 48*, 941–948.

Simpson, H. B., Zuckoff, A., Page, J., Franklin, M. E., & Foa, E. B. (2008). Adding motivational interviewing to exposure and ritual prevention for obsessive–compulsive disorder: An open pilot trial. *Cognitive Behaviour Therapy, 37*, 38–49.

Sookman, D., & Steketee, G. (2007). Directions in specialized cognitive behavior therapy for resistant obsessive–compulsive disorder: Theory and practice of two approaches. *Cognitive and Behavioural Practice, 14*, 1–17.

Swartz, H. A., Frank, E., Zuckoff, A., Cyranowski, J. M., Houck, P. R., Cheng, Y., et al. (2008). Brief interpersonal psychotherapy for depressed mothers whose children are receiving psychiatric treatment. *American Journal of Psychiatry, 165*, 1155–1162.

West, D. S., DiLillo, V., Bursac, Z., Gore, S. A., & Greene, P. G. (2007). Motivational interviewing improves weight loss in women with type 2 diabetes. *Diabetes Care, 30*(5), 1081–1087.

Westra, H. A., Arkowitz, H., & Dozois, D. J. A. (2009). Adding a motivational interviewing pretreatment to cognitive behavioral therapy for generalized anxiety disorder: A preliminary randomized controlled trial. *Journal of Anxiety Disorders, 23*, 1106–1117.

Westra, H. A., & Dozois, D. J. A. (2006). Preparing clients for cognitive behavioral therapy: A randomized pilot study of motivational interviewing for anxiety. *Cognitive Therapy Research, 30*, 481–498

Zuckoff, A., & Daley, D.C. (2001). Engagement and adherence issues in treating persons with nonpsychosis dual disorders. *Psychiatric Rehabilitation Skills, 5*, 131–162.

Zuckoff, A., & Hettema, J. E. (2007, November). Motivational interviewing to enhance engagement and adherence to treatment: A conceptual and empirical review. In H. B. Simpson (Chair), *Using motivational interviewing to enhance CBT adherence.* Paper presented at the 41st annual convention of the Association for Behavioral and Cognitive Therapies, Philadelphia, PA.

Zweben, A., & Zuckoff, A. (2002). Motivational interviewing and treatment adherence. In W. R. Miller & S. Rollnick, *Motivational interviewing: Preparing people for change* (2nd ed., pp. 299–319). 2nd edition. New York: Guilford Press.

CHAPTER 4

• • • • • •

Integrating Motivational Interviewing into the Treatment of Anxiety

Henny A. Westra
Adi Aviram

The application of motivational interviewing (MI; Miller & Rollnick, 2002, 2013) to anxiety disorders is a relatively recent development. Common treatments for anxiety such as cognitive-behavioral therapy (CBT) typically require a high level of motivation for change since the individual is required to take active steps toward recovery, such as exposure to fear-provoking stimuli. Yet, many individuals, even those presenting for treatment, are ambivalent about change and implementing change strategies. Given the focus on helping individuals move through ambivalence about change, applications of MI for anxiety hold promise for complementing existing effective treatments (see Westra, 2012). In this chapter, we begin by briefly discussing existing treatments for anxiety and making a case for applying MI to the treatment of anxiety disorders. The bulk of the chapter then presents an overview of this approach along with clinical illustrations. Finally, we outline the clinical challenges of this work and present a summary of the research assessing the use of MI in the treatment of anxiety.

Usual Treatments

Various treatment guidelines currently recommend CBT as the first-line approach to treating anxiety disorders. Although CBT typically consists of multiple intervention strategies (e.g., breathing retraining, self-monitoring), exposure to feared situations and/or stimuli is considered a critical ingredient. The specific focus of exposure varies depending on the type of anxiety that is being treated, but the theoretical principle remains the same, namely, by facing anxiety-provoking stimuli, fears can become extinguished, new coping skills may be developed, and adaptive cognitive changes occur. In particular, change in threat-related cognitions occurs as new evidence that is discrepant from one's catastrophic beliefs is accumulated, thereby providing an opportunity for new learning to take place. The efficacy of CBT for a variety of anxiety disorders is well established. For example, in a recent review of 269 meta-analyses examining CBT efficacy for a wide range of presenting problems, anxiety disorders emerged as a class of mental health difficulties where in which support for CBT was consistently strong (Hofmann, Asnaani, Vonk, Sawyer, & Fang, 2012).

Rationale for Using MI for Anxiety

Although effective treatments have been developed for anxiety, client resistance to change and nonadherence to recommended treatment procedures are formidable problems limiting the benefits of these treatments (e.g., Antony, Ledley, & Heimberg, 2005). Homework noncompliance and limited client engagement are commonly acknowledged problems among CBT practitioners (e.g., Helbig & Fehm, 2004; Sanderson & Bruce, 2007). For example, in a survey of practitioner-identified obstacles to the implementation of empirically supported treatments for panic disorder, client unwillingness to engage in treatment was reported by 61% of therapists, and minimal client motivation at the outset of therapy was identified as a problem by 67% of the therapists surveyed (American Psychological Aaaociation, 2010). Similarly, in a recent survey of therapists on their clinical experiences conducting CBT for generalized anxiety disorder (GAD), the majority of respondents identified client resistance to the directiveness of treatment as a barrier to treatment efficacy (Szkodny, Newman, & Goldfried, 2014). Moreover, there is strong and consistent evidence that the effectiveness of psychotherapy is associated with the relative absence of resistance (e.g., Beutler, Harwood, Michelson, Song, & Holman, 2011). Indeed, despite being relatively rare as compared to client cooperation, resistance even as early as the first session of therapy is a very strong predictor of reduced subsequent engagement in CBT (i.e., in-session task involvement, Jungbluth & Shirk, 2009; homework compliance, Aviram & Westra, 2011) as well as poorer treatment outcomes (Westra, 2011). And, importantly, receiving MI prior to CBT for anxiety has been shown to substantially reduce resistance within CBT (Aviram & Westra, 2011).

Much of what is thought of as resistance or noncompliance in psychotherapy may be a reflection of ambivalence about change (Engle & Arkowitz, 2006). As just one example, although clients with GAD see their worry as a problem, they also hold *positive* beliefs about worry (e.g., worry is motivating) and are therefore ambivalent about relinquishing it (Borkovec & Roemer, 1995). In addition, recent research suggests that the way a therapist responds to client ambivalence may be critical to treatment outcomes. In general, more supportive strategies have been indicated in the presence of resistance, while directive strategies are contraindicated in this context (Beutler et al., 2011). In fact, studies on interpersonal process in therapy have underscored the disruptive nature of therapists' directiveness in rigidly adhering to CBT techniques at times in which clients voice concerns about the therapy or the therapist (Aspland, Llewelyn, Hardy, Barkham, & Stiles, 2008; Castonguay, Goldfried, Wiser, Raue, & Hayes, 1996). Such findings underscore the need for flexibly moving between supportive and directive responses to client readiness for change. A combination of MI and CBT may thus be promising in the treatment of anxiety, with MI directed at increasing motivation and resolving ambivalence about change and CBT directed at helping clients achieve desired changes (Westra, 2012).

Clinical Application

Miller and Rollnick (2013) define MI as a collaborative goal-oriented style of communication that gives particular attention to the language of change. It is designed to strengthen personal motivation for and commitment to a specific goal by eliciting and exploring the person's own reasons for change within an atmosphere of acceptance and compassion. In essence, the goal of MI is to help people move through ambivalence and toward change. Four overlapping processes are identified within

MI, including engaging, focusing, evoking, and planning. After a brief discussion of MI spirit, the application of MI to the treatment of anxiety is discussed and elaborated within these four processes.

The "Spirit" of MI

Any discussion of MI should begin with the underlying spirit of the approach. At its core, MI rests on a particular view of human nature, the change process, and the therapist's role in facilitating that change. Any therapist behavior, no matter how much it may resemble MI, is not considered MI unless it is congruent with this underlying attitude (Miller & Rollnick, 2002, 2013). Thus, there is an onus on the counselor practicing MI to know, cultivate, and nurture MI spirit—and to monitor any deviations from it.

In MI, the client is not viewed as deficient or lacking in expertise that the therapist then supplies. Instead, clients are seen as already possessing all they need to resolve ambivalence and accomplish change. The clinician practicing MI trusts this fundamental notion, thus seeking to identify and mobilize the client's intrinsic resources to stimulate behavior change. Since motivation is seen as coming from within and can never be supplied from without, the MI therapist consistently communicates the message "I don't have what you need, but *you* do. And I will help you to find it." Thus, the MI therapist operates as a guide or consultant to the client (Miller & Rollnick, 2002, 2013).

Elements of this underlying spirit include partnership, acceptance (including empathy), compassion, and evocation (Miller & Rollnick, 2013). MI therapists strive to create a safe atmosphere that enables clients to work productively toward resolving ambivalence and mobilizing resolve and resources for change. In this sense, one is not so much an expert on the content of the problems or their resolution (as that is the client's domain); rather, one is an expert on the process (Westra, 2012).

MI therapists seek to work in harmony with clients at all times. They avoid coercion, argumentation, persuasion, and confrontation. The latter styles of interacting emerge from a therapist-as-expert perspective and run the risk of engendering client resistance and opposition. Importantly, MI is not coercive or "strategic." The MI therapist recognizes that choices always reside with the individual and can never be appropriated by another. At moments of disharmony, MI therapists avoid pejorative perceptions of clients as unmotivated, obstructive, or difficult. They seek to reframe client opposition by reflecting it, working with it, and understanding it.

As noted by Westra (2012), MI therapists also bring themselves—their humanity—to the encounter. They bring their curiosity, compassion, understanding, and validation. They bring faith in the process and in the capacity of everyone to be free from suffering and live a meaningful, satisfying life that is congruent with his or her values. They protect their clients' right to self-determination and freedom from coercion and offer themselves as confident companions and guides in clients' journeys of self-discovery and, ultimately, behavior change.

Engaging

Client engagement with the process of treatment has been identified as a central component of effective psychotherapy (Orlinsky, Grawe, & Parks, 1994). Regardless of the approach used, clients must be actively involved in the process and tasks of treatment in order to achieve good outcomes, and active engagement is a necessary prerequisite at all stages in therapy. Accordingly, client disengagement should be of significant concern for therapists. Within MI, listening and empathy are identified as being among the skills necessary for establishing a solid working alliance. Below we discuss two key elements of engagement, providing a credible treatment rationale and expressing empathy.

Providing a Rationale

In workshops, participants sometimes ask if they should tell their clients that they are stuck or low on motivation and are thus in need of MI. What participants are really getting at here is the issue of providing a rationale for your approach. Indeed, a critical part of engaging clients is to provide a credible rationale for the selected approach. This may be particularly true in the case of MI when applied to anxiety disorders, given that it is more exploratory or conversational in style, whereas clients may expect a more directive interaction where the therapist operates as an expert. It is thus incumbent on the therapist not only to be prepared to explain his or her approach and provide a treatment rationale but also to actively solicit client process expectations and negotiate the approach to be taken in accordance with the client's preferences (Constantino, Ametrano, & Greenberg, 2012).

Communicating your view of the importance and relevance of ambivalence and how exploration of this can be an important component of the treatment of anxiety is likely to increase client receptivity to this way of working. When introducing MI into the treatment of anxiety, Westra

(2012) outlines several points that can be communicated to enhance client receptivity to this approach, including noting that ambivalence about change is normal and omnipresent ("even though people know that they shouldn't worry or avoid feared situations, another part of them argues for continued worry and avoidance"), that change is difficult ("while change may be desirable, the process of change is not and is typically quite difficult"), that therapy offers an important space to explore different parts of self (e.g., "parts of yourself one day insist on change and the next day try to talk you out of it"), and that change involves not only taking action but also thinking about resolving conflicted feelings and preparing for change.

Expressing Empathy

Expressing empathy involves striving to understand and experience the world from the client's perspective without judgment or criticism and continually reflecting this emergent and evolving understanding back to the client (Rogers, 1951). It means far more than a kind, friendly attitude toward the client; rather, it is a highly active, complex, and multilayered process that is critically important in helping clients with anxiety understand and work through ambivalence about change. To be empathic also requires therapists to actively put aside their own hopes, biases, values, agendas, and the like in order to "experience" the client and the uniqueness of the client's reality (Geller & Greenberg, 2002).

Moreover, as a vehicle for promoting self-awareness and encouraging self-confrontation, empathic listening can play a central role in accomplishing this vital task of treatment. That is, empathy serves to more fully understand and deconstruct anxious clients' dominant views of themselves, others, and the world by bringing that which has been marginalized and silenced to center stage. In the service of this objective, the therapist strives to be neither behind the client (e.g., simply parroting or restating client statements) nor too far ahead of the client (e.g., making reflections that are too far outside of the client's immediate awareness or that the client is not likely to accept), given that neither of these positions will facilitate movement in the client's developing understanding or awareness Rather, the therapist strives to capture the implicit meanings that are immediately outside of the client's awareness, but are nonetheless contained within it (Sachse & Elliott, 2002).

While empathy is central to engaging the client, it can also serve many functions that go well beyond maintaining a positive working alliance. For instance, empathic responding facilitates clients' self-reflection in therapy and acknowledges that they can know themselves, evaluate their beliefs and behaviors, and make choices about how to best enhance the quality of their lives or change (Rogers, 1951). Moreover, empathic listening also promotes self-acceptance. That is, empathy is a major vehicle through which the therapist is able to convey the underlying attitudes of MI to his or her client. Such experiences of being regarded by another in this accepting and nonjudgmental manner can serve as a catalyst for greater client self-regard and self-acceptance. Moreover, such experiences are especially important for clients with anxiety and depression, who suffer from chronic self-criticism and low self-regard.

CLINICAL EXAMPLE OF USING EMPATHY IN THE CONTEXT OF WORKING WITH AMBIVALENCE

Consider a young woman with social anxiety who articulated ambivalence about managing conflict. She characterized her approach as "immature" and noted that she often sulks for a protracted period of time and is passive–aggressive (e.g., indirectly indicating displeasure, such as by slamming doors and giving others "the silent treatment"). The client noted that, although she knew what a better strategy would be, she was consistently unable to navigate these situations in a more "mature" manner.

THERAPIST: I hear that you are displeased with yourself for acting in an "immature" manner. If you are willing, can you say what are you attempting to get or hoping to get by dragging out your displeasure at the other person.

CLIENT: (C): (pause) I think I want them to notice me—and to know that they hurt me.

THERAPIST: So, this is a way of communicating very important feelings, things you don't want people to overlook or just pass over. And that sounds important, given that you've said that you often feel invisible or unimportant to others—it's hard to get their attention. [Garnered from previous sessions with the client; the therapist is attempting to reframe "negative" behavior during conflict.]

CLIENT: Right. Like, I try and try to get my parents to take me seriously but usually I feel like I might as well just talk to the wall.

THERAPIST: So, it goes nowhere, and that's what you're used to. And you've had to develop creative ways to get noticed—to be taken seriously. If I hear you right, you have tried the "more mature" approach, probably quite a few times, and it hasn't worked.

CLIENT: Absolutely. Being rational and reasonable never accomplishes anything with them.

THERAPIST: So, it may not be ideal, in an ideal world, and there are some things you don't like about how you're acting—but it works! And it certainly sounds better than the alternative of just giving up.

CLIENT: That's true. But why can't they just listen to reason? Why do I have to resort to this?

THERAPIST: You sound frustrated with the situation and with yourself for having to act in ways that another part of you—the mature part—really dislikes. I'm curious. What happens when you act this way with your parents?

CLIENT: Well, my dad, who just ignores me most of the time, comes around. Like when I'm mad, I usually say "I don't want to eat supper"—which is a big deal because of my diabetes. Then he actually goes out of his way to come up to my room. And then he is very sweet and kind and asks me to calm down. And then I usually draw it out—my anger—some more.

THERAPIST: And what is it like when he comes to you and is kind?

CLIENT: It feels really good. Like he talks with me and notices me (*pause*), and I feel powerful.

THERAPIST: So, quite a nice change from feeling helpless and powerless with him! And it sounds like those are the rare moments where you feel connected with him—feel like he cares.

CLIENT: Yes, absolutely.

THERAPIST: So, it makes a lot of sense then that you would act this way. If I'm hearing it right, it sounds like a smart and necessary strategy to get some control and feel close to others. [The therapist prizing and validating]

CLIENT: I never thought about it that way. But it actually does feel really good. Even though I know I'm being stubborn and difficult, I like it in some ways.

THERAPIST: And you learned that people are like that—that they can only hear you when you are stubborn and withdraw. So, naturally, you would keep acting that way.

CLIENT: But I don't think that everyone is like that though.

THERAPIST: So, there's another part of you that thinks that the world, or others, may operate with different rules or ways of conducting themselves. What makes you say that? [The client, having further uncovered and heard what she thinks, then begins to challenge her assumption. The therapist hears this protesting voice and invites the client to expand further, thereby inviting change talk. Importantly, the protest has arisen from the client and not from the therapist].

CLIENT: Well, my boyfriend. He really cares about me and how I'm feeling. He often asks me how I'm doing, even when I'm not angry with him but I seem upset or like I've had a bad day.

THERAPIST: So, if I hear you right you are saying, "I don't have to be this way in order for him to take an interest. I learned to be this way; it's well practiced—and it works, at least with some people. But I may not have to be this way with everyone in order to be taken seriously or to get others interested in me." Is that right?

Through the process of empathic reflection aimed at understanding ambivalence and the motives underlying seemingly negative behaviors, clients can then more freely make decisions about how well the behavior is working to meet these vital needs and contemplate whether there are other ways of meeting these core needs that are less self-destructive. When the therapist reframes problematic views and reactions in this way, it not only assists in helping clients become more aware of and able to deconstruct these reactions, but it also reduces clients' pejorative perceptions of ambivalence. Such pejorative perceptions are very common among individuals with anxiety, with clients frequently expressing frustration with themselves or becoming overtly self-critical as a result of continuing to think and/or act in ways that they are painfully aware are self-defeating. Therefore, the therapist holding and reflecting a more compassionate view of resistance to change as understandable and informative can be a powerful antidote to the client's pejorative, self-critical attitudes and can provide potent modeling for enhancing positive client self-regard.

Caveat: A Deviation from MI as Originally Conceived

As MI has evolved, and the mechanisms underlying its effectiveness have largely yet to be determined, various hypotheses have emerged to explain its impact. This has led to differing prescriptions about how MI should be practiced (see Arkowitz, Miller, Westra, & Rollnick, 2008). Miller and Rollnick (2013) argue that clients talk themselves into change, and so the focus, from this perspective, should be on change talk rather than sustain talk. The way of working with MI described above reflects our experience in adapting MI to the treatment of anxiety and related problems, but it differs from MI as currently conceived (Miller & Rollnick, 2013) in that *both* sides of a client's ambivalence—including arguments for the status quo (or "sustain talk")—are explored. From this perspective, MI can be conceptualized as a type of conflict resolution between competing aspects of the self. Thus, in our approach, the therapist helps the client explore both sides of his or her ambivalence about change: resistance to change and reasons to change. Unlike in MI as described by Miller and Rollnick (2013), the client is encouraged to voice and elaborate counterchange positions and not exclusively or predominantly change positions. That is, the therapist helps the client explore both sides of his or her ambivalence about change: resistance to change and reasons to change. Most significantly, this means that the client is encouraged to voice and elaborate counterchange positions, and not exclusively or predominantly change positions. When exploring the part of the person that argues against change, such conversations should exemplify the spirit of rolling with resistance (Miller & Rollnick, 2002, 2013); and one employs all the methods for coming alongside opposition that are so beautifully outlined in MI.

Focusing

In anxiety disorders, comorbid problems are the norm rather than the exception, with common comorbidities such as mood disorders, substance abuse, interpersonal problems, and other anxiety disorders. Each of these areas of concern may be a focus for the person, and there may be varying levels of motivation to address each problem. Further, the client-centered nature of MI, with its focus on the client as the expert and evoking client agency in treatment, suggests that a rigid predetermined focus on the part of the clinician is not appropriate. Moreover, the client's focus may shift—and in fact frequently does—in clinical practice.

We have found it helpful and most consistent with MI spirit to consider common foci for work with anxiety (as noted above) but to allow the specific focus to be fluid and determined by the client. With respect to anxiety-specific foci, we consider that an individual could be ambivalent on two levels: (1) change in anxiety itself (i.e., "What would life look like without panic or worry?" "Who would I be?" "Would there be other demands?"); and (2) change in the use of existing avoidant coping methods or, conversely, the implementation of alternative means of managing anxiety (e.g., exposure, reducing reassurance-seeking, reducing overprotective behavior, taking interpersonal risks). Consequently, although the focus remains on exploring ambivalence and enhancing motivation, this breadth in focus permits a freedom or flexibility that is important in working with comorbid populations while also striving for a client-centered interaction.

As Miller and Rollnick (2013) note, one can be engaged in a conversation but not necessarily focused within it, and focusing or steering the conversation is a critical task of the therapist. The client-centered model on which MI is based can often lead to difficulties among therapists in assuming responsibility for guiding the conversation since this can seem (to the inexperienced trainee) as interfering with a client's process or as antithetical to trusting the client. Alternatively, beginning therapists may attempt to "reflect everything," mistakenly assuming that everything a client says is of equal significance. Since reflection has a natural amplifying function (it focuses the client's attention) and carries a natural invitation to expand on what was reflected, one must choose what to reflect (and what to ignore). If one tries to reflect everything or refuses to "direct" or guide the client, that is also a choice, one that essentially gives the client permission to meander, sometimes aimlessly. Such conversations often have the feeling of "not moving" or not going anywhere.

Thus, a major component of expertise in therapy is knowing what to reflect and how to steer the conversation. Accordingly, a major component of your expertise is recognizing that not all moments are equally significant, and thus, watching for the markers that indicate significant moments requiring differential focus and expansion. What the therapist watches for is based on his or her theoretical model, and with experience therapists may develop multiple lenses that guide them and tell them what is significant and key in a therapy session. In the case of MI, this involves client motivational language (change talk, counterchange or sustain talk, ambivalence), moments of disharmony or disagreement, and signals of readiness for change. Moreover, in our experience, clients expect the therapist to guide and steer the conversation and to be informed about best therapy practices and processes. Rather than being affronted by a therapist who guides the process of therapy, clients typically welcome this.

Evoking

Informed by recent research on the role of client language in MI, close attention is paid to client speech and therapist behavior in shaping it (Miller & Rose, 2009). The proficient use of MI should ultimately increase clients' in-session "change talk" (talk in the direction of change) and decrease their "sustain talk" (talk in favor of not changing). Emerging process research in MI supports the importance of client language within MI (see the review in Miller & Rollnick, 2013). Interestingly, recent research examining client motivational language in the context of CBT for anxiety also suggests that early client statements regarding change have important predictive value. In these studies, while early change talk has been found to be unrelated to outcomes, early client arguments against change (counterchange talk or sustain talk) are highly significant predictors. Specifically, a greater frequency of arguments against change in the first session of CBT for GAD has been found to be a substantive predictor of lower homework compliance and poorer treatment outcomes across two randomized controlled trials (Button, Westra, & Hara, 2014; Lombardi, Button, & Westra, 2014). Moreover, a higher frequency of early arguments against change differentiated those who went on to experience an alliance rupture later in therapy (major disruption in the therapeutic alliance as defined by significant drops in client alliance ratings) from those who did not experience an alliance rupture (Hunter, Button, & Westra, 2014).

The Case for Observation

Thus, a necessary prerequisite for the use of MI skills, including or especially evoking clients' own motivations, is the identification of key moments and markers. Research on client language and resistance has indicated that not all moments are equally significant. Indeed, some moments, although relatively rare (e.g., arguments against change, signs of readiness for change, disagreements and other signals of disharmony in the therapy relationship), have important predictive significance. Moreover, such markers are not only relevant within MI but also generalize to other standard models of therapy such as CBT. In general, psychotherapy training and research have largely focused on intervention more than observation. However, in models such as MI that are predicated on responsivity (Stiles, Honos-Webb, & Surko, 1998; i.e., what you do depends on the immediate and ever changing moment-to-moment context), the ability to accurately observe key moments and markers becomes vital.

Moreover, Hara, Westra, Aviram, Constantino, Antony, et al. (2015) recently reported that accurate observation of important phenomena such as resistance cannot be assumed. In particular, we found that CBT therapists' postsession ratings of resistance (degree of opposition to the therapist/therapy) among clients with GAD were not related to either client postsession alliance scores or posttreatment outcomes. In contrast, the ratings of trained observers of resistance in these same sessions were highly predictive of outcomes (Hara et al., 2014). Such findings suggest that therapist observation is a particular (and trainable) skill. In essence, a therapist that is trained to be a good participant-observer is constantly getting feedback on a moment-to-moment basis (i.e., How engaged is this person? Are there markers of ambivalence or, alternatively, signals of readiness to begin planning for change? Is there any change talk? Is there any evidence that the client is receptive to the therapist's suggestion? Are there signals of disharmony or opposition?) Notably, collecting and providing therapists with feedback on client progress has been found to enhance performance, particularly in the case of negative outcomes (e.g., Lambert, Harmon, Slade, Whipple, & Hawkins, 2005). Of direct relevance to MI however, where therapists must shift and interpolate between more supportive and more directive counseling styles, gathering this feedback on client engagement and ambivalence on an ongoing basis is especially vital in guiding effective intervention. Moreover, this feedback is particularly crucial to the evocation skills that distinguish MI from other client-centered approaches.

Clinical Illustration of Evoking Motivation for Change

In the proficient use of MI, it is the client rather than the therapist who articulates the reasons for change. Thus, when hearing change talk, therapists facilitate the client's exploration and elaboration of the arguments for change, thereby addressing both the downsides of anxiety/avoidance and the possible benefits to change. Increasing change talk (or talk in the direction of change) is the proximal goal of MI here.

Consider the following example of elaborating emergent change talk with a young mother with GAD whose son was nearly injured in a sledding accident. She reported that she kept ruminating over the incident and criticizing herself for not being a better mother, given that she was unable to prevent the accident.

CLIENT: I would do anything for him. It scares me so much to know that there are things out there that could hurt him, and I just want to do everything I can to protect him from that. And it's so hard to do what we have been talking about . . . to just accept that bad stuff happens, you know, . . . and to be OK with that.

THERAPIST: Absolutely. And I'm guessing that doing that, accepting that, might leave you feeling helpless. But by worrying about it, by keeping it alive in your mind, then at least you're doing *something*, exerting some control . . . because it's just so awful to think that you don't always have control, especially over crucial things like the safety of your son. Would that be right?

CLIENT: Yes. (*pause*) But then I think *I* pay the price, you know. Like, he's OK, but I still end up thinking about it (*laughing*). [Change talk emerges.]

THERAPIST: Oh, I see. It hurts you to dwell on this—is that right? And you're laughing as you say that—what's the laughter about? [The therapist is also attuned to the way the client's statement is uttered, hearing the entire message; i.e., the laughter implies thinking that likely comes from the change position.]

CLIENT: Well (*smiling*), it's quite ridiculous. The world didn't end, we coped, and he was all right. It's so silly that I continue to dwell on it.

THERAPIST: It doesn't sound silly to me at all. And I hear another part of you talking, maybe the real you or at least another voice that says "The anxiety tells me it's the end of the world, but *I* don't agree—*I* think differently." Would that be right? Say, more from that other voice.

CLIENT: (*indignant, disgusted*) Yes, like he was fine, and when we came home I was the one who cried and had a meltdown!

THERAPIST: Ouch! I'm hearing, all this worry causes you a lot of stress and overreacting to things. And I'm hearing "I don't like myself when I do that. It turns me into someone that I am not and that I don't want to be." Would that be true?

CLIENT: (*quietly, tearfully*) Yes. And I don't want to model that for my son.

THERAPIST: That really touches you. That sounds important. You don't want him to suffer like you do. You don't want him to be anxious like you are sometimes. Talk from the tears.

CLIENT: There's more to life than worry.

THERAPIST: I see. You're saying, "I want him to know that there are other priorities in life—that you don't have to be worried all the time." Is that right? If you're willing, say more.

The emergence of change talk, or the protest of the status quo position, is an important process marker that the therapist seeks to nurture and expand in order to allow the client to more fully hear herself and elaborate incentives for change. Moreover, the change voice can often be quite muted, secondary to a highly dominant anxious voice. As such, gently encouraging further expansion of the protest voice is key to facilitating movement away from the status quo and toward change (Westra, 2012). Moreover, repeated articulation of the arguments for change often results in experiencing mounting or increasing pressure to change. Importantly, while enhancing internal advocacy and momentum for change in the client is a focus of MI, given the potential of this process to evoke resistance to change (i.e., retreat to the status quo position), it is imperative to be prepared to "roll with resistance" in this process. We now turn our attention to this important phenomenon of resistance.

Two Ways to Argue against Change

In the third edition of *Motivational Interviewing* (Miller & Rollnick, 2013), the authors note that they had confounded two different phenomena within the term "resistance." That is, they had lumped together sustain talk (counterchange talk) with the notion of discord in the therapeutic relationship. Elaborating on this distinction, Sijercic, Button, Westra, and Hara (in press) noted that a client may argue against change in a therapy session for two reasons. The first reason is that the client is merely expressing the part of him- or herself that is conflicted or ambivalent about change and in that moment favors the status quo. In GAD for example, this might involve statements such as "Worrying keeps me in control and motivated." Interpersonally, this would merely reflect a *disclosure* that presents one component of a client's ambivalence about change. And there is nothing inherently pathological about such ambivalence.

However, another reason for arguing against change may potentially be more disruptive since it may reflect disharmony in the therapeutic relationship (Miller & Rollnick, 2013; Sijercic et al., 2015). That is, a client may argue against change in order to disagree with or otherwise *oppose* the therapist's direction. For example, the therapist makes a suggestion and the client argues that this would not be worthwhile to attempt, putting forth the reasons for this position. And in general therapists who more strongly argue for change, or push the client in a direction he or she is not amenable to, may expect such disagreement to occur as a result (Miller & Rollnick, 2013).

Data presented by Sijercic et al. (in press) confirm the importance of this distinction between sustain talk as ambivalence and sustain talk as reflecting opposition. In this study, two process coding systems were utilized simultaneously to code the first session of CBT for GAD: client motivational language (change talk vs. sustain or counterchange talk) and resistance (client opposition to the therapist or therapy). Client statements made in order to oppose the therapist (i.e., in the context of interpersonal disharmony or resistance) were then separated from those uttered outside of resistance (i.e., when no evidence of opposition or disharmony was present). Findings indicated that a higher number of statements against change representing opposition or disharmony were highly toxic to subsequent homework compliance and posttreatment worry outcomes, even up to 1 year posttreatment. However, arguments against change that occurred when opposition and disharmony were not present (i.e., mere disclosures of ambivalence) bore no significant relationship to outcomes. Sijercic and colleagues concluded that the interpersonal context of arguments against change is crucial to understanding their predictive value. Moreover, client ambivalence may only be a problem when it leads to opposition and disagreement. Such findings also suggest that learning to listen for client motivational language is important in a CBT context and not just within MI, since such statements have a strong ability to predict what will happen later in therapy.

Given the strong capacity of disharmony to predict outcomes, the presence of early arguments against change uttered in order to oppose the therapist/therapy (e.g., disagreement, ignoring, interrupting) should serve as critical process markers in therapy. Thus, it becomes incumbent on the therapist to continually gauge the level of harmony and collaboration in the process and be alert to signs of disengagement and discord. Moreover, given that these process markers are strong predictors of subsequent engagement (e.g., later homework compliance), CBT therapists do not have to wait until the client fails to complete homework to appreciate that there is a problem with client engagement. Once identified, the manner in which the therapist responds to resistance plays a major role in perpetuating or diminishing it.

Thus, a major contribution of MI to clinical practice is providing for an alternative nonpejorative framework (with accompanying clinical strategies) for effectively managing such discord or disharmony in the therapeutic relationship. This discord communicates vitally important information about engagement and collaboration, namely, that the therapist is not appreciating something important that the client is attempting to communicate or bring into the conversation. Rather than persisting with his or her own agenda, the therapist needs to shift in order to effectively hear the message that the client is communicating. Fortunately, the data are very clear that resistance or disharmony is quite malleable and highly responsive to clinician style (Aviram & Westra, 2011;

Beutler et al., 2011). Moreover, Miller and Rollnick (2013) note that the way one responds to sustain talk (counterchange talk) is similar to that for responding at moments of discord.

In general, the approach in MI is to roll with or get alongside of opposition rather than confronting it directly. Specific strategies for rolling with opposition are outlined in MI and include various forms of reflection (e.g., double-sided, amplified), reframing opposition (i.e., seeing the wisdom in it), and emphasizing choice and autonomy. Below we outline an example of opposition to the therapist for an OCD client seeking therapy to reduce chronic tendencies toward excessive organization and orderliness. In the example, signals of client disengagement and discord in the relationship are noted. Following this illustration, we outline how the same interaction could have proceeded, had it been conducted in an MI style, using MI strategies for reflecting and rolling with opposition and sustain talk.

MI-INCONSISTENT APPROACH

THERAPIST: So, if you were to begin changing this problem, where would you start?

CLIENT: (*quickly*) I don't know. I have no idea. [Passivity reflecting disengagement]

THERAPIST: Is there anything from your previous experience of getting over the fear of driving that could be useful here?

CLIENT: (*Interrupts, states abruptly.*) I don't think that's the same at all. [The client is objecting to the therapist's suggestion.]

THERAPIST: Well, actually strategies for overcoming anxiety can have a lot in common, even though the situation is different. It sounds like in the past, when you overcame your fear of driving, you let go of some of the specific behaviors that the anxiety told you were necessary to stay safe—like not driving fast, not venturing too far. . . . For being overly organized, a similar strategy might involve letting go of some of the organizing and not having everything in its place all the time. It will make you more anxious in the short term—just like the driving did—but you might find out whether or not the anxiety eventually goes down as you change things up. How does that . . .

CLIENT: (*Interrupts.*) I don't want people to think I'm lazy, though, if I don't clean up right away. [Interrupting, disagreeing, articulating arguments for not changing]

THERAPIST: Would people think that, though? Is there a chance they wouldn't think that?

CLIENT: (*passively*) Well, maybe not, but it's important to me to be impressive to others. Like, when we get together with other parents and my kids will talk about all the fun things we do, people say, "Gosh, you do a lot of stuff with your kids!" And that makes me feel good. It makes me feel like I'm a great mom.

THERAPIST: I could be wrong about this, but I also seem to recall that one of the reasons you wanted to work on the problem is because you're concerned about how it might affect your kids. Is that right?

CLIENT: Yes, I do worry that I might be pushing them too hard, but I worry too about letting things go. [Yes, butting]

THERAPIST: I wonder if the best thing for your kids would be for you to be less perfect—less organized. [Note here that the therapist, not the client, is the one who is making the arguments for change.]

CLIENT: I do want them to have a terrific childhood though, and so I have to push myself to do more. [Ignoring and disagreeing]

THERAPIST: And it sounds like your anxiety says that a perfect childhood is one that is completely stimulating. I wonder if another version of a terrific childhood is one in which you do things with your kids but it's more balanced—where you let go of some stuff.

CLIENT: I'd like my kids to have more freedom, but I have a hard time letting go. [Yes, butting]

As illustrated in this segment, by repeatedly placing demands on the ambivalent client, the therapist creates a tense and conflictual interpersonal climate. That is, persisting with his or her agenda for the client to change and see/do things differently, and failing to hear the client's objections, places the client in the position of further articulating her objections to change in order to oppose the therapist. Importantly, the client in this case is merely articulating that there is an important part of her that resists or fears change, and is seeking to have this part heard and understood. If this important information is not acknowledged, the client may persist (e.g., by turning up the volume, making repeated attempts to communicate objections). In essence, this results in the client and therapist *acting out* the client's ambivalence rather than helping the client process and *work through* her ambivalence. In order to work more harmoniously and reestablish collaboration, the therapist integrating MI would be alert for such signals of disharmony and shift from a directive to a more supportive, exploratory, and empathic stance, as illustrated in the following example:

MI-CONSISTENT APPROACH

THERAPIST: So, if you were to begin changing this problem, where would you start?

CLIENT: (*quickly*) I don't know. I have no idea. [Passivity, reflecting disengagement]

THERAPIST: It's hard to know even where to begin. And only you can know whether it makes sense right now to start changing this. It might not. What are your thoughts?

CLIENT: Well, I do worry that I'm setting a bad example for my kids. I feel like I push them too hard and I need to let go of some of that. But, at the same time, I worry about letting go too. [Note here that the therapist's support of the client's autonomy allows the client to merely disclose her ambivalence rather than placing her in the position of having to disagree or oppose the therapist in order to do so.]

THERAPIST: It sounds like you feel conflicted about changing this. And I'm also hearing that you might be afraid of what would happen if you do let up more. Is that right? [The therapist reflects sustain talk and aims to help the client further understand her ambivalence.]

CLIENT: Yes. Like I worry a lot about what other people think of me. It's important to me that people look up to me. Like when people say, "Gosh, you do a lot of fun stuff with your kids," I feel really proud as a mom.

THERAPIST: Naturally, who wouldn't! So, this is an important way of feeling good about yourself. [Validating underlying positive intentions of the existing behavior.]

CLIENT: Right. Like, other parents look up to me. They ask me for advice. They admire me.

THERAPIST: And that feels good. And it sounds like it's important not to risk losing that . . . because you're thinking, "If I weren't the perfect mom, people might not respect me . . . and I might damage my kids too. I would feel worse, and they would feel worse." [Amplified reflection]

CLIENT: As I hear you say that, the way I am thinking sounds extreme actually. [Change talk]

THERAPIST: Maybe that's not really true. Can you say more?

CLIENT: Well, I know that I overdo it with my kids, and I need to let up sometimes. And as much as I like working hard to be a great parent, I think going overboard also sets a bad example for them too. Like, I already see my son getting flustered when his things are out of order. He gets really upset about it and he's five! [Notice here as well that the therapist's rolling with opposition allows the client rather than the therapist to articulate the arguments for change.]

THERAPIST: So, while being a perfect mom is really gratifying in many ways, there's a sense that there is a significant cost to this—this could hurt my kids. [Reflecting in order to elaborate]

When the therapist gets alongside of the client's objections to change and fosters the client's autonomy in making choices, the client can then freely and unobstructedly process his or her ambivalence. Were the therapist not to adopt this style of responding in the presence of critical markers of opposition and disharmony, it is easy to see how therapeutic communication could easily deteriorate into argument or lead to the client's shutting down. In our experience, these are among the most difficult skills to master. Indeed, it is much easier to be warm and experience positive regard for the client when things are going well. The trickier terrain involves continuing to prize and seek to understand the client when encountering opposition. Identifying and effectively navigating (rolling with) such moments is a key skill in MI and as such may hold promise in helping therapists develop confidence and competence in responding to commonly occurring critical events in CBT such as client opposition (e.g., disagreement, challenging, sidetracking, ignoring) and noncompliance.

Planning

When reduced resistance to change and increased interest in achieving change are present, the therapist needs to shift with the client and support him or her in planning for, experimenting with, and supporting the efforts to change. Essentially, the focus shifts from *why* to change to *how* to change (Miller & Rollnick, 2013). At this stage, there is often a palpable shift in the client, with greater interest in specifically envisioning change and experimenting with ways to achieve desired changes.

In terms of integrating MI with more directive approaches such as CBT in the treatment of anxiety, Westra (2012) has noted that MI can be used as a foundational platform from which any specific change-oriented approach can be practiced. That is, the underlying spirit and methods of MI do not have to be abandoned when clients are planning for and taking steps to change. For example, a central aspect of MI is the belief that clients have inherent expertise, not only to resolve ambivalence but also to initiate and accomplish change. Trusting this, the MI therapist is primarily concerned with creating a safe collaborative space that is conducive to uncovering, discovering, calling forth, and helping clients realize and apply this inherent expertise.

Integrating the foundational spirit and methods of MI has much to offer in terms of informing the *process* of therapy and facilitating sensitivity to the contextual influences (client receptivity and engagement) inherent in it. Moreover, integrating MI does not inform one as to *what* techniques or methods of promoting change to use; rather, it can significantly inform *when* and *how* to support clients in selecting and implementing methods for achieving change. Here, therapists informed by MI can operate as guides or consultants to clients in developing, implementing, and processing their plans for change (Miller & Rollnick, 2013).

When planning for change, therapists can continually evoke client ideas, preferences, and proposed solutions (e.g., "If you did decided to make a change, where would you start?" "If you imagined your anxiety greatly diminished in future, what would have happened to get you there?"; Westra, 2012). Importantly, the therapist actively works to refrain from imposing his or her own ideas and preferred methods about how change should be accomplished, in order to avoid coercing clients to conform to their agenda.

In addition, Westra (2012) outlines how the spirit of tentativeness that is inherent in empathic reflections can be generalized to support clients' autonomy and underscore client expertise and authority when offering feedback, providing psychoeducation, planning for change, and making suggestions. Such valuable guidance and additions to clients' efforts to change can be introduced and processed in a way that enhances the probability of client engagement with such offerings. Of particular significance is protecting and reinforcing client autonomy and freedom of choice. Also, explicit monitoring of client receptivity and level of engagement with such offerings is critically important. Contributing your perspective using MI spirit means recognizing that it is *your* perspective and not currently the client's, thus "holding it lightly" (tentatively) with an attitude of "information for the client to possibly consider, should they choose to do so." Moreover, such underlying spirit involves being prepared to back off from your suggestion, idea, or position if the client rejects it or is not prepared to engage with it. This is similar to the style of elicit–provide–elicit as outlined by Miller and Rollnick (2013). Consider the following clinical illustration of this style.

THERAPIST: Sometimes when other people criticize, it can say more about them than the person they're criticizing. Does that fit for you at all? It might not.

CLIENT: That's true.

THERAPIST: You seem to agree. Say more.

CLIENT: Like, it could just be a reflection of their need to be critical or their insecurity.

THERAPIST: And, if I'm hearing you right, it might be important to consider where it's coming from—rather than seeing it as all equally valid. Would that be true? I might be off on that, though.

CLIENT: Yes. Like, right now I just think anything negative anyone has to say about me is true.

THERAPIST: And you're saying that it might not be.

CLIENT: Right. In fact, most of the time I think it's not valid at all.

THERAPIST: So, there are times—even a lot of them—when criticism is not valid. Assuming that all criticism is right might be the way to go, and only you can know if it's helpful or necessary to make that kind of assumption. What do you think?

Problems and Suggested Solutions

Over the years, we have identified that a major difficulty in implementing MI is the seamless movement between promoting acceptance and facilitating action (Westra, 2012). Working with this dialectic is particularly challenging if one is more experienced with action-oriented and structured methods for facilitating anxiety management. In these cases, one has the dual task of making the MI-consistent response but also of inhibiting the MI-inconsistent response. If this is not effectively accomplished, therapists can find themselves saying the right words (e.g., "you get to decide") while communicating the very opposite message.

Empathy and related concepts such as alliance have garnered much empirical support in contributing to positive psychotherapy outcomes. As such, they hold great promise as points of fuller integration through methods such as MI with action- or change-based models. Yet, greater integration of these ideas is not always smooth or easy. That is, substantial integration of the "spirit" of MI can be a source of challenge to foundational assumptions about how change emerges, the source of change, processes and mechanisms of change, the role of the therapist, and so on. Being truly empathic requires a fundamental shift that is not always easily accomplished. Put differently, using MI as a clever technology to facilitate change is antithetical to the very foundations of the model. In a reciprocal manner, it is often difficult for therapists from empathy-based models to seamlessly integrate action-based methods. Although this dialectic of acceptance and change, ways of being and technique, directive and nondirective, may be worthwhile to contend with, it is important to recognize that it is also precarious terrain.

Studies Evaluating the Efficacy of MI for Anxiety

The diversity of the ways in which MI and other related procedures that include elements of MI (often known as motivational enhancement therapy [MET]) have been used in the treatment of anxiety disorders is striking (for a review, see Westra, Aviram, & Doell, 2011). Within this growing body of literature, MI has been most commonly used as a prelude to other therapies or as an approach that is integrated into standard assessment and intake procedures, or, alternatively, integrated throughout treatment as one part of a larger multicomponent treatment package. Beyond these uses, MI has also been applied to increase treatment seeking and problem recognition among those who are not yet seeking or who refuse treatment and for early prevention among individuals deemed at risk for developing anxiety disorders (see Westra et al., 2011).

Although preliminary studies investigating the use of MI in the treatment of anxiety have shown that it may be applied flexibly, research has only recently begun to examine the value of adding MI to existing treatments for anxiety. Consistent with the early stages of this work, this research includes uncontrolled case studies and controlled pilot studies, which have generally been supportive of the use of MI (Westra et al., 2011). In small randomized controlled studies comparing MI to psychoeducational, supportive, or no-treatment control conditions, MI is demonstrating promise in increasing treatment seeking, increasing problem recognition and treatment attendance, enhancing receptivity to recommended exposure-based treatments, and improving response to CBT for anxiety. For example, in a larger randomized controlled trial (RCT) comparing four sessions of MI pretreatment to no intervention prior to CBT for GAD, MI was associated with greater homework compliance and symptom reduction during the CBT phase, particularly for those with severe worry at the outset of treatment (Westra, Arkowitz, & Dozois, 2009). Among those with high worry severity, those who received MI, as compared to those who did not, showed substantially lower levels of resistance (i.e., higher receptivity to change) in CBT, and this accounted for their higher levels of worry reduction in treatment (Aviram & Westra, 2011).

While promising, the methodological limitations of these studies are significant. Small sample sizes, single-subject designs, and lack of control conditions are some of the limitations that characterize the research. Future studies using rigorous controlled designs are needed to determine the value of adding or integrating MI with other treatments for anxiety. Most notably, few studies have examined adjunctive MI use relative to a control group that received equivalent additional therapist contact. For example, Korte and Schmidt (2013) randomized participants with elevated anxiety sensitivity, a known risk factor in the development and maintenance of anxiety psychopathology, into an MET or health-focused psychoeducation control group. Results revealed that participants in the MET condition showed a significant reduction in anxiety sensitivity as compared to those in the psychoeducational group and that this effect was mediated by changes in motivation (i.e., the confidence to change).

While MI is associated with increased attendance and engagement with treatment (Westra et al., 2011), more research from well-controlled studies is required to identify whether such effects mediate the impact of adding MI on clinical outcomes. Additionally, quantitative and qualitative research methods are required to identify major active ingredients within MI. For example, Marcus and colleagues reported that client accounts of their experiences of MI as a pretreatment for GAD reflected increased motivation, the importance of therapist empathy, and creation of a safe climate to explore feelings about change (Marcus, Westra, Angus, & Kertes, 2011). The delineation of such mechanisms has important implications for understanding how MI works and for effective training in MI (Miller & Rose, 2009).

Conclusions

Given the prevalence of ambivalence about change in individuals with anxiety, MI holds promise as an adjunct to, or a fundamental context for, existing and effective methods in the treatment of anxiety (Westra, 2012). Although existing early data are promising, more rigorous investigation of this integration is clearly required. One of the major advantages of investigating MI in the treatment of anxiety and other related disorders is that MI is conceptually and methodologically complementary to existing treatments. Moreover, the diversity of ways that MI can and has been used in the treatment of anxiety suggests that this model is very transportable to various clinical populations and can be adapted to many different treatment contexts.

While interest in and research on MI for anxiety and related problems are still in the early stages, existing evidence is consistent in supporting the potential of MI to enhance engagement with and response to other treatments for a wide range of anxiety disorders. It is particularly promising that MI is demonstrating efficacy with populations (e.g., those who refuse treatment, those reluctant to seek care) and subsets of populations (e.g., high severity, comorbid presentation) that typically do not respond well to treatment or are otherwise difficult to engage (Westra et al., 2011). Such findings speak to the promise of MI in the treatment of people with anxiety disorders who often experience significant ambivalence regarding change as well as difficulty engaging with treatment and completing therapeutic tasks that require them to confront their fears and abandon avoidance strategies.

References

American Psychological Association. (2010). Division 12 Committee on building a two-way bridge between research and practice: Clinicians' experiences in using an empirically supported treatment for panic disorder. *The Clinical Psychologist, 64*, 10–20.

Antony, M. M., Ledley, D. R., & Heimberg, R. G. (Eds.). (2005). *Improving outcomes and preventing relapse in cognitive-behavioral therapy*. New York: Guilford Press.

Arkowitz, H., Miller, W. R., Westra, H. A., & Rollnick, S. (2008). Motivational interviewing in the treatment of psychological problems: Conclusions and future directions. In H. Arkowitz, H. A. Westra, W. R. Miller, & S. Rollnick (Eds.), *Motivational interviewing in the treatment of psychological problems* (pp. 324–342). New York: Guilford Press.

Aspland, H., Llewelyn, S., Hardy, G. E., Barkham, M., & Stiles, W. (2008). Alliance ruptures and rupture resolution in cognitive-behavior therapy: A preliminary task analysis. *Psychotherapy Research, 18*, 699–710.

Aviram, A., & Westra, H. A. (2011). The impact of motivational interviewing on resistance in cognitive behavioural therapy for generalized anxiety disorder. *Psychotherapy Research, 21*, 698–708.

Beutler, L. E., Harwood, T. M., Michelson, A., Song, X., & Holman, J. (2011). Resistance/reactance level. *Journal of Clinical Psychology, 67,* 133–142.

Borkovec, T. D., & Roemer, L. (1995). Perceived functions of worry among generalized anxiety disorder subjects: Distraction from more emotionally distressing topics? *Journal of Behavior Therapy and Experimental Psychiatry, 26,* 25–30.

Button, M., Westra, H. A., & Hara, K. (2014, April). *Ambivalence and homework compliance in cognitive behavioral therapy: A replication.* Paper presented at the annual meeting of the Society for the Exploration of Psychotherapy Integration, Montreal, Canada.

Castonguay, L. G., Goldfried, M. R., Wiser, S., Raue, P. J., & Hayes, A. M. (1996). Predicting the effect of cognitive therapy for depression: A study of unique and common factors. *Journal of Consulting and Clinical Psychology, 64,* 497–504.

Constantino, M. J., Ametrano, R. M., & Greenberg, R. P. (2012). Clinician interventions and participant characteristics that foster adaptive patient expectations for psychotherapy and psychotherapeutic change. *Psychotherapy, 49,* 557–569.

Engle, D., & Arkowitz, H. (2006). *Ambivalence in psychotherapy: Facilitating readiness to change.* New York: Guilford Press.

Geller, S., & Greenberg, L. (2002). Therapeutic presence: Therapists experience of presence in the psychotherapy encounter in psychotherapy. *Person-Centered and Experiential Psychotherapies, 1,* 71–86.

Hara, K. M., Westra, H. A., Button, M. L., Aviram, A., Constantino, M. J., & Antony, M. M. (2015). Therapist awareness of client resistance in cognitive-behavioral therapy for generalized anxiety disorder. *Cognitive Behavior Therapy, 44,* 162–174.

Helbig, S., & Fehm, L. (2004). Problems with homework in CBT: Rare exception or rather frequent? *Behavioral and Cognitive Psychotherapy, 32,* 291–301.

Hofmann, S. G., Asnaani, A., Vonk, I. J. J., Sawyer, A. T., & Fang, A. (2012). The efficacy of cognitive behavioral therapy: A review of meta-analyses. *Cognitive Therapy and Research, 36,* 427–440.

Hunter, J. A., Button, M. L., & Westra, H. A. (2014). Ambivalence and alliance ruptures in cognitive behavioral therapy for generalized anxiety. *Cognitive Behavioral Therapy, 43,* 201–208.

Jungbluth, N. J., & Shirk, S. R. (2009). Therapist strategies for building involvement in cognitive-behavioral therapy for adolescent depression. *Journal of Consulting and Clinical Psychology, 77,* 1179–1184.

Korte, K. J., & Schmidt, N. B. (2013). Motivational enhancement therapy reduces anxiety sensitivity. *Cognitive Therapy and Research, 37,* 1140–1150.

Lambert, M. J., Harmon, C., Slade, K., Whipple, J. L., & Hawkins, E. J. (2005). Providing feedback to psychotherapists on their patients' progress: Clinical results and practice suggestions. *Journal of Clinical Psychology, 61,* 165–174.

Lombardi, D. R., Button, M. L., & Westra, H. A. (2014). Measuring motivation:

Change talk and counter-change talk in cognitive behavioral therapy for generalized anxiety. *Cognitive Behavior Therapy, 43*, 12–21.

Marcus, M., Westra, H. A., Angus, L., & Kertes, A. (2011). Client experiences of motivational interviewing for generalized anxiety disorder: A qualitative analysis. *Psychotherapy Research, 21*, 447–461.

Miller, W. R., & Rollnick, S. (2002). *Motivational interviewing: Preparing people for change.* New York: Guilford Press.

Miller, W. R., & Rollnick, S. (2013). *Motivational interviewing: Helping people change* (3rd ed.). New York: Guilford Press.

Miller, W. R., & Rose, G. S. (2009). Toward a theory of motivational interviewing. *American Psychologist, 64*, 527–537.

Orlinsky, D. E., Grawe, K., & Parks, B. K. (1994). *Process and Outcome in Psychotherapy: Noch einmal.* Oxford, UK: Wiley.

Rogers, C. R. (1951). *Client-centered therapy.* Boston: Houghton Mifflin.

Sachse, R., & Elliott, R. (2002). Process-outcome research on humanistic therapy variables. In D. J. Cain (Ed.), *Humanistic psychotherapies: Handbook of research and practice* (pp. 83–115). Washington, DC: American Psychological Association.

Sanderson, W. C., & Bruce, T. J. (2007). Causes and management of treatment-resistant panic disorder and agoraphobia: A survey of expert therapists. *Cognitive and Behavioral Practice, 14*, 26–35.

Sijercic, I., Button, M. L., Westra, H. A., & Hara, K. M. (in press). The interpersonal context of client motivational language in cognitive behavioral therapy. *Psychotherapy.*

Stiles, W. B., Honos-Webb, L., & Surko, M. (1998). Responsiveness in psychotherapy. *Clinical Psychology: Science and Practice, 5*, 439–458.

Szkodny, L. E., Newman, M. G., & Goldfried, M. R. (2014). Clinical experiences in conducting empirically supported treatments for generalized anxiety disorder. *Behavior Therapy, 45*, 7–20.

Westra, H. A. (2011). Comparing the predictive capacity of observed in-session resistance to self-reported motivation in cognitive behavioral therapy. *Behaviour Research and Therapy, 49*, 106–113.

Westra, H. A. (2012). *Motivational interviewing in the treatment of anxiety.* New York: Guilford Press.

Westra, H. A., Arkowitz, H., & Dozois, D. J. A. (2009). Adding a motivational interviewing pretreatment to cognitive behavioral therapy for generalized anxiety disorder: A preliminary randomized controlled trial. *Journal of Anxiety Disorders, 23*, 1106–1117.

Westra, H. A., Aviram, A., & Doell, F. (2011). Extending motivational interviewing to the treatment of major mental health problems: Current directions and evidence. *Canadian Journal of Psychiatry, 56*, 643–650.

CHAPTER 5

• • • • • •

Enhancing Motivation in Individuals with Posttraumatic Stress Disorder and Comorbid Substance Use Disorders

David Yusko
Michelle L. Drapkin
Rebecca Yeh

Posttraumatic stress disorder (PTSD) is a significant public health challenge owing to its substantial impact on mental health, physical health, and interpersonal, social, and occupational problems. The military engagements in Iraq and Afghanistan have brought greater awareness to the public of the health significance of PTSD. Exposure to trauma has been a relatively common experience. Epidemiological studies in the United States estimate that between 37 and 92% of respondents (depending on the sample; see Breslau, 1998) report experiencing at least one traumatic event as defined by Criterion A1 of the *Diagnostic and Statistical Manual of Mental Disorders* (4th ed., text rev. [DSM-IV-TR]; American Psychiatric Association, 2000). Despite the prevalence of trauma, only a relatively small proportion of people who experience it will develop PTSD. For example, the National Comorbidity Survey found that only 20.4% of female trauma survivors and 8.2% of male trauma survivors developed PTSD during their lifetime (Kessler, Sonnega, Bromet, Hughes, & Nelson, 1995). Notwithstanding a lifetime prevalence of PTSD of around 8.7% in the population at large (Kessler et al., 2005), these symptoms may persist for years following the traumatic event. PTSD is also highly comorbid with such other psychiatric illnesses as anxiety disorders, depression, and substance use disorders (Holbrook, Hoyt, Stein, & Sieber, 2001; Kessler et al., 1995), causing further diminished functioning and low quality of life (e.g., Kessler, 2000). For example, the prevalence of severe impairments in quality of life in PTSD (59%) was comparable to that associated with major depressive disorder (63%; Rapaport, Clary, Fayyad, & Endicott, 2005). PTSD is also linked to poor health outcomes, including cardiovascular, neurological, and gastrointestinal disorders (Breslau & Davis, 1992; McFarlane, Atchison, Rafalowicz, & Papay, 1994; Shalev, Bleich, & Ursano, 1990). Furthermore, there is strong evidence that PTSD is associated with marked economic costs. For example, an analysis of PTSD and depression in veterans of the conflicts in Iraq and Afghanistan showed that the social costs (lost productivity, mental health treatment, and suicides) during a 2-year period totaled approximately $925 million (Kilmer, Eibner, Ringel, & Pacula, 2011). Results of several studies suggest that the reduction of PTSD symptoms leads to marked improvements in quality of life (Foa et al., 1999; Schnurr, Hayes, Lunney, McFall, & Uddo, 2006), and Kilmer et al. (2011) estimated that evidence-based treatments would result in a savings of some $138 million (approximately a 15% reduction) of the aforementioned $925 million in social costs attributable to PTSD and depression.

Given the significant negative consequences of PTSD, along with the potential for successfully reducing PTSD symptoms and their consequences via evidence-based treatments, it is critical to better understand this disorder and maximize our interventions to prevent and treat its occurrence. In this chapter, we first provide an overview of the conceptualization of PTSD, specifically highlighting the unique comorbidity of PTSD and substance use disorders; briefly review the efficacy of empirically supported interventions for the disorder; we then discuss the potential for motivational interviewing (MI) to improve treatment outcomes with this often challenging clinical population.

Clinical Population

In the current version of the *Diagnostic and Statistical Manual of Mental Disorders* (DSM-5; American Psychiatric Association, 2013), PTSD is now designated a "trauma- and stressor-related disorder," defined as a disorder that encompasses severe and persistent stress reactions after exposure to a traumatic event. A PTSD diagnosis requires the experience of a traumatic event, defined as exposure to death, threatened death, actual or threatened serious injury, or actual or threatened sexual violence (Criterion A). PTSD is also composed of four additional symptom clusters. The first of these symptom clusters involves intrusion symptoms, like intrusive memories of the trauma, trauma-related nightmares, flashbacks, intense emotional reactions to trauma reminders, and intense physical reactions to trauma reminders. The second symptom cluster involves avoidance symptoms, including active avoidance of thoughts, feelings, and/or situations that are reminders of the trauma. The third symptom cluster involves negative changes in cognitions and mood, including symptoms like excessive self-blame, inappropriate levels of guilt and/or shame, negative beliefs about oneself and/or the world, significantly diminished interest in activities, and diminished access to positive emotions. The fourth symptom cluster involves arousal and reactivity symptoms, including irritable or aggressive behavior, impulsive or self-destructive behavior, hyper-vigilance, exaggerated startle response, concentration difficulties, and sleep disturbance. A PTSD diagnosis requires the presence of symptoms for at least 1 month after the traumatic experience.

As a disorder, PTSD usually follows a typical course. While individuals often report posttraumatic stress reactions in the first days after experiencing a trauma, most of these reactions are transient (Bryant, 2003). For example, 94% of rape survivors reported PTSD symptoms 1 week posttrauma, and this rate dropped to 47% 11 weeks later (Rothbaum, Foa, Riggs, Murdock, & Walsh, 1992). In another study, 70% of women and 50% of men were diagnosed with PTSD at an average of 19 days after an assault; at 4-month follow-up the rate of PTSD dropped to 21% for women and zero for men (Riggs, Rothbaum, & Foa, 1995). Similar observations exist for people following motor vehicle accidents (Blanchard, Hickling, Barton, & Taylor, 1996) and other catastrophes and traumas (Galea et al., 2002; Galea et al., 2003; van Griensven et al., 2006).

It is important to note that PTSD is often associated with other psychiatric disorders. Lifetime comorbidity with PTSD has been reported as ranging between 62 and 92% (de Girolamo & McFarlane, 1996; Kessler et al., 1995; Perkonigg, Kessler, Storz, & Wittchen, 2000; Yehuda & McFarlane, 1995). PTSD is most commonly comorbid with depression, other anxiety disorders, and substance abuse. This comorbidity may involve the individual's developing a primary psychiatric disorder first, rendering him or her vulnerable to developing PTSD after a trauma (Breslau, Davis, Peterson, & Schultz, 1997; Perkonigg et al., 2000), or PTSD developing first, thereafter increasing the likelihood of developing other disorders (Perkonigg et al., 2000). Of particular concern is the comorbidity between PTSD and substance use disorders (SUD), with data suggesting that as many as 62% of those with an SUD have comorbid PTSD (Chilcoat & Menard, 2003; Dore, Mills, Murray, Teesson, & Farrugia, 2012). Similarly, up to as many as 65% of patients with PTSD also have a comorbid SUD (Pietrzak, Goldstein, Southwick, & Grant, 2011). The combination of PTSD and substance use is especially problematic, given how PTSD can uniquely limit the effectiveness of substance use treatment (Ouimette, Ahrens, Moos, & Finney, 1997). These findings highlight the overriding importance of treating PTSD, because it typically presents with other disorders and can contribute to a broader range of psychopathology.

Evidence-Based Treatments for PTSD

Prolonged Exposure Therapy

Prolonged exposure (PE) is a form of cognitive-behavioral therapy (CBT) that is based primarily on emotional processing theory (EPT; Foa & Kozak, 1985, 1986). According to EPT, fear is represented in memory as a cognitive structure that includes information about fear stimuli and fear responses. In a pathological fear structure, fear is overgeneralized such that objectively safe stimuli and responses (e.g., fireworks and one's heart beating fast) are erroneously associated with meanings of incompetence (e.g., "I am a weak person"), danger (e.g., "Nobody can be trusted"), and self-blame (e.g., "I am responsible for what happened"). A pathological fear structure is maintained when a trauma victim avoids confrontation with trauma-related stimuli in daily life. Thus, PE aims to help the patient disconfirm these irrational cognitions through direct exposure to trauma-related stimuli discussion of trauma memories in safe settings.

PE, which typically consists of 8–15 individual 90-minute sessions, is distinguished by three main components: *in vivo* exposure to trauma-related stimuli, imaginal exposure to the trauma memories, and processing of the imaginal exposure. *In vivo* exposure consists of the deliberate presentation of trauma-related situations that the client normally avoids because they cause him or her distress. Exercises are selected from a hierarchical list of avoided situations that are ranked by how anxious the patient would be if he or she normally approached the situation. During *in vivo* exposures, the patient is instructed to remain in the situation for at least 30 minutes or until his or her anxiety decreases by at least 50%. The exposure is repeated until the situation no longer produces significant distress, at which point the patient proceeds to confront the next challenging situation on the hierarchy. Patients are expected to complete *in vivo* exposures on their own between sessions. The remaining sessions are primarily focused on conducting imaginal exposures, in which the patient revisits the traumatic experience by verbally describing thoughts, feelings, and physical sensations experienced at the time of the trauma and imagining him- or herself revisiting the traumatic event. The patient is encouraged to remain in the imaginal exposure for about 45 minutes. Each imaginal exposure is audio recorded so that patients can listen to the trauma narrative as daily homework assignments. After each exposure, the therapist helps the patient process the experience by asking open-ended questions about thoughts and feelings that arose during the session and commenting on any learning that was observed either within or between sessions. By engaging in the memory rather than avoiding it, the patient may gain insights about the trauma and is able to modify irrational cognitions. PE has been repeatedly shown to be efficacious in reducing PTSD symptoms in various study samples, including patients with co-occurring PTSD and SUD (Foa, Gillihan, & Bryant, 2013), victims of sexual assault (Foa & Rauch, 2004; Foa et al., 1999), and victims of combat or terror (Nacasch et al., 2011; Schnurr et al., 2007).

Cognitive Processing Therapy

Cognitive processing therapy (CPT; Resick & Schnicke, 1993) focuses on how individuals incorporate trauma information into existing schemas about safety, trust, power/control, esteem, and intimacy. According to CPT, distorted cognitions develop when trauma is recalled inaccurately in order to preserve preexisting schemas or when beliefs about the self and world are modified too drastically in order to account for trauma information. These distorted interpretations lead individuals to experience "manufactured" and unrealistic emotions (e.g., guilt) that interfere with natural recovery from a trauma. The goal of CPT is to help patients modify distorted interpretations, known as "stuck points," that contribute to manufactured emotions so that patients develop more realistic beliefs about the trauma and allow natural recovery to occur.

During CPT, the patient is asked to write an "impact statement" in which he or she describes what caused the trauma and how it impacted the patient's perspectives on him- or herself and the world. The purpose of the impact statement is to help identify stuck points. Using this impact statement, the therapist teaches the patient to label thoughts and emotions and understand how distorted beliefs could influence or intensify the experience of unrealistic emotions. The therapist also introduces cognitive therapy techniques to address stuck points, such as brainstorming alternative explanations of events, gathering evidence to challenge existing beliefs, or identifying areas of problematic thinking (e.g., self-blame, hindsight bias, survivor's guilt). At home, the patient is asked to write elaborate accounts of the trauma that describe in detail the events that took place and the natural emotions that they produced. These accounts are read aloud in sessions to further identify and challenge stuck points. For exposure purposes, the patient is also asked to read the narrative on a daily basis in order to call up natural emotions and allow their expression. According to many CPT therapists, natural emotions dissipate if they are expressed and can run their course. Repeated exposure to natural emotions is not necessary for habituation. Several studies have demonstrated both the efficacy and effectiveness of CPT among samples of sexual assault victims and victims of child sexual abuse (Chard, 2005; Resick & Schnicke, 1992), refugees (Schulz, Resick, Huber, & Griffin, 2006), military veterans (Alvarez et al., 2011; Forbes et al., 2012; Macdonald, Monson, Doron-Lamarca, Resick, & Palfai, 2011), and female victims of interpersonal violence (Resick et al., 2008).

Eye Movement Desensitization and Reprocessing

The goal of eye movement desensitization and reprocessing (EMDR; Shapiro, 1995, 2001) is to help the patient reprocess various elements of a trauma memory so that those elements become associated with more adaptive emotions, beliefs, and behaviors. EMDR follows a three-pronged protocol that targets past experiences, present situations, and future behaviors for reprocessing. Depending on the complexity of the trauma, treatment can range from as few as 3 sessions to 12 or more sessions, with each session typically lasting 90 minutes. The protocol consists of eight phases. In the first three phases (i.e., history and treatment planning, preparation, and assessment), the therapist identifies "target events" from the past trauma and present situations that require reprocessing and determines skills that will be useful for guiding future behaviors. The patient is asked to visualize a scene that best represents the target event and to formulate statements that express negative beliefs associated with the target (e.g., "I am helpless"). Afterward, the patient is asked to formulate opposing statements that are more adaptive (e.g., "I am in control") and to rate the extent to which he believes the statement to be true on a Validity of Cognition (VOC) scale ranging from 1 (not true) to 7 (very true). The patient also identifies any emotions or physiological sensations associated with the target event. The next three phases (i.e., desensitization, installation, and body scan) focus on reprocessing target memory networks so that elements of the target are associated with adaptive cognitions identified in previous phases. Future behaviors are also discussed so that they are aligned with these adaptive cognitions. During sessions, the patient engages in bilateral stimulations that last 15–30 seconds each repetition, usually in the form of eye movements, tones, and taps. Successful reprocessing results in decreased negative emotions, reduced physiological reactivity, and increased endorsement of adaptive cognitions on the VOC scale. In the last two phases (i.e., closure and reevaluation), the therapist ensures that the patient leaves the session feeling calmer and reevaluates the patient at the start of the subsequent session to confirm that treatment gains were maintained. Treatment is completed when all identified targets have been reprocessed and the patient no longer experiences anxiety when reminded of the trauma. Although few randomized controlled trials have rigorously evaluated the efficacy of EMDR, results from existing studies have shown improvements in adults and children receiving this type of treatment (Ahmad, Larsson, & Sundelin-Wahlsten, 2007; Lee, Gavriel, Drummond, Richards, & Greenwald, 2002; Rothbaum, Astin, & Marsteller, 2005; Scheck, Schaeffer, & Gillette, 1998; Taylor et al., 2013).

Rationale for Employing MI for PTSD and Comorbid SUD

As reviewed above, research has made it abundantly clear that there are several treatments that are highly effective in ameliorating the symptoms and associated difficulties stemming from PTSD. However, there is a significant proportion of PTSD patients who have difficulties engaging in these evidence-based approaches. One of the most commonly cited critiques of evidence-based treatments for PTSD is the unexplained percentage of patients that drop out. For example, PE is the treatment with the largest amount of research supporting its efficacy, but it has up to a 20.5% dropout rate (Hembree, Rauch, & Foa, 2003; Hembree et al., 2003). Similarly, the dropout rates are considerable for other empirically supported PTSD treatments (e.g., CPT, 22.1%, and EMDR, 18.9%). Given that most treatments incorporate some kind of traumatic memory revisiting, it can be hypothesized that those who struggle to engage in PTSD treatment are ambivalent about this element of treatment and possibly the therapy as a whole and either drop out or do not engage in interventions that help the most. Unfortunately, there is no decisive research about what factors are related to treatment responders and nonresponders.

An MI approach may help resolve ambivalence related to engaging in trauma-focused therapies. Avoidance of traumatic memories and reminders has been associated with a habit of coping that ultimately serves to maintain symptoms of PTSD over time (Riggs, Cahill, & Foa, 2006). Problematic drug and alcohol use often accompany PTSD and may also be maintained by a similar pattern of maladaptive avoidant behaviors. Therefore, research on how to change drug and alcohol behaviors could also be applied to PTSD avoidance behaviors. For example, commitment to change has been found to predict outcomes for drug and alcohol use treatments (Amrhein, Miller, Yahne, Palmer, & Fulcher, 2003), and retrospective studies that examined patient language in treatment sessions found that commitment language is the strongest predictor of future behavior (Moyers et al., 2007; Moyers, Martin, Houck, Christopher, & Tonigan, 2009). Therefore, it is possible that PTSD treatment dropout and other lack of response to treatment might be associated with a deficit in commitment language during PTSD treatment sessions. MI is particularly adept at eliciting commitment language (Amrhein, 2004; Amrhein et al., 2003; Moyers et al., 2007) and therefore may be particularly helpful in increasing patient engagement efficacy in PTSD treatments (Miller & Rollnick, 2013).

Similarly, given the high comorbidity between PTSD and substance use disorders, MI may be applicable in helping with both. There is a growing body of literature supporting concurrent treatment for these disorders (Foa et al., 2013; Hien et al., 2009; Mills et al., 2012). To date, the most commonly utilized concurrent treatment program is Seeking Safety (Najavits, 1999). While this is not based in an MI approach, Seeking Safety has demonstrated the ability to address the comorbidity of PTSD and substance use at the same. However, Seeking Safety has also not demonstrated an ability to produce better treatment outcomes in either the short or long term when compared to treatment as usual (Hien et al., 2009). Other approaches to therapy have incorporated prolonged exposure therapy for PTSD concurrent with other treatments for substance use disorders. For example, Mills et al. (2012) combined MI and CBT for substance dependence with PE for PTSD and compared that to treatment as usual only for substance use alone. While adding PE produced improved PTSD outcomes, substance use outcomes were no different as compared to those with treatment as usual. In a similar study, Foa et al. (2013) compared concurrent delivery of PE therapy and naltrexone to a sequential treatment of offering naltrexone prior to PTSD treatment. The benefits of this study suggested that combined treatment of PE plus naltrexone, compared to either treatment alone, helped reduce relapse after treatment ended. As the evidence suggests, concurrent treatment models could become the treatment of choice for this population, but it isn't yet clear what kinds of interventions will create the most effective treatment program. Given the effectiveness of MI for substance use treatment, it seems natural that MI could also be utilized as a component of combined treatments.

In particular, the new four-processes approach in MI is a good fit to the treatment of both PTSD and comorbid PTSD/SUD (Miller & Rollnick, 2013). Engagement is a key process for individuals suffering from these disorders. It is defined as "the process of establishing a mutually trusting and respectful helping relationship" (p. 40). PTSD treatments require a solid working relationship, mutual respect, and collaboration between the therapist and the patient. One of the more common "traps" in the treatment of these disorders is the "premature focus trap," where "the counselor presses too quickly to focus the discussion, discord results and the person may be put off, becoming defensive" (p. 43). Using an MI approach can facilitate a more effective engagement process to reduce discord and increase the willingness to focus on one or both of the targets (i.e., PSTD and/or PTSD/SUD).

Clinical Applications

At present, the Philadelphia and the Minneapolis Veterans Affairs Medical Centers are conducting a research study that we hope will provide us with some insight into these challenges (Drapkin et al., 2014). This multisite study is designed to examine the efficacy and effectiveness of an integrated versus a sequential treatment approach for comorbid SUD and PTSD. The treatment strategies used in the trial are motivational enhancement therapy (MET, which is MI with feedback about the problem) for SUD as well as PE for PTSD. Both treatments involve 16 weekly 90-minute individual psychotherapy sessions that are conducted over a 20-week period. The integrated treatment is designed to incorporate

MET and PE within the session by the same therapist. MET follows the protocol described by Miller, Zweben, DiClemente, and Rychtarik (1994) and is most heavily incorporated into the first three sessions of treatment. Each session begins with MET, and then the focus of the session transitions to a standard PE protocol, ending with an integration of the two. The sequential treatment is also delivered by one therapist, with the important distinction that the first four sessions involve the MET protocol only, coupled with a health education component as a control condition for time not being dedicated to PE content. Therefore, the first four sessions of the sequential treatment do not have any PE; at Session 5 a standard 12-session PE protocol commences with little or no MET treatment from Sessions 5–16. Participants are randomly assigned at each site to either the integrated or sequential treatment.

The primary hypothesis of the study is that the integrated treatment will show greater overall symptom improvement (for both PTSD and SUD) for the participants than in the sequential treatment. Symptom improvement is defined by at least a 50% reduction in PTSD symptoms as measured by the PTSD Checklist (PCL) and the number of abstinence days from substance use. Secondary hypotheses will examine the degree of symptom improvement in each symptom domain separately. Specifically, it is hypothesized that participants in the integrated treatment will demonstrate greater PTSD symptom improvement than those in the sequential treatment during the 16 weeks of treatment and will also show greater rates of abstinence from substance use than participants in the sequential treatment. Additionally, exploratory analyses will examine whether participants in the integrated treatment sustain greater improvements in PTSD and SUD symptoms over 6 months as compared to participants in the sequential treatment and, moreover, lower rates of treatment dropout and greater treatment satisfaction.

Another similarly designed study is currently being conducted by the Center for the Treatment and Study of Anxiety at the University of Pennsylvania. The participants in this study are current cigarette smokers who are also diagnosed with PTSD. The design of this study is focused on examining how to maximize smoking cessation interventions within a PTSD population. All participants in this study receive varenicline (Chantix), a U.S. Food and Drug Administration-approved medication for smoking cessation. Subjects are randomly assigned to either an MI intervention designed to assist with smoking cessation alone or to a combined MI and PE treatment protocol designed to address both smoking cessation and PTSD symptoms concurrently. The MI treatment is a brief intervention consisting of 15-minute sessions delivered over 12 weeks as an adjunct to the varenicline. The goal of the treatment is to assist participants in attaining smoking cessation goals by helping to resolve ambivalence over quitting smoking, increasing motivation to reach smoking cessation goals, and problem-solving difficulties associated with reaching smoking goals. In the combined MI and PE treatment, the same 15-minute MI intervention is added to a standard 12-session PE protocol. Given that this is primarily a smoking cessation study, the goals of this research are to determine whether a combined treatment for smoking cessation and PTSD is a more successful approach than addressing smoking symptoms alone.

These two treatment research studies are the first to incorporate an MI intervention along with an evidence-based treatment for PTSD. We hope they will help us better understand the potential benefits of integrated versus sequential, and singular versus combined, treatment modalities. Additional benefits of these projects include testing the feasibility of therapists who are primarily trained in either MI or PE and are challenged to learn and implement both MI and PE. These studies will begin to help us understand how MI can be incorporated into PTSD treatment for comorbid populations that need more effective treatments to address their challenging clinical presentations. That being said, there currently remain no published treatment research studies that involve MI in a PTSD-only population. While theoretically it seems apparent that MI could help enhance treatment commitment and compliance, there are no data supporting this theory or guiding clinicians about how this could be most effectively accomplished.

Previous Research on MI for Treatment of PTSD

Increasing motivation, enhancing commitment to change, and increasing treatment engagement are specific components targeted for improvement in evidence-based treatments for PTSD. Trauma victims are often ambivalent about seeking treatment because they view their existing coping strategies as adaptive responses to daily events rather than seeing those behaviors as ones that need to be changed. For example, a veteran who perceives his extreme irritability as a normal response to an "unjust world" may believe that he does not need treatment and becomes frustrated when family members feel upset by his behaviors. Furthermore, some trauma victims are also skeptical about psychotherapy and/or feel ashamed about starting treatment. Lastly, fear of revisiting traumatic events of the past is a powerful motivator to avoid treatment and significantly adds to the ambivalence felt toward engaging in treatment.

The PTSD Motivation Enhancement (ME) Group (Murphy, 2008; Murphy, Rosen, Cameron, & Thompson, 2002) is a seven-session intervention that has primarily been implemented in Veterans Affairs PTSD treatment programs. The PTSD/ME group aims to help patients identify problematic behaviors, make decisions to change these behaviors, and follow through with plans to change. Patients first generate three separate lists of problems that they "definitely have," "might have," or "don't have." They then categorize problems that they "might have" into two additional categories: "problems you have wondered if you have" and "problems other people say you have but you disagree." The goal of all subsequent group sessions is to help patients evaluate the severity of problems they "might have." To do so, patients compare the frequency, severity, and purpose of "might have" problems to age-appropriate norms, weigh the pros and cons of these behaviors, and identify distorted beliefs that interfere with their willingness to acknowledge these problems.

The PTSD/ME group referenced above has been integrated into PTSD treatment programs in several ways. For instance, the intervention can be conducted concurrently with other treatment components of a comprehensive PTSD treatment program. This approach can be advantageous in that it allows patients to address ambivalence issues throughout the entire course of treatment. However, if this group treatment is introduced along with other treatment techniques, the patients may not be fully engaged in skills that are taught early in the program before any ambivalence is resolved. Thus, some treatment programs prefer to integrate the intervention during a preliminary phase of treatment so that patients actively participate in the remainder of treatment. The intervention can also be delivered as an occasional component of ongoing supportive therapy groups.

To date, only one randomized controlled trial of the PTSD/ME group has been conducted (Murphy, Thompson, Murray, Rainey, & Uddo, 2009). This trial found evidence that the intervention increased treatment engagement (defined as readiness to change, perceived treatment relevance, and PTSD program attendance) among veterans receiving outpatient CBT. Further research on interventions for enhancing motivation will be required to understand how to increase engagement among patients receiving treatment for PTSD and the potential impact of MI on PTSD treatment outcomes.

Clinical Illustration

The first difficulty to overcome is simply getting an individual with PTSD to entertain the possibility of treatment. Therefore, from the very first assessment appointment, efforts to increase engagement in treatment begin. Jerry was a 26-year-old veteran of Operation Iraqi Freedom, having been twice deployed to Iraq. He reported experiencing several traumatic events during his deployments. Jerry was resistant to come in for the evaluation but was under pressure from his wife to address the difficulties associated with his PTSD as well as alcohol use symptoms. Jerry made it clear during the initial evaluation that the only reason he was there was because of his family, and while he did recognize that things were not going well, he was clearly ambivalent about undertaking treatment. By the end of the 2-hour evaluation, enough information had been gathered to counsel Jerry that he met the criteria for PTSD as well as having alcohol dependence and major depressive disorder. The therapist explained to Jerry how those diagnoses were obtained, and he was given the opportunity to ask questions about them and what treatment options were available to him, including not doing anything. Therefore, from the very first encounter with Jerry, assessment feedback was utilized to engage him in the evaluation and treatment decision-making process.

What appeared particularly helpful to Jerry was providing him with information. This included discussing with him the research about the unique interaction between trauma and substance use issues, how recent concurrent treatment programs had had success in ameliorating both symptoms, and that if nothing were done, the research indicated that his symptoms would likely persist despite his hope that all of this would eventually go away. Jerry's decision making was reinforced, and he was informed about the treatment options, which included alcohol treatment only, sequential treatment for alcohol use first followed by PTSD treatment, concurrent treatment for alcohol use and PTSD, or no treatment. Jerry was encouraged to take this information home, think it over, discuss it with people close to him, and contact the clinic in 1 week with his decision about treatment. Jerry decided to pursue concurrent treatment for PTSD and alcohol dependence involving MET and PE. He continued to express ambivalence about the treatment program, especially the ideas of talking about his traumas and making changes in his drinking. At the same time, Jerry was not happy with the severity of his symptoms and the associated problems these symptoms caused.

All treatment sessions were weekly individual 90-minute sessions that incorporated both MET and PE in each visit. The agenda for the first session was to provide an overview of the concurrent treatment program and describe the an initial rationale for a treatment program similar to that in PE but emphasizing the unique comorbidity of PTSD and substance use, to discuss and gather information about Jerry's alcohol use, and finally to use the MI methods of open-ended questions, affirmations, reflective listening, and summaries (OARS) to elicit and reinforce change talk and strengthen his commitment change.

Jerry and his therapist discussed his traumatic experiences and selected one where Jerry was part of a convoy that was struck by a roadside bomb as his "index trauma" (i.e., the most disturbing or haunting memory according to Jerry that was driving the majority of his PTSD symptoms). They used this trauma to talk further about Jerry's strategies for coping (including alcohol use) that typically focus on avoidance of the traumatic memory, trauma triggers, and other thoughts and feelings associated with the trauma. As Jerry shared his examples of avoidance, the therapist focused on how these avoidance strategies entailed short- and long-term consequences. The goal of this conversation was to segue into the rationale for why PE utilizes *in vivo* and imaginal exposure interventions to break the cycle of relying on avoidance (including alcohol use) for its short-term benefits, and thereby achieve long-term resolution of his symptoms. The hope was that providing him with the reasoning behind the treatment would help him better understand what he was being encouraged to do, thereby increasing his motivation to engage in treatment. While the rationale for treatment was not described explicitly in MI language, an MI approach can be applied in the delivery. This is very consistent with MI information exchange approaches (asking permission, reflecting, asking open-ended questions, etc.).

The second half of the session focused on MET content. Jerry and his therapist completed an assessment of his alcohol use pattern, discussing the consequences he had experienced related to his alcohol use, the risk factors associated with alcohol use problems, and posing and answering any questions related to his readiness for change (including its importance o him and confidence rulers). This assessment was used in the next session as part of a personalized feedback report. Using open-ended nonjudgmental questions, the therapist engaged Jerry in a conversation about his alcohol use. He reported enjoying both the social aspects of drinking and the numbing component that helped him sleep at night and avoid negative emotions. As Jerry discussed the pros and cons of his alcohol use, the therapist asked him what, if anything, he wanted to change about his drinking. Jerry wasn't sure what he wanted to do, but he did feel he needed to change something. The session ended with a breathing retraining exercise (consistent with PE) and discussion of homework.

The agenda for Session 2 was set collaboratively and included homework review, examination of Jerry's personal feedback report regarding his alcohol use, psychoeducation around the common reactions to trauma, discussion of the rationale for *in vivo* exposure, and construction of an *in vivo* exposure hierarchy. After reviewing Jerry's homework, therapy moved on to his personalized feedback report. This began with a summary of his typical alcohol consumption over an average week and included normative feedback based on his age and sex. Jerry averaged over 30 standard drinks a week, typically consumed over 4 days of drinking per week. His peak BAC level was 0.25, and he was drinking more than 99% more than of his peers. The primary negative consequences for drinking were related to his family and job. His spouse was threatening separation, he felt bad about being irritable and impatient with his children, and his work supervisors had recently warned him about his poor performance and excessive use of sick days. Finally, his family history of alcohol use problems, along with his symptoms of PTSD and mild traumatic brain injury, were identified as risk factors for alcohol use disorders. This report provided an honest, accurate, and objective reflection of Jerry's alcohol use and related problems for him to consider while avoiding an adversarial or confrontational counseling stance. Jerry and his therapist were able to engage in a collaborative review of the assessment results focused on eliciting his reactions to this information without the therapist's opinions or interpretations about his alcohol use. Reflections of both verbal and nonverbal behavior were used throughout. Lastly, this report was a mirror that enabled Jerry to see his own behavior, consider whether he had a potential problem, and begin to discuss options for change. By the end of the conversation, Jerry stated that he wanted to decrease his alcohol use and set a goal of limiting himself to three standard drinks per drinking episode during the coming week.

Then, the session transitioned to concentrating on the PE components of reviewing common reactions to trauma and developing an *in vivo* exposure hierarchy. The purpose of discussing common reactions to trauma was to help Jerry better understand his symptoms as normative common experiences for someone with trauma and to provide hope that most of these reactions would improve since he was now receiving a trauma-focused therapy. Some of his most common reactions included fear and anxiety being easily triggered; reexperiencing the trauma via memories and flashbacks; nightmares; hyperarousal; hypervigilance; depression; feelings of guilt and/or shame; increased alcohol/drug use; increased anger and irritability; increased negative thinking about oneself/others/the world; and disrupted relationships. This conversation was designed to allow Jerry to tell the therapist how each of these common reactions was or was not experienced by him. The therapist elicited information and permission by using open-ended questions, reflected empathy and support, and encouraged his client by reinforcing how PE would help improve these issues.

The remainder of the session was focused on implementation of *in vivo* exposure. This began with a conversation about the treatment rationale, followed by a discussion of how Jerry had been avoiding and coping with trauma triggers in his environment. In short, this discussion reviewed how *in vivo* exposure helps to block avoidance and thus prevent the short-term benefits of that coping strategy (specifically the concept of negative reinforcement). *In vivo* exposure helps disconfirm beliefs of what might happen if one is exposed to trauma triggers; disconfirms the belief that anxiety or distress lasts forever (process habituation); and increases the client's confidence, helping to instill and a sense of competence. As in the previous session, the review of the treatment rationale was designed to increase Jerry's understanding of why this is being asked of him and how this intervention could help him feel better. The remainder of the session was spent generating items for the hierarchy, with the goal of identifying low-, moderate-, and high-difficulty items to practice over the course of treatment. Some typical hierarchy items for veterans of the war in Iraq include being in crowded places like shopping malls or movie theaters, driving (especially under bridges or on roads with debris on the shoulder), dealing with Middle Eastern people/places/things, going somewhere alone at night, stopping at red lights while driving, and reading about a similar event or seeing it on television or movies. Jerry's first homework assignment was an *in vivo* exposure. We collaboratively discussed what he felt relatively comfortable and confident doing. For him, that was going to the gym in the evening, even when it was more crowded than usual.

The agenda for Session 3 was to review homework, discuss alcohol use, review the rationale for imaginal exposure, do imaginal exposure, process the exposure, and assign homework. Jerry came to this session having done relatively well with his alcohol goal, drinking four standard drinks per drinking episode. He did exceed that drinking goal on one occasion, and this prompted a discussion of what had happened. The therapist continued to use the MI strategies of OARS and attempts to elicit preparatory change talk (DARN: statements of Desire, Ability, Reasons and Need for change) along with mobilizing change talk (CAT: Commitment, Activation, and Taking steps to change). Jerry expressed an overall commitment to continue to change his drinking habits while also identifying some ambivalence around certain social drinking occasions in which he was less committed to his four standard drink goal. Ample time was devoted to exploring Jerry's motivation as it relates to drinking and arriving at a goal that he is comfortable with. After more discussion, Jerry agreed to eliminate nonsocial drinking during the coming week and to limit himself to six standard drinks in social situations.

This also was the last session where the planned rationale for exposure was discussed. Revisiting traumatic memories can be very difficult for trauma survivors. Therefore, invoking a specific rationale for imaginal exposure is very important. This process begins by validating how difficult and painful remembering the trauma can be, how Jerry feels about remembering, and how he has relied on avoidance to cope. Once again, the short-term benefits of avoidance were reviewed along with the long-term consequences of this approach. Very often an analogy is helpful in illustrating how imaginal exposure helps process and digest traumatic experiences. The goals of imaginal exposure were reviewed: to process and organize the traumatic memory; to increase the differentiation between "remembering" the trauma and being "retraumatized"; to learn to appreciate that memories of the trauma are not dangerous; to promote differentiation and decrease generalization between the traumatic event and other similar but safe events, to bring about habituation (i.e., with repetition, anxiety and distress decrease); and to enhance a sense of personal competence, mastery, and confidence over the memory. Jerry was ambivalent about this procedure but understood the consequences of continuing to avoid and the potential benefits of exposure. He agreed to imaginal exposure try and spent 45 minutes revisiting his memory in session. While the process was difficult for him, he began to realize that he could do it and became more personally invested in the rationale rather than just intellectually understanding how it could help.

The remaining sessions followed the same agenda. Jerry eventually settled on a drinking goal of four standard drinks during one social drinking episode per week and was able to reach this goal successfully. By not forcing a goal of abstinence on Jerry, he was able to discuss his drinking openly and honestly with the therapist each week until he found a goal that he was motivated to accomplish. Jerry struggled at times with the PTSD treatment. He skipped several sessions early on in the treatment, along with avoiding some of the PE-focused homework. However, the therapist was able to discuss with him the reasons he skipped sessions and opted out of homework assignments. Since the beginning of treatment focused so much on rationale as well as eliciting Jerry's personal reasons for avoidance and what he had to gain by engaging in therapy, these problems were resolved by revisiting those conversations as ambivalence about therapy waxed and waned over the course of treatment. This flexibility enabled Jerry to explore his struggles with the treatment, to problem-solve his difficulties, and ultimately to end treatment no longer meeting the criteria for PTSD, major depression, or alcohol dependence.

Problems and Suggested Solutions

The most substantial problem related to the integration of MI into PTSD treatment is the glaring lack of research. There are currently no randomized controlled trials on how MI could be used in conjunction with evidence-based PTSD treatments (PE, CPT, or EMDR) and therefore no data indicating that MI should increase the efficacy of treatments. Theoretically, it makes sense that MI could increase PTSD treatment engagement, enhance PTSD treatment compliance, decrease PTSD treatment dropout, and therefore improve PTSD treatment outcomes. Unfortunately, however, currently these are just educated guesses, and therapists have no guidelines on whether this expectation is realistic and, if so, how best to incorporate MI into PTSD treatment manuals. The research that does exist, utilizing the PTSD ME group, suggests that an MI-based intervention may be effective in increasing treatment engagement. However, this research does not demonstrate that treatment outcomes are enhanced or inform us about how this group would work with the most commonly used evidenced-based treatments for PTSD (PE, CPT, and EMDR). Similarly, current research with comorbid substance use and PTSD populations does not examine how MI could be used within the PTSD treatment, as MI is only being utilized within the substance abuse intervention. These studies will help us better understand whether integrated treatments for both disorders can be conducted within the session by the same therapist, but the treatments themselves remain separate. MI is being used for the substance use, and PE is being used for PTSD. The notion that these two things can be done at the same time is certainly an advance in the treatment literature, but unfortunately it will not help us learn more about how MI could be used in PTSD therapy. Therefore, the obvious solution here is to conduct more specific research that tests whether MI could enhance PTSD treatment outcomes. Until we have more data, the perspective that "good" therapists are already adhering to an MI style in PTSD treatment—and that therefore specific MI training is unnecessary—will likely persist in the PTSD treatment field.

Beyond the need for more research, there are also some potential conflicting aspects of MI and PTSD interventions. MI is predicated on certain values, such as abandoning labels, allowing for client choice, avoiding the expert stance, and maintaining a client-centered attitude. While these values do not preclude the use of MI in PTSD treatments, they complicate the balance of going back and forth between styles by the same therapist. PTSD treatment is often at the opposite end of the spectrum from MI with regard to several of these values. Inclusion for PTSD treatment is predicated on a diagnosis and the presence of certain symptoms. The PTSD therapist is taught to be the expert and wants to teach the patient a set of skills that he or she currently does not posseass or is not using, and the need for treatment is based on the idea that natural recovery has failed. Therefore, the patient "needs" these skills in order to recover from the label (PTSD). PTSD therapists are often more directive than those who use MI, adhere to a more strict session-by-session structure, and attempt to convince patients why treatment is necessary. Incorporating MI more formally into the protocol, could be uncomfortable for a PTSD therapist, as well as confusing for therapists and patients. However, it may be possible to conduct the PTSD treatment within an MI framework.

Potential solutions to these problems appear to be a function of education and training. MI has been successfully incorporated into cognitive-behavioral treatments for substance use, which often tend to be skills-based, expert-driven interventions (Bien, Miller, & Tonigan, 1993; Heather, Rollnick, Bell, & Richmond, 1996). However, this could be a product of the training of substance use therapists, who are taught early on how to use MI in the treatment. There are no such training programs that currently teach PTSD therapists how to flexibly apply MI and integrate an MI-oriented therapeutic approach into a PTSD-focused treatment approach. Additionally, the training of therapists in evidenced-based approaches, both MI and PTSD interventions, varies across programs and disciplines. Just as with any attempt to change behavior, there are significant barriers to changing a therapist's style. Therefore, one potential solution is to increase the training for evidence-based treatments such as MI and PE early on during the educational process, as students are learning to become therapists. Such an increase in training might well make it easier to then teach therapists how to integrate the two treatments when working with a comorbid PTSD/SUD individual.

Mental health organizations may also face several challenges when seeking to integrate MI into treatments for PTSD. The first challenge for an organization is a willingness to concurrently treat substance use disorders and PTSD. Despite a growing body of literature supporting the efficacy of a concurrent treatment approach, the general practice is still to address substance use disorders before treating trauma. It would take a strong commitment from an organization's leadership to make this systemic change. The second organizational challenge is related to the separation of mental health and substance use treatment facilities. In many states an organization is chartered to be either a mental health or a substance abuse treatment facility—but typically not both. Therefore, clinical staff members are typically trained for just one of these treatment modalities. This pattern highlights a related challenge regarding the feasibility of training clinicians and disseminating evidence-based treatments to clinical providers already working in their respective fields.

Despite the availability of several well-known effective treatments for PTSD, most patients continue to receive treatment of unknown efficacy (Foa et al., 2013). The additional challenge of incorporating MI into evidence-based treatment for PTSD requires the acquisition of another therapeutic strategy. To complicate the training needs further, an individual clinician seeing a comorbid substance use disorder and PTSD patient would need to be knowledgeable about substance use disorders and proficient in MI and PTSD treatments. One potential solution would be to have different providers for substance use problems and PTSD symptoms, but there are limitations to this approach. This increases obstacles around coordination of treatment, differences of opinion between providers, extra treatment visits, and rapport building with multiple providers.

This set of circumstances raises the broader issue of the dissemination of evidence-based treatments in general. Given that most patients do not receive an evidence-based treatment for PTSD, the challenge of properly training therapists in both MI and PTSD treatment interventions is something experts need to start addressing. The Veterans Affairs Health System has taken this need seriously and has implemented evidence-based treatment "rollouts" (e.g., Karlin et al., 2010) that undertake to train therapists across the entire system on MI and PTSD treatments (PE and CPT in particular). But this initiative requires the leadership of an organization to mandate such training and its implementation. Until there are more incentives (and substantive consequences for not acting) interventions like MI and evidence-based PTSD treatments will continue to be underutilized.

Conclusions

The incorporation of MI strategies into evidence-based treatments for PTSD remains in an early stage of development. Each strategy by itself has an abundance of literature supporting its efficacy, but taken together there is only one randomized controlled trial to date. The hopeful news is that we already have highly effective treatments for PTSD that, when given a chance, have already helped countless victims of trauma. However, these treatments are not universally effective and have limitations that could be significantly minimized or reversed by integrating the treatments with MI. Specifically, treatment retention is a problem that needs to be better understood in order to see if MI strategies would help keep patients engaged in treatment after they make that difficult decision to schedule an appointment. Furthermore, enhancing treatment engagement could be another way that MI can increase PTSD treatment effectiveness. Given that we have a sense of what does work in PTSD treatment, the problem seems more related to not knowing how to increase our ability to engage our patients in that process. MI would seem to be an obvious partner for PTSD therapists, given the inherent difficulty involved in helping patients commit to changing these patterns of behavior and perspective that maintain symptoms over time.

Many clients go through trauma treatment by willingly facing difficult experiences from the past. At the same time, their ambivalence about overcoming the past and being unsure about facing their fears is understandable. MI offers the opportunity to help those courageous individuals to take advantage of the treatments that can deliver the relief they deserve.

References

Ahmad, A., Larsson, B., & Sundelin-Wahlsten, V. (2007). EMDR treatment for children with PTSD: Results of a randomized controlled trial. *Nordic Journal of Psychiatry, 61,* 349–354.

Alvarez, J., McLean, C., Harris, A. H. S., Rosen, C. S., Ruzek, J. I., & Kimerling, R. (2011). The comparative effectiveness of cognitive processing therapy for male veterans treated in a VHA posttraumatic stress disorder residential rehabilitation program. *Journal of Consulting and Clinical Psychology, 79,* 590–599.

American Psychiatric Association. (2000). *Diagnostic and statistical manual of mental disorders* (4th ed., text rev.). Washington, DC: Author.

American Psychiatric Association. (2013). *Diagnostic and statistical manual of mental disorders* (5th ed.). Arlington, VA: Author.

Amrhein, P. C. (2004). How does motivational interviewing work? What client talk reveals. *Journal of Cognitive Psychotherapy, 18,* 323–336.

Amrhein, P. C., Miller, W. R., Yahne, C. E., Palmer, M., & Fulcher, L. (2003). Client commitment language during motivational interviewing predicts drug use outcomes. *Journal of Consulting and Clinical Psychology, 71,* 862–878.

Bien, T. H., Miller, W. R., & Tonigan, J. S. (1993). Brief interventions for alcohol problems: A review. *Addiction, 88,* 315–335.

Blanchard, E. B., Hickling, E. J., Barton, K. A., & Taylor, A. E. (1996). One-year prospective follow-up of motor vehicle accident victims. *Behaviour Research and Therapy, 34,* 775–786.

Breslau, N. (1998). Epidemiology of trauma and posttraumatic stress disorder. In R. Yehuda (Ed.), *Psychological trauma* (pp. 1–29). Arlington, VA: American Psychiatric Association.

Breslau, N., & Davis, G. C. (1992). Posttraumatic stress disorder in an urban population of young adults: Risk factors for chronicity. *American Journal of Psychiatry, 149,* 671–675.

Breslau, N., Davis, G. C., Peterson, E. L., & Schultz, L. (1997). Psychiatric sequelae of posttraumatic stress disorder in women. *Archives of General Psychiatry, 54,* 81–87.

Bryant, R. A. (2003). Acute stress disorder: Is it a useful diagnosis? *Clinical Psychologist, 7,* 67–79.

Chard, K. M. (2005). An evaluation of cognitive processing therapy for the treatment of posttraumatic stress disorder related to childhood sexual abuse. *Journal of Consulting and Clinical Psychology, 73,* 965–971.

Chilcoat, H. D., & Menard, C. (2003). Epidemiological investigations: Comorbidity of posttraumatic stress disorder and substance use disorder. In P. Ouimette & P. J. Brown (Eds.), *Trauma and substance abuse: Causes, consequences, and treatment of comorbid disorders* (pp. 9–28). Washington, DC: American Psychological Association.

de Girolamo, G., & McFarlane, A. C. (1996). The epidemiology of PTSD: A comprehensive review of the international literature. In A. J. Marsella, M. J. Friedman, E. T. Gerrity, & R. M. Scurfield (Eds.), *Ethnocultural aspects of posttraumatic stress disorder: Issues, research, and clinical applications* (pp. 33–85). Washington, DC: American Psychological Association.

Dore, G., Mills, K., Murray, R., Teesson, M., & Farrugia, P. (2012). Posttraumatic stress disorder, depression and suicidalit in inpatients with substance use disorders. *Drug and Alcohol Review, 31,* 294–302.

Drapkin, M. L., Kehle-Forbes, S. M., Polusny, M., Foa, E. B., Oslin, D., & Blasco, M. M. (2014, June). *Integrated vs. sequential treatment for comorbid PTSD/addiction among veterans.* Poster presented at the 37th annual meeting of the Research Society on Alcoholism, Bellevue, WA.

Foa, E. B., Dancu, C. V., Hembree, E. A., Jaycox, L. H., Meadows, E. A., & Street, G. P. (1999). A comparison of exposure therapy, stress inoculation training, and their combination for reducing posttraumatic stress disorder in female assault victims. *Journal of Consulting and Clinical Psychology, 67,* 194–200.

Foa, E. B., Gillihan, S. J., & Bryant, R. A. (2013). Challenges and successes in dissemination of evidence-based treatments for posttraumatic stress: Lessons learned from prolonged exposure therapy for PTSD. *Psychological Science in the Public Interest, 14,* 65–111.

Foa, E. B., & Kozak, M. J. (1985). Treatment of anxiety disorders: Implications for psychopathology. In A. H. Tuma & J. D. Maser (Eds.), *Anxiety and the anxiety disorders* (pp. 421–452). Hillsdale, NJ: Erlbaum.

Foa, E. B., & Kozak, M. J. (1986). Emotional processing of fear: Exposure to corrective information. *Psychological Bulletin, 99,* 20–35.

Foa, E. B., & Rauch, S. A. M. (2004). Cognitive changes during prolonged exposure versus prolonged exposure plus cognitive restructuring in female assault survivors with posttraumatic stress disorder. *Journal of Consulting and Clinical Psychology, 72,* 879–884.

Foa, E. B., Yusko, D. A., McLean, C. P., Suvak, M. K., Bux, D. A., Oslin, D., et al. (2013). Concurrent naltrexone and prolonged exposure therapy for patients with comorbid alcohol dependence and PTSD: A randomized clinical trial. *JAMA, 310,* 488–495.

Forbes, D., Lloyd, D., Nixon, R. D. V., Elliot, P., Varker, T., Perry, D., et al. (2012). A multisite randomized controlled effectiveness trial of cognitive processing therapy for military-related posttraumatic stress disorder. *Journal of Anxiety Disorders, 26,* 442–452.

Galea, S., Ahern, J., Resnick, H., Kilpatrick, D., Bucuvalas, M., Gold, J., et al. (2002). Psychological sequelae of the September 11 terrorist attacks in New York City. *The New England Journal of Medicine, 346,* 982–987.

Galea, S., Vlahov, D., Resnick, H., Ahern, J., Susser, E., Gold, J., et al. (2003). Trends of probable post-traumatic stress disorder in New York City after the September 11 terrorist attacks. *American Journal of Epidemiology, 158,* 514–524.

Heather, N., Rollnick, S., Bell, A., & Richmond, R. (1996). Effects of brief counseling among male heavy drinkers identified on general hospital wards. *Drug and Alcohol Review, 15,* 29–38.

Hembree, E. A., Foa, E. B., Dorfan, N. M., Street, G. P., Kowalski, J., & Tu, X. (2003). Do patients drop out prematurely from exposure therapy for PTSD? *Journal of Traumatic Stress, 16,* 555–562.

Hembree, E. A., Rauch, S. A. M., & Foa, E. B. (2003). Beyond the manual: The insider's guide to prolonged exposure therapy for PTSD. *Cognitive and Behavioral Practice, 10,* 22–30.

Hien, D. A., Wells, E. A., Jiang, H., Suarez-Morales, L., Campbell, A. N. C., Cohen, L. R., et al. (2009). Multisite randomized trial of behavioral interventions for women with co-occurring PTSD and substance use disorders. *Journal of Consulting and Clinical Psychology, 77,* 607–619.

Holbrook, T. L., Hoyt, D. B., Stein, M. B., & Sieber, W. J. (2001). Perceived threat to life predicts posttraumatic stress disorder after major trauma: Risk factors and functional outcome. *Journal of Trauma, 51,* 287–292.

Karlin, B. E., Ruzek, J. I., Chard, K. M., Eftekhari, A., Monson, C. M., Hembree, E. A., et al. (2010). Dissemination of evidence-based psychological treatments for posttraumatic stress disorder in the Veterans Health Administration. *Journal of Traumatic Stress, 23,* 663–673.

Kessler, R. C. (2000). Posttraumatic stress disorder: The burden to the individual and to society. *Journal of Clinical Psychiatry, 61,* 4–14.

Kessler, R. C., Berglund, P., Demler, O., Jin, R., Merikangas, K. R., & Walters, E. E. (2005). Lifetime prevalence and age-of-onset distributions of DSM-IV disorders in the National Comorbidity Survey Replication. *Archives of General Psychiatry, 62,* 593–602.

Kessler, R. C., Sonnega, A., Bromet, E., Hughes, M., & Nelson, C. B. (1995). Posttraumatic stress disorder in the National Comorbidity Survey. *Archives of General Psychiatry, 52,* 1048–1060.

Kilmer, B., Eibner, C., Ringel, J. S., & Pacula, R. L. (2011). Invisible wounds, visible savings?: Using microsimulation to estimate the cost and savings associated with providing evidence-based treatment for PTSD and depression to veterans of Operation Enduring Freedom and Operation Iraqi Freedom. *Psychological Trauma: Theory, Research, Practice, and Policy, 3,* 201–211.

Lee, C., Gavriel, H., Drummond, P., Richards, J., & Greenwald, R. (2002). Treatment of PTSD: Stress inoculation training with prolonged exposure compared to EMDR. *Journal of Clinical Psychology, 58,* 1071–1089.

Macdonald, A., Monson, C. M., Doron-Lamarca, S., Resick, P. A., & Palfai, T. P. (2011). Identifying patterns of symptom change during a randomized controlled trial of cognitive processing therapy for military-related posttraumatic stress disorder. *Journal of Traumatic Stress, 24,* 268–276.

McFarlane, A. C., Atchison, M., Rafalowicz, E., & Papay, P. (1994). Physical symptoms in posttraumatic stress disorder. *Journal of Psychosomatic Research, 38,* 715–726.

Miller, W. R., & Rollnick, S. (2013). *Motivational interviewing: Helping people change* (3rd ed.). New York: Guilford Press.

Miller, W. R., Zweben, A., DiClemente, C. C., & Rychtarik, R. G. (1994). *Motivational enhancement therapy manual: A clinical research guide for therapists treating individuals with alcohol abuse and dependence*)Project MATCH Monograph Series, Vol. 2. NIH Pub. No. 94-3723). Rockville, MD: National Institute on Alcohol Abuse and Alcoholism.

Mills, K. L., Teesson, M., Back, S. E., Brady, K. T., Baker, A. L., Hopwood, S., et al. (2012). Integrated exposure-based therapy for co-occurring posttraumatic stress disorder and substance dependence: A randomized controlled trial. *JAMA, 308,* 690–699.

Moyers, T. B., Martin, T., Christopher, P. J., Houck, J. M., Tonigan, J. S., & Amrhein, P. C. (2007). Client language as a mediator of motivational interviewing efficacy: Where is the evidence? *Alcoholism: Clinical and Experimental Research, 31,* 40S–47S.

Moyers, T. B., Martin, T., Houck, J. M., Christopher, P. J., & Tonigan, J. S. (2009). From in-session behaviors to drinking outcomes: A causal chain for motivational interviewing. *Journal of Consulting and Clinical Psychology, 77,* 1113–1124.

Murphy, R. T. (2008). Enhancing combat veterans' motivation to change post-traumatic stress disorder symptoms and other problem behaviors. In H. Arkowitz, H. A. Westra, W. R. Miller, & S. Rollnick (Eds.), *Motivational interviewing in the treatment of psychological problems* (pp. 54–87). New York: Guilford Press.

Murphy, R. T., Rosen, C. S., Cameron, R. P., & Thompson, K. E. (2002). Development of a group treatment for enhancing motivation to change PTSD symptoms. *Cognitive & Behavioral Practice, 9*, 308–316.

Murphy, R. T., Thompson, K. E., Murray, M., Rainey, Q., & Uddo, M. M. (2009). Effect of a motivation enhancement intervention on veterans' engagement in PTSD treatment. *Psychological Services, 6*, 264–278.

Nacasch, N., Foa, E. B., Huppert, J. D., Tzur, D., Fostick, L., Dinstein, Y., et al. (2011). Prolonged exposure therapy for combat- and terror-related post-traumatic stress disorder: A randomized control comparison with treatment as usual. *Journal of Clinical Psychiatry, 72*, 1174–1180.

Najavits, L. M. (1999). Seeking Safety: A new cognitive-behavioral therapy for PTSD and substance abuse. *National Center for Post-traumatic Stress Disorder Clinical Quarterly, 8*, 42–45.

Ouimette, P. C., Ahrens, C., Moos, R. H., & Finney, J. W. (1997). Posttraumatic stress disorder in substance abuse patients: Relationship to 1-year posttreatment outcomes. *Psychology of Addictive Behaviors, 11*, 34–47.

Perkonigg, A., Kessler, R. C., Storz, S., & Wittchen, H. (2000). Traumatic events and posttraumatic stress disorder in the community: Prevalence, risk factors and comorbidity. *Acta Psychiatrica Scandinavica, 101*, 46–59.

Pietrzak, R. H., Goldstein, R. B., Southwick, S. M., & Grant, B. F. (2011). Prevalence and Axis I comorbidity of full and partial posttraumatic stress disorder in the United States: Results from Wave 2 of the National Epidemiologic Survey on Alcohol and Related Conditions. *Journal of Anxiety Disorders, 25*, 456–465.

Rapaport, M. H., Clary, C., Fayyad, R., & Endicott, J. (2005). Quality-of-life impairment in depressive and anxiety disorders. *The American Journal of Psychiatry, 162*, 1171–1178.

Resick, P. A., Galovski, T. E., Uhlmansiek, M. O., Scher, C. D., Clum, G. A., & Young-Xu, Y. (2008). A randomized clinical trial to dismantle components of cognitive processing therapy for posttraumatic stress disorder in female victims of interpersonal violence. *Journal of Consulting and Clinical Psychology, 76*, 243–258.

Resick, P. A., & Schnicke, M. K. (1992). Cognitive processing therapy for sexual assault victims. *Journal of Consulting and Clinical Psychology, 60*, 748–756.

Resick, P. A., & Schnicke, M. K. (1993). *Cognitive processing therapy for sexual assault victims: A treatment manual.* Newbury Park, CA: Sage.

Riggs, D. S., Cahill, S. P., & Foa, E. B. (2006). Prolonged exposure treatment of posttraumatic stress disorder. In V. M. Follette & J. I. Ruzek (Eds.), *Cognitive-behavioral therapies for trauma* (2nd ed., pp. 65–95). New York: Guilford Press.

Riggs, D. S., Rothbaum, B. O., & Foa, E. B. (1995). A prospective examination of symptoms of posttraumatic stress disorder in victims of nonsexual assault. *Journal of Interpersonal Violence, 10,* 201–214.

Rothbaum, B. O., Astin, M. C., & Marsteller, F. (2005). Prolonged exposure versus eye movement desensitization and reprocessing (EMDR) for PTSD rape victims. *Journal of Traumatic Stress, 18,* 607–616.

Rothbaum, B. O., Foa, E. B., Riggs, D. S., Murdock, T., & Walsh, W. (1992). A prospective examination of post-traumatic stress disorder in rape victims. *Journal of Traumatic Stress, 5,* 455–475.

Scheck, M. M., Schaeffer, J. A., & Gillette, C. (1998). Brief psychological intervention with traumatized young women: The efficacy of eye movement desensitization and reprocessing. *Journal of Traumatic Stress, 11,* 25–44.

Schnurr, P. P., Friedman, M. J., Engel, C. C., Foa, E. B., Shea, M. T., Chow, B. K., et al. (2007). Cognitive behavioral therapy for posttraumatic stress disorder in women: A randomized controlled trial. *JAMA, 297,* 820–830.

Schnurr, P. P., Hayes, A. F., Lunney, C. A., McFall, M., & Uddo, M. (2006). Longitudinal analysis of the relationship between symptoms and quality of life in veterans treated for posttraumatic stress disorder. *Journal of Consulting and Clinical Psychology, 74,* 707–713.

Schulz, P. M., Resick, P. A., Huber, L. C., & Griffin, M. G. (2006). The effectiveness of cognitive processing therapy for PTSD with refugees in a community setting. *Cognitive and Behavioral Practice, 13,* 322–331.

Shalev, A., Bleich, A., & Ursano, R. J. (1990). Posttraumatic stress disorder: Somatic comorbidity and effort tolerance. *Psychosomatics: Journal of Consultation and Liaison Psychiatry, 31,* 197–203.

Shapiro, F. (1995). *Eye movement desensitization and reprocessing: Basic principles, protocols, and procedures.* New York: Guilford Press.

Shapiro, F. (2001). *Eye movement desensitization and reprocessing: Basic principles, protocols, and procedures* (2nd ed.). New York: Guilford Press.

Taylor, S., Thordarson, D. S., Maxfield, L., Fedoroff, I. C., Lovell, K., & Ogrodniczuk, J. (2003). Comparative efficacy, speed, and adverse effects of three PTSD treatments: Exposure therapy, EMDR, and relaxation training. *Journal of Consulting and Clinical Psychology, 71,* 330–338.

van Griensven, F., Chakkraband, M. L. S., Thienkrua, W., Pengjuntr, W., Cardozo, B. I., Tantipiwatanaskul, P., et al. (2006). Mental health problems among adults in tsunami-affected areas in southern Thailand. *JAMA, 296,* 537–548.

Yehuda, R., & McFarlane, A. C. (1995). Conflict between current knowledge about posttraumatic stress disorder and its original conceptual basis. *The American Journal of Psychiatry, 152,* 1705–1713.

CHAPTER 6

• • • • • •

Motivational Interviewing as a Prelude to Psychotherapy for Depressed Women

Allan Zuckoff
Holly A. Swartz
Nancy K. Grote

Mothers of psychiatrically ill children and economically disadvantaged pregnant women are two groups that have especially high rates of depression and low rates of treatment. Swartz and colleagues (2005) found that 61% of mothers bringing their children to a pediatric mental health clinic met DSM-IV (American Psychiatric Association, 1994) criteria for a current Axis I disorder, most commonly depression (35%); two-thirds of those with a psychiatric diagnosis were not receiving psychiatric treatment. Most pregnant (Flynn, Blow, & Marcus, 2006; Marcus, Flynn, Blow, & Barry, 2003) and low-income (Levy & O'Hara, 2010; Lorant et al., 2003; Miranda, Azocar, Komaromy, & Golding, 1998) women suffering from depression go untreated despite being at high risk for depression (as compared with the general population).

Practical barriers to treatment participation by depressed and vulnerable women include cost, clinic inaccessibility, and problems with child care. Depressed people suffer, by definition, from low energy, hopelessness, and cognitive slowing, symptoms that may make them more vulnerable to the "time and hassle" factors associated with participating in treatment. Worry or embarrassment about acknowledging depression and doubts that treatment could be helpful (Scholle, Hasket, Hanusa, Pincus, & Kupfer, 2003) as well as previous negative experiences with mental health services (McKay & Bannon, 2004) inhibit initial engagement, and feeling misunderstood or unhelped predicts premature discontinuation (Garcia & Weisz, 2002). Mismatches between the type of treatment offered and that desired (McCarthy et al., 2005), incompatible views of the nature of the problem, negative attitudes about the legitimacy of accepting help, disclosing private experiences, or taking care of oneself (e.g., Mackenzie, Knox, Gekoski, & Macaulay, 2004), and negative relationship expectancies are also inhibitory. Cultural insensitivity or ignorance on the part of therapists may also present a significant barrier (Miranda, Azocar, Organista, Muñoz, & Lieberman, 1996). Low perceived need for services, especially among those with mild to moderate depression (Mojtabai et al., 2011), suggests that some may feel resigned, assuming that there is nothing to be done about their low mood.

Usual Treatments

Interventions to improve engagement in mental health treatment include psychotherapy preparation strategies such as role induction, vicarious therapy pretraining, experiential pretraining, and use of cognitive therapy techniques (Pollard, 2006; Walitzer, Dermen, & Connors, 1999). Case management has been employed to engage depressed women in primary care into depression treatment (Miranda, Azocar, Organista, Dwyer, & Areane, 2003). None of these approaches has been widely used.

Rationale for Adapting Motivational Interviewing to Enhance Engagement in Depression Treatment

Treatment preparation interventions have rarely attended to clients' agendas—including a wish to tell their story, understand the nature of their problems, and specify the kind of help they wish to receive—or to the psychological and cultural barriers they might face. Motivational interviewing (MI; Miller & Rollnick, 2013) emphasizes the meeting of the treatment aspirations of client and therapist within a client-centered relationship. Furthermore, many barriers to treatment can be understood in terms of ambivalence about change, participating in treatment, or both. As a counseling style for resolving ambivalence in the context of an accepting, compassionate, and autonomy-supportive understanding of individuals' perspectives, hopes, and concerns, MI provides a promising framework for engagement intervention. A substantial body of research supports the use of MI for this purpose (Lundahl, Kunz, Brownell, Tollefson, & Burke, 2010; Zuckoff & Hettema, 2007), with the evidence suggesting that the effects of adding MI to lengthier or more intensive treatments are meaningful and lasting (Hettema, Steele, & Miller, 2005).

Clinical Applications

Development of the Engagement Session

Seeking effective yet feasible ways to reach out to difficult-to-engage populations, Swartz, who had developed a brief form of interpersonal psychotherapy for depressed mothers of psychiatrically ill children (IPT-B; Swartz et al., 2004; Swartz, Grote, & Graham, 2014), and Grote, who adapted IPT-B for depressed socioeconomically disadvantaged pregnant women (Grote, Bledsoe, Swartz, & Frank, 2004), initiated a collaboration with Zuckoff (Grote, Swartz, & Zuckoff, 2008; Swartz et al., 2007), who with colleagues had described (Daley & Zuckoff, 1999; Zuckoff & Daley, 2001; Zweben & Zuckoff, 2002) and pilot-tested (Daley, Salloum, Zuckoff, Kirisci, & Thase, 1998; Daley & Zuckoff, 1998) an MI-based approach to adherence intervention targeting motivation for treatment as well as motivation for change. From ethnographic interviewing (Schensul, Schensul, & LeCompte, 1999), we incorporated an emphasis on the potential for interviewers' culturally specific values, ways of understanding others, and judgments about what constitutes "rational" behavior to interfere with their ability to grasp and support the culturally specific values, understandings, and judgments of the interviewee. From IPT, we incorporated psychoeducation about depression, provided in an MI-consistent style: remaining sensitive to the potential for the discord-triggering "labeling trap" but also recognizing that the diagnostic language of "major depression" can provide the client some relief by conveying that changes in behavior are attributable not to personal weaknesses or moral failings but to an illness for which clients are not to blame and which can be effectively treated.

The "engagement session" we developed is a single-session pretherapy intervention focused on communicating the therapist's understanding of clients' individual and culturally embedded perspectives, helping them see how the potential benefits of treatment align with their own priorities and concerns, facilitating the identification and resolution of ambivalence, and problem-solving barriers to engagement. We named our intervention prior to the development of the "four processes" model of MI (Miller & Rollnick, 2013), which describes "engaging" as one MI process. While the goal of the intervention is to increase engagement of depressed persons into an effective therapy for that condition, the provider of the intervention employs all four MI processes: engaging the client, developing a collaborative focus for the session, evoking talk in favor of participating in treatment for depression, and planning for the initiation of treatment.

Research on the Engagement Session

In an open prospective pilot study (Swartz et al., 2006), a group of depressed, nonsuicidal mothers of adolescents receiving mental health treatment was offered the engagement session and eight sessions of IPT-B. Of 13 mothers who met DSM-IV criteria for major depressive disorder and were not in treatment, 11 received an engagement session. Following the session, all completed the Client Satisfaction Questionnaire (CSQ), an eight-item instrument assessing subjective satisfaction with treatment, with possible scores ranging from 8 to 32 (Attkisson & Greenfield, 2004). The mean CSQ score for the engagement session was 27.2 (±4.0), indicating high levels of satisfaction. All 11 participants subsequently scheduled an initial treatment appointment, and all but 1 completed a full course of therapy. The one noncompleter, who attended seven of the eight sessions, had also clearly "engaged."

In the randomized controlled trial that followed (Swartz et al., 2008), depressed mothers of youth in psychiatric treatment ($n = 47$) attended twice as many sessions at the 3-month treatment endpoint (9.0 vs. 4.5, $p < .05$) when randomly assigned to receive the engagement session and eight sessions of IPT-B ("ES+IPT-MOMS") versus referral to treatment as usual in the community. Clients receiving ES+IPT-MOMS also showed superior depression outcomes at treatment completion and 9-month follow-up.

In a randomized pilot study in the public obstetrics clinic of a large urban women's hospital (Grote, Zuckoff, Swartz, Bledsoe, & Geibel, 2007), 64 depressed socioeconomically disadvantaged pregnant women (63% African American) who were not seeking depression treatment but agreed to accept treatment through the study were offered either the engagement session and eight sessions of IPT-B provided by the same therapist in the prenatal clinic ("Engagement and IPT-B") or a referral for standard depression treatment by a community mental health provider in the prenatal clinic or their neighborhood ("Enhanced Usual Care," EUC). Of 31 women assigned to Engagement and IPT-B, 25 entered the study and received an engagement session; 24 women (96%) attended an initial treatment session, and 17 (68%) completed a full course of IPT-B. Of 33 women assigned to EUC, 28 entered the study, 10 (36%) attended an initial treatment session, and 2 (7%) completed a course of standard depression treatment. Treatment entry and retention were significantly superior in Engagement and IPT-B as compared to EUC ($p < .001$). Clients receiving Engagement and IPT-B also showed superior depression outcomes before childbirth (3 months postbaseline) and at 6 months postpartum (Grote et al., 2009).

In a pilot randomized controlled trial (O'Mahen, Himle, Fedock, Henshaw, & Flynn, 2013), 55 racially diverse and low-income pregnant women with major depressive disorder were offered either 12 sessions of modified cognitive-behavioral therapy that included an engagement session (mCBT) or referral for treatment as usual (TAU) in the community. Of women assigned to mCBT, 83% attended the engagement session, 72% returned for the second session, and 60% attended at least four sessions. Of women assigned to TAU, 17% received some psychotherapy. Women assigned to mCBT showed a greater decrease in depressive symptoms than those assigned to TAU at posttreatment and 3-month follow-up, although there were no differences in reliable and clinically significant change.

Description of the Engagement Session

The engagement session is semistructured, with five phases: Eliciting the Story; Providing Feedback and Psychoeducation; Exploring the History of Distress, Coping, and Treatment, and Hopes for Treatment; Problem-Solving Practical, Psychological, and Cultural Treatment Barriers; and Eliciting Commitment or Leaving the Door Open. We describe each phase and provide an annotated transcript with a prototypical client.

Eliciting the Story

The goals of the initial phase are to ensure that the client feels understood and to elicit talk about the importance of change. The therapist begins by inquiring how the client has been feeling and what things have been like for her lately. If she responds by talking solely about how she feels, the therapist also asks about her situation: "You've been feeling so hopeless lately. . . . What has been going on in your life that might be affecting you?" Similarly, if she responds by talking solely about the circumstances of her life, the therapist also asks about how she has been feeling: "You're stuck with all these bills and busy all the time. . . . Tell me about how you're being affected by the lousy situation you're in." The therapist listens for the client's perspective on how she is suffering, what she believes is contributing to her suffering, and how it interferes with her daily life, attending specifically to the social and interpersonal context.

In almost all cases, the client's "story" can be framed as a *dilemma*, a problem that is unsolvable in principle because each potential solution would exact intolerable costs. This both reflects and is a source of feelings of hopelessness inherent to depression. A successful conclusion to this phase usually results in a summary that both *crystallizes* the client's dilemma and highlights her wishes for help in escaping from it.

THERAPIST: Tell me how things have been going and how you've been feeling lately.

Beginning with an open-ended question to draw out the story.

CLIENT: My son Johnny is a terror. He is getting on my nerves so bad. I feel like I'm really going to hurt him. He's been getting into trouble at school. He won't let me alone at home. I don't know what to do.

The client focuses on how her troubled child is affecting her and conveys her sense of helplessness and distress.

THERAPIST: You're starting to worry about the way you feel around him—you might lash out and do something that you'd regret.

The therapist reflects meanings and feelings.

CLIENT: It's affecting my whole life. I'm irritable at work and snapping at my coworkers.

THERAPIST: It affects you when you're not with him, too. What else have you noticed about how you've been feeling and acting that's different from the way you usually feel or act?

Reflection.
Asking for elaboration to elicit problem recognition, a contributor to increased importance of change.

CLIENT: I'm not enjoying my free time. I'm always angry. I don't want to talk to anyone. I'm never happy.

The client describes symptoms of depression.

THERAPIST: It doesn't matter where you are or who you're with or what you're doing, you feel the same way . . . this angry, unhappy feeling, and it's really hard because you are trying to deal with Johnny, and no matter what you do it doesn't seem to get any better.

Summary of the client's expressions of dissatisfaction with the status quo.

CLIENT: Yeah. Anything I try just doesn't work with him. It's getting worse and worse.

The client confirms that she feels understood.

THERAPIST: It's been incredibly frustrating for you.

Reflection of feeling.

CLIENT: I'm frustrated with everything.

THERAPIST: And this is a big change from the way things were before.

Looking back.

CLIENT: Yeah, it's just over the past year that he's gotten worse. His father left, and now he's living across the street with his girlfriend.

Focusing on the context of her child's problems, she describes sources of current distress.

THERAPIST: That's a difficult situation.

Supportive statement.

CLIENT: And before that things weren't too good between his father and me, and he saw a lot of that, but it's been worse since his father left. It seems like he's escalating. He's on the verge of being expelled. I've had conferences with his teachers and his guidance counselor, and they make it seem like it's all my fault.

Is she afraid she will be blamed by this therapist and/or a future therapist as well?

THERAPIST: You're doing everything you can think of to get Johnny to come around, and not only is it not

Affirmation and complex reflections; highlighting an aspect of her dilemma and

working, which is really hard for you, but you're feeling blamed by other people who you're looking to for help. (*Client nods.*) And you're really angry about this.

identifying a possible barrier to engagement.

CLIENT: I am. Nobody seems to understand what is going on.

She's beginning to feel understood.

THERAPIST: You feel pretty much alone in all of this. (*Client nods.*) No one seems to be able to help, no one seems to really get it.

Reflecting meaning and feelings.

CLIENT: Even my mother blames me for the break-up. She thinks I should've stuck it out.

THERAPIST: How did you make that decision? What happened between you?

Drawing out more about her dilemma . . .

CLIENT: I couldn't take it anymore. He was going to kill me. I felt really bad because Johnny saw all of this. I would try to have him go upstairs, but he'd sneak down and sometimes he'd see his father beating on me.

. . . which she describes in terms of her situation and the reasons for her actions.

THERAPIST: You felt like you had no choice. You *had* to leave. (*Client nods vigorously.*) Let me see if I'm understanding.
You've been dealing with these problems for a while now, but things were getting worse. So, you decided you had to get away before something horrible happened, and you made that decision for yourself but also for Johnny because you were worried about what he was seeing and how that was affecting him. You're trying to do the best

Empathizing with her choice in the face of her dilemma.

Transitional summary, including understanding of her view of how she came to be in her current problematic situation . . .

thing you know how to do, make the best decision you can, and the result has been that things have seemed to get worse.

. . . affirmation of her good intentions and efforts . . .

CLIENT: That's right!

THERAPIST: Instead of feeling or acting better, Johnny seems to be acting worse, and you don't know how to get through to him or how to help him or what to do for him. It's like you took this incredibly difficult step, and things have just gone downhill.

. . . crystallizing her dilemma . . .

CLIENT: No matter what I do, I can't win.

THERAPIST: And now you don't know where to turn, you don't know what to do, and you're worried about what you might be capable of if things don't get better.

. . . and reflecting her fears about what will happen if she doesn't get help.

CLIENT: Yeah, I'm afraid I'm going to lose control or at work I'm going to lose my job.

Implicit recognition of the need for change.

THERAPIST: And that's really scary because the bottom could really drop out.

CLIENT: Yeah. And I don't know how to get out of this by myself.

First approach to talk in favor of treatment (engagement talk).

Providing Feedback and Psychoeducation

The goal of this phase is to offer the client a different perspective on her current difficulties. The therapist reframes the problems as comprising a recognizable medical condition for which effective treatment is available rather than a hopeless situation or a failure of will or ability. This is not intended to minimize the importance of the contextual factors but rather to suggest that alleviating the mood disorder will allow the client to cope with these factors more effectively.

The client is given individualized feedback on her current condition. Examples of assessment tools include standardized self-assessments of depressive symptoms such as the Quick Inventory of Depressive Symptoms (Rush et al., 2003) or the nine-item Patient Health Questionnaire (Kroenke, Spitzer, & Williams, 2001). The therapist then elicits what the client already knows about depression, offers (with permission) psychoeducation tailored to the client's individual concerns and current knowledge, and then elicits her reaction. The elicit–provide–elicit format helps to ensure that the client is open to what the therapist has to say and reduces the likelihood of discord, which often emerges when people are given education they're not interested in. It also communicates respect for her views and acknowledges that it will be her interpretation of this information that will ultimately determine what she does with it.

The psychoeducation offered by the therapist includes the ideas that depression is a "no-fault" illness and thus that the depressed person is not to blame for the troubles she is having; that depression negatively affects people's ability to solve interpersonal problems or manage difficult situations; that depression can be effectively treated; and that when depression is treated successfully, people often begin to see alternative solutions to what had seemed like unsolvable life problems. Should the client object to diagnostic language, express uncertainty as to whether she is really "depressed" (rather than, for example, "stressed out" or "overwhelmed") or feel reluctant to acknowledge that she needs "treatment," the therapist accepts the status quo side of the client's ambivalence and responds nondefensively. Inquiring about the client's perspective and emphasizing its legitimacy, the therapist at the same time looks for opportunities to connect troubles the client describes—painful feelings, problematic thinking patterns, difficulty functioning—to the therapist's ability to help: "As you see it, stress is very different from depression, and you're sure that you're stressed rather than depressed. You've also told me that your new situation has been a big source of stress. Would a therapy that could help you find and use some better ways of managing the situation be something you'd find worthwhile?"

This phase, in which the therapist shifts focus from the client's perspective to a professional one, is one place where racial, cultural, or gender-related barriers may arise. Understanding the client's cultural context and allowing the client to educate the therapist about unique elements of her background and identity are crucial. However, it is often very difficult for individuals of different backgrounds to frankly discuss issues of mistrust and misunderstanding. Therefore, the therapist should invite and even encourage clients to voice concerns related to aspects of the psychiatric view of depression and its treatment that may be considered culturally unacceptable. These concerns may include reluctance to confide in a therapist of a different race or gender or to reveal sensitive information in a professional treatment context.

THERAPIST: I'd like to review the depression questionnaire we gave you to let you know what we make of your responses and see what your thoughts are. Is that OK?

Introduction of feedback.

Asking permission.

CLIENT: Yes, it sounds good.

THERAPIST: Let me know if anything I say doesn't sound right to you—because I really want to know that—as well as anything that does make sense to you. This is the Patient Health Questionnaire. It asks about markers that we use to tell us if somebody is depressed or not, and of the seven markers you agreed with five. For example, you said you had noticed some changes in your sleep. Tell me what you've noticed about how your sleep has changed.

Inviting her to be active in the discussion to promote collaboration.

Characterizing the source of feedback, explaining how the assessment was arrived at, and providing feedback.

Asking for elaboration.

CLIENT: I'm waking up a lot in the middle of the night. I'll have a nightmare about something that I'm worried about, and when it wakes me up, I stay awake.

THERAPIST: So, it's harder to stay asleep, and it's harder to get back to sleep. You also said your appetite is not as good.

Clarifying symptoms.

CLIENT: I've been living on junk food. I eat, but not regular meals like I usually do.

THERAPIST: Changes in sleep and appetite are two physical changes we often see when people are depressed. Depression affects people's bodies as well as their thoughts and feelings. You've also been feeling much less interested in things, you don't have the energy you usually have, and you've had some thoughts of wanting to die. Tell me about that.

Offering information, in terms of the model of depression.

CLIENT: Well, Johnny really acts out, and I don't have anybody to talk to. I feel like the reason I am living now is to take care of him, and then when he acts out it makes me feel like there is nothing really worth living for.

THERAPIST: You're exhausted all the time trying to deal with this, and you can't sleep well or eat right and that's taking a toll also. So, you sometimes reach this point where you want to give up, like there's no point in going on.

Collecting summary.

CLIENT: Yeah, why should I do it for him if he's going to treat me like that?

THERAPIST: So, there is an angry part, too. Like, "The hell with you . . . if you're going to act this way, I don't even want to be here."

Reflection of feeling.

CLIENT: Exactly. Isn't that terrible to feel that way toward your son?

THERAPIST: When people have these kinds of problems with sleeping, appetite, energy, interest, and feeling like giving up, we say they have

With implicit permission to provide information, reframing her mood and behavioral changes, and

depression. So, from our perspective it looks like you are depressed and that's why you're feeling and acting in ways that aren't normal for you. What are your thoughts about that?

her self-blame, in terms of the medical model of depression.

Eliciting her reaction.

CLIENT: I don't think I'd be depressed if it wasn't for everything going on in my life.

A little defensiveness (discord) arises.

THERAPIST: It's having a big impact on how you feel and how you're doing.

Defusing discord via reflection.

CLIENT: Yeah, if Johnny wasn't acting out, if his father wasn't living across the street with his girlfriend, if I wasn't trying to scrape to get by, I don't think I would feel this way.

THERAPIST: That makes sense. People in stressful situations are more vulnerable to becoming depressed and feeling the way you've been feeling. I think that is very consistent with the way we see things. Do you have any o ther thoughts about that? (*Client shakes her head, looking uncertain.*) You're sure?

Reframing in line with the model of depression.

Eliciting her reaction.

Checking for unspoken disagreement.

CLIENT: So, is depression something inside me? Is it like a disease?

THERAPIST: You're wondering what I mean by "depression." When you hear the word "depression," what is your understanding?

Eliciting the client's understanding, and the concern she's hinting at.

CLIENT: Just feeling sad. Like when my friend broke up with her boyfriend, she was down and she said she was feeling depressed.

THERAPIST: People can use the word "depression" to talk about times when they feel kind of down or sad—that will probably pass on their own. It sounds like that's how you're thinking about it. Our understanding is that depression is a medical illness that people can suffer from but, fortunately, also something that's treatable and that we know how to help people with. (*Client looks thoughtful.*) We also think that once someone is depressed, stressful situations are more difficult to deal with. So, each affects the other. The stress and difficulties can trigger a depression. Then, once you're depressed, the difficulties are harder to deal with. You don't have the same energy and focus to handle the stressful situations in your life. Does that sound like what's been happening?

Providing psychoeducation . . .

. . . and offering hope.

Eliciting her reaction to the psychoeducation.

CLIENT: So, what you're saying is that the way I'm feeling is because of everything going on, and once I feel this way it is going to make everything seem like it is worse than it really is?

Is she suspicious that the therapist is implying that her complaints are exaggerated?

THERAPIST: Not that it seems worse than it really is, but probably more *hopeless* than it is. I believe your situation is very difficult and that it feels really bad. We find that when someone is depressed it becomes very hard to see any kind of solution to difficult situations. Everything looks sort of bleak. As people become less depressed,

Being careful not to minimize the difficulty of her situation . . .

. . . and reframing in terms of the model of depression, which offers hope.

it doesn't make the situation get better right away, but they're more able to see ways to improve the situation and to use the things that they know how to do to deal with difficult situations. Does that make sense?

CLIENT: Yes. I could definitely use some help dealing with some of the things that are going on—because I can't fix them myself.

Engagement talk—the discord seems defused.

THERAPIST: The good news is that if we can provide that help for you, you will probably start to feel a little more like you can deal with the situation, and that's actually going to help the depression as well. How does that sound?

Conveying optimism.

CLIENT: Good. That would be good.

Exploring the History of Distress, Coping, and Treatment, and Hopes for Treatment

The therapist's goals in this phase include understanding the client's current difficulties in the context of her relevant history; uncovering potential barriers to engagement related to negative experiences with or beliefs about treatment; understanding her past and present coping efforts and affirming the strengths she has called on in coping; and eliciting talk about the possibility of positive change (i.e., hope).

The therapist begins by asking whether the client has previously felt the way she feels now. Discussion of the client's experience with depression is followed by questions about how she coped with these feelings (if she has been depressed previously) as well as about what she has tried recently to help herself feel better and manage her situation. The therapist looks for opportunities to affirm the client for her efforts and to support self-efficacy as well as to understand the kinds of interventions she is likely to find plausible or desirable.

If the topic has not come up already, the therapist then asks about the client's perceptions of treatment. These may derive from personal or vicarious (e.g., children's or other family members') experience or from media portrayals. It is crucial to elicit discussion of both positives and negatives—the former, because they constitute "engagement talk," and the latter, because they potentially constitute the most potent sources of ambivalence or barriers to engagement. The therapist employs empathic reflection to communicate nonjudgmental understanding of negative feelings and/or beliefs about treatment, strategies such as shifting focus and emphasizing personal choice and control if such negativity generalizes to the current therapist or treatment, and reframing to emphasize the potential for the proposed treatment to be more helpful.

Finally, the therapist asks about the client's hopes and fears for treatment now. Encouraging the client to describe what she does and does not want from the treatment and from the therapist is both an unusual thing to do and, we believe, among the elements of the session that have the most powerful engagement effect. Looking forward—"What would you like to be different at the end of this treatment?" or "If this treatment were to work exactly the way you hope, what would your life be like 2 months from now?"—can further evoke hope that things can be better and that treatment could play an important role in the improvement.

During this discussion, the therapist looks for opportunities to help the client see how the treatment on offer can provide what she is looking for. This typically involves briefly describing the treatment's basic principles and noting consistencies between the treatment approach and the client's wishes. We have found IPT to be a good match for the women with whom we work; the idea that depression is linked to transitions, disputes, or losses in our interpersonal world seems to make intuitive sense to them and almost always fits with the focus of the discussion. Similarly, the stance of the IPT therapist—warm, active, encouraging, moving flexibly between more and less directive interventions—has great appeal. The effectiveness of the engagement session is tied in part to the acceptability of the treatment in which clients are being asked to engage.

THERAPIST: Were there times in the past when you've felt like you're feeling now?	*Asking for history of depression.*
CLIENT: When my dad passed. It only lasted about a month and gradually it got better. This time it seems to be getting worse.	*Recognition that the current problem is different and could require professional help.*

THERAPIST: You expect to have difficult periods in your life and then things get back to normal. But it's not getting back to normal.

Highlighting this recognition through reflection.

CLIENT: Yeah, usually I am able to kind of get myself back up.

THERAPIST: How have you done that?

Asking about past success in coping.

CLIENT: Well, Johnny's father was there for me. Johnny wasn't as bad when he was around. And when my dad was around, if I felt this way I could talk to him. Then after my dad passed, I could talk to my mom. Now it just seems like I'm taking care of Johnny all by myself, and no one really cares or understands. They can't understand what's going on.

Identifying interpersonal contributors to current depressive episode.

THERAPIST: You feel like you don't have anyone to turn to when you're feeling down and when you need someone to understand you or offer a little support. That's the big difference between now and before— you don't have anyone to turn to who could help.

Reflection of meaning . . .

. . . and a subtle reframe.

CLIENT: I hadn't thought about it that way. I don't have anyone now who I can talk to.

THERAPIST: And you miss that, and you're really feeling the need for it now.

OK—but it would be better to elicit this from the client.

CLIENT: I've got to do something. I just can't go on feeling like this any more.

Preparatory engagement talk.

THERAPIST: Have you ever been able to talk to someone outside the family or friends?

Asking about previous treatment experience.

CLIENT: I used to talk to Johnny's pediatrician. She understood the problems he was having. But she seemed to understand me, too. We talked about how hard it was for me to deal with him. I always felt better after that.

Describing what she wants from a "helper" by recalling positive experiences of being helped.

THERAPIST: What was it about her that made you feel understood?

Asking for elaboration.

CLIENT: Even though the focus was on Johnny, she would take time to ask how I was dealing with things and listen to me. I feel like I'm taking care of everyone else all the time, and she was interested in how I was feeling.

Positive talk about help from a professional.

THERAPIST: You didn't have to worry about taking care of her. You could let her take care of you a little bit, be concerned about you.

Reflection of meaning.

CLIENT: Yeah. I mean, she wasn't family, so she never really talked about her problems.

THERAPIST: She listened, she seemed to understand, and she wanted to help. She seemed to care about you and wanted to help you feel better and deal with Johnny better.

Interim (collecting) summary.

CLIENT: She would help me deal with Johnny and tell me what to do with the problems he was having—not like I was a bad mom, but just suggestions.

Key point about what she wants and doesn't want from a helper.

THERAPIST: That was a very positive experience. Were there times when you had less positive experiences with doctors or therapists?

A specific reflection could have highlighted the key point about not feeling blamed.

CLIENT: That's the only time I ever talked to anyone outside of friends or family. I always felt like I could handle it myself. My girlfriend went to see someone, and they put her on this medicine, and then she wasn't herself. I'd rather feel like myself than be on the medication and change like she did. I tried to talk to my doctor once, and he wanted to put me on medicine.

Revealing a barrier: negative treatment expectations.

THERAPIST: And that was not something you felt comfortable with at all.

Reflection of feeling.

CLIENT: Yeah, he gave me a prescription, but I didn't have it filled.

She will not follow a course of treatment just because a professional tells her to.

THERAPIST: It was scary for you to see the change in your friend. (*Client nods.*) There are two kinds of help you've seen people get. One is medication, which you are not comfortable with. It wasn't helpful when your doctor gave you medication, because you didn't feel it was right for you. On the other hand, having somebody to talk to, who understands you and seems to care and want to help—somebody you don't have to worry about taking care of—*that* feels like it could be a helpful thing. At least that was a helpful thing before.

Reflection of feeling.

Linking summary and reframe.

CLIENT: Yes, a very helpful thing.

Preparatory engagement talk.

THERAPIST: What we offer is called "interpersonal therapy." It's a talking therapy that focuses on relationship problems to help relieve

Introducing the treatment.

depression. The therapist will be in
your corner, listening to you and
helping you figure out what you
can do to make things better.

CLIENT: That sounds good. Those are
the kinds of problems I have.

Preparatory engagement talk.

THERAPIST: Looking down the road
months from now, if the therapy
works and is helpful for you, how
will things be different?

Looking forward.

CLIENT: What I would really like to
be different is the situation with
Johnny, but I don't see how that
could change because it takes
everything I have to keep my cool
at work and get through the day
and take care of him.

Expressing her wish but also her pessimism—i.e., her ambivalence.

THERAPIST: A change with Johnny is
one thing that you would really
like, yet you can't quite see how
that would happen.

Double-sided reflection.

CLIENT: Maybe, if I could get a break
or have a little time for myself, I
wouldn't be so short with him. I
spend my whole day working,
and then I have to come home
in the evenings and take care
of everything there and fight
with Johnny, and I never get a
break.

Thinking about possible steps toward change and the barriers to taking them.

THERAPIST: If things could go well
with the therapy, one change
would be that you would somehow
find a way to get some help with
Johnny so that you could have a
break to focus more on yourself
and take care of yourself instead
of just taking care of everyone
else.

Highlighting a source of hope through reflection.

CLIENT: And I would like to have the energy to do that. I can barely drag myself out of bed to go to work and take care of Johnny.

Reason for change.

THERAPIST: The way you're feeling it doesn't seem like there's any way you could do this, but if things went well and you had the energy again, you could figure out how to get some additional help or handle situations with Johnny more con-structively or get a break to take care of yourself. Those would be some really positive changes.

Reframing in terms of the model of depression, from pessimism to hope.

CLIENT: Yeah. It would be really great if therapy could help with that.

Envisioning change through engagement.

Addressing Practical, Psychological, and Cultural Treatment Barriers

As the focus of the session shifts from evoking to planning (building and strengthening commitment to treatment), the therapist's goal moves to drawing out, exploring, and problem-solving remaining barriers to engagement. Practical reasons why it will be hard to come for treatment are usually the first ones offered; they are safe—socially appropriate and not too revealing. The therapist takes these at face value and works to resolve them; if they are the only barriers, that will soon become apparent, and if there are other concerns, these will emerge once the practical barriers are addressed.

Underlying psychological barriers include disagreement with the diagnosis of depression, desire for a different kind of treatment, negative mental health treatment experiences, discomfort with self-disclosure, or generally negative relationship expectations (e.g., anticipation of being controlled, neglected, or exploited). In particular, many mothers express feelings of guilt about taking care of their own needs rather than thinking only of their family members. Culturally-related concerns may include doubts as to whether someone of a different race, gender, ethnicity, religion, age, sexual orientation, or social status can really understand their lives or anticipation of being judged negatively for their differences. Alternatively, some clients from small minority communities may fear recognition and stigmatization by another member of the same community and prefer a therapist from a different ethnic or religious background.

In some cases the client will not spontaneously offer any barriers; she may even initially deny that any exist. This may be true, but to ensure that important barriers are not going unspoken the therapist should suggest some. For example: "Some people have told me that, even though they wanted to come for therapy, it might be hard to find the time or money. Others have worried about what it would be like, or felt guilty about taking time for themselves instead of putting all their effort into taking care of their families, or had other concerns. It wouldn't be unusual if you had some doubts like these . . . " Trying to elicit the direct expression of these potential unspoken barriers, remaining nondefensive and open to client's worries, and placing the client in the role of teacher can often diffuse such concerns.

THERAPIST: What could make it hard for you to come for treatment?	*Open-ended question to elicit barriers.*
CLIENT: I don't have much energy, and that makes it hard to do anything.	*A psychological barrier.*
THERAPIST: No energy to get here.	*Reflection of meaning.*
CLIENT: It takes all the energy I have to take care of Johnny and make it to work. I had trouble coming here today.	
THERAPIST: It takes energy to get help so that you can have more energy.	*Acknowledging the apparent paradox.*
CLIENT: If I could see someone on Monday, I could probably come. That's my afternoon off. The rest of the week I have to be at work and take care of Johnny.	*A potential practical barrier.*
THERAPIST: The last thing we want to do is to put one more thing on you that's going to make your life more difficult. I'm certain we'll be able to work out the schedule so that you can come on your afternoon off. It sounds like that would clear one potential hurdle out of the way.	*Reflection of meaning.* *Problem-solving the practical barrier first . . .*

That doesn't necessarily solve the energy problem, though. When you imagine yourself coming to the next session, what kinds of thoughts go through your mind?

. . . then returning to the psychological barrier, asking for specifics.

CLIENT: I know it will be hard to get here—I'll just want to go home and shut myself in my room. If I come, someone might try to tell me how to feel better, but I don't know if it's going to work. They might try to tell me that I should do this and that to feel better, but it's hard for me to do anything right now.

"Low energy" is revealed to be related to concerns about what the therapist will expect of her and how much control the therapist will seek to exert.

THERAPIST: You are imagining yourself getting ready to come in, and part of you will be wondering "How is this going to go?"

Reflection—a bit general.

CLIENT: I may not be able to do what they're going to tell me to do. If I didn't have the energy to do those things and someone didn't understand that, then it wouldn't help.

Trying again to get the therapist to understand her concerns.

THERAPIST: I'm *sure* it wouldn't help. It would be very important for your therapist to understand how hard it is for you right now to get yourself to do the things you need to do, and not have unrealistic expectations. If you felt the therapist was going to be critical and give you things to do that you couldn't handle, it would be very discouraging for you.

Joining, empathizing, and subtly reframing.

Implying the counterfactual: "If this were to happen, it would feel bad . . . (but it won't happen here)."

CLIENT: Yeah, or things I didn't want to do, like "Take this pill."

An underlying concern.

THERAPIST: You're wondering if the therapist might tell you to do things that didn't feel right to you.

Still too general for the client to feel understood.

CLIENT: I want to make sure that they would understand certain things about my life. I need them to not be telling me things about work or Johnny or his father that I can't do.

She really wants this therapist to understand, concretely.

THERAPIST: What would not be helpful would be for someone to say, "Just tell your boss you need time off, and tell your son's father that he has to help you"—things like that.

The therapist "gets it," concretely.

CLIENT: Because that would just make things worse—create problems at work and more arguments with Johnny and his dad.

THERAPIST: Right. You're in this delicate situation. The therapist needs to understand and respect that. I'm wondering if you have any thoughts about how you could make sure the therapist understands?

Eliciting her ideas for solving the problem.

CLIENT: I guess I need someone who will listen to me—someone who understands my situation. My mom doesn't even understand. She doesn't know what it's like to have no one who is really there just for you, to listen to you.

The client says what she wants from therapy— though not how to get it.

THERAPIST: So, imagine a therapist who is first going to sit down and listen to you and try to understand your situation, not offer advice or suggestions right away, but take the time to understand how difficult things are for you and the delicate situation you're in. If you knew you were coming to see a therapist like that, would that make it easier to make it here?

The therapist implicitly offers her what she is ask-ing for . . .

. . . and then asks if this resolves the barrier.

CLIENT: Yeah, because I don't know how to get the energy to come to see someone if it isn't going to help. My situation is difficult. I'm not just making a big deal out of nothing.

Indirectly expressing recurring concern about being blamed or criticized.

THERAPIST: It's a bad situation and a delicate one. You feel like you're right at the edge and if you're not careful you could fall off.

Validates her perspective . . . but could have spoken to her anxious anticipation of being blamed.

CLIENT: Yeah, and I've got to do something to keep from doing that because I have to take care of Johnny.

Preparatory engagement talk.

THERAPIST: I'm hearing both things: it does feel important to get help with this, to find something that is going to help you feel better; and, if there is something that you really believe is going to help you feel better, you'll probably be able to find the energy you need to get there.

Reframing summary, with the implication that "energy" is a metaphor for willingness or motivation.

CLIENT: I have to, because Johnny is difficult enough to handle when I am feeling good, and I'm afraid of what I might do.

Engagement talk.

THERAPIST: And what would take your energy away would be feeling like you were coming to someone who doesn't get your situation and understand how difficult it is.

Using her language.

CLIENT: Like that doctor who tried to give me pills.

A potent potential barrier to engagement.

THERAPIST: You probably didn't feel like going back to see him at all.

CLIENT: No, I haven't gone back to him.

THERAPIST: What else can you think of that might keep you from coming in?

Asking for more barriers.

CLIENT: Nothing, really.

THERAPIST: Some mothers we've worked with have identified some things that make it difficult for them to come in. Would it be all right if I mention these things just to see if they apply to you? (*Client nods.*)

Asking permission to explore other possible barriers.

One thing that sometimes comes up is concern about whether a therapist *can* understand you because of differences between you and the therapist or between the therapist's life and your life. Has that thought crossed your mind at all?

Probing for cultural barriers (which the client has not raised spontaneously).

CLIENT: No. I just need somebody who will listen. As long as they are willing to listen, I think they could understand.

THERAPIST: It's not so important who the therapist is—their background, if they're a man or woman, white or black, rich or poor. What matters is how interested and willing they are to hear you and understand your situation and not impose their ideas on you.

Reflecting meaning . . .

. . . though also reflecting her wish to be heard without being blamed would have added to the impact.

CLIENT: Yeah, like Johnny's pediatrician. She didn't have a life like mine. We didn't really talk about her life. She would just listen to me.

THERAPIST: It didn't look like you had similar lives. But that didn't matter because she cared and was willing to listen.

CLIENT: Yeah, and I guess I didn't really think about the rest of it.

Eliciting Commitment or Leaving the Door Open

The therapist's final goal is to elicit commitment to treatment. This begins with a recapitulation: the client's perceived dilemma and change talk; the strengths she has shown in coping with challenges; objective evidence of "no-fault" depression and expressed ambivalence about seeing herself as depressed or coming for treatment; what the client most wants from treatment and the therapist and anything she does not want; and identified barriers to treatment participation and potential solutions. After providing information about the next steps in the treatment process, the therapist asks a "key question"—"How does this sound to you? Is this what you want to do?"—and listens for the opportunity to highlight commitment talk.

Whether or not the client expresses commitment to treatment, the therapist seeks to end the session on a positive note: taking a positive and inviting stance regarding the client's ability to participate in and gain benefits from treatment, should she choose to participate; normalizing occasional struggles with treatment attendance; and offering hope by affirming the client's participation, reiterating the view of depression as a treatable condition, and expressing the belief that the client has already taken a first step toward feeling and functioning better.

THERAPIST: [Following the recapitulation] Is that a fair summary?	
CLIENT: Yeah, I think it is. (*Pause*) I would be taking a chance, I guess.	*Not quite a commitment.*
THERAPIST: How are you feeling about taking that chance right now?	*Key question.*
CLIENT: I need to find a way to deal with some of the problems I'm having. If it gets any worse, I might do something I'd regret. It's at least worth trying therapy to see if it will help.	*Preparatory engagement talk.* *Mobilizing (commitment) talk.*
THERAPIST: There's a part of you that feels "I'm taking a chance here," and at the same time it feels like not taking that chance might be even more risky for you.	*Double-sided reflection, ending with a gentle reframe.*

CLIENT: Right. I can't afford not to do something, so it's worth taking a chance.

THERAPIST: Got it. I can schedule you an appointment. Is that what you want to do?

Asking for commitment to treatment . . .

CLIENT: Yeah. I think it would be good.

. . . and getting it.

THERAPIST: I'd like to mention a couple of things before we end. If you can't keep the appointment, we'd like you to call to let us know so that we can reschedule. At the same time, we know that sometimes things come up at the last minute and you might not be able to call. We understand that when people's lives are as stressful as yours, these things can be unavoidable. I don't want you to feel like you can't call later to reschedule.

Recalling the practical barrier and its solution.

Emphasizing the nonpunitive stance.

CLIENT: That's good. I do have a very busy life, and things change at the last minute.

She appreciates this stance.

THERAPIST: I guess this seems especially important because there is every reason to think that we will be able to help you. We have had a lot of success in helping moms like you in the past. And, as you said, our therapy tackles just the kinds of problems you're having. And you're already working hard to make things better. So, we don't want you to miss this chance. (*Client nods, smiles.*) Is there anything else you'd like to ask about before we stop?

Expressing optimism about treatment success.

Affirming her efforts.

Eliciting questions/ reactions.

CLIENT: No. I think I've got it.

THERAPIST: I'm glad you came in today. It's not always easy talking with a stranger about such personal things. I appreciate your trust. I think this went well, and that's a good sign for what's to come.   *Ending with affirmation and optimism.*

Problems and Potential Solutions

Semistructured Intervention

A challenge in conducting semistructured interventions is to find the balance between adhering to the structure too rigidly or too loosely. The outline we provide represents an "ideal" form of the engagement session, and the structure is intended to ensure that the therapist accomplishes a set of tasks designed to enhance commitment to treatment. At the same time, the session should be delivered flexibly to meet the specific needs of each client. If a particular area does not seem relevant to a given client, it should be noted briefly and skipped; if the client seems to be addressing topics in an order that differs from that specified here, therapists should follow the client and not the outline. Being flexible may also mean that, in rare cases, the therapist may determine that the need for a given client to tell her story and be heard is so great that the bulk of the session must be given over to simply listening empathically. Delivering the engagement session in a rigid or "cookbook" fashion is likely to undermine its purpose of meaningfully engaging the client being interviewed.

Intervention Duration

The engagement session takes 45–60 minutes to complete. Factors that drive the duration of the interview include client style (loquacious vs. taciturn), mood disorder symptoms (psychomotor agitation vs. retardation), the number of treatment barriers, and the extent of client ambivalence about treatment. If pressed for time, the therapist should focus primarily on those aspects of the session that seem most relevant for a given client. For example, a client may come for therapy already well educated about the nature of depression, making extended psychoeducation redundant; another may have had positive treatment experiences for another condition, yet may never have been depressed before, requiring more focus on understanding depression than on ambivalence about treatment. It is also important to explain the intervention duration to clients so that they allot enough time in their schedules to complete the interview.

Engagement Session versus Psychotherapy

Although the engagement session may be therapeutic for the client, it is not intended as psychotherapy but as a "pretherapy" intervention. Therapists who are unaccustomed to starting this way may be tempted to revert to a more familiar initial agenda—for example, taking a thorough history, making a final diagnosis, and establishing a treatment plan. The rationale for conducting an engagement session is simple: clients who are ambivalent about treatment may be more likely to drop out; in such cases, history taking, diagnosis, and treatment planning are premature. Investing a session in engaging the client prior to initiating the formal treatment process has the potential to get the treatment started on a more solid footing.

The Suicidal, Psychotic, or Agitated Client

Good clinical judgment supersedes all protocols. If the therapist observes acute suicidal ideation, psychosis, uncontrollable agitation, or another critical condition, the intervention should be abandoned in favor of making arrangements for the client's immediate safety and an appropriate level of care. Zerler (2008) provides guidance on how to engage suicidal individuals using an MI-consistent approach.

When the Engagement Session Therapist Is Not the Psychotherapist

In some settings, the individual conducting the engagement session may not become the client's therapist. Although it is optimal to arrange for continuity of care, it may not always be practical. In these cases, the therapist conducting the interview should align him- or herself with the prospective therapist (e.g., "It will be very important for us both to keep in mind that you felt intimidated by your previous therapist") and emphasize that he or she will communicate the important aspects of the session with the individual's consent. It goes without saying that ensuring such communication is essential.

When the Engagement Session Is Not the First Encounter with the Client

In some settings, the first encounter with the client must follow external guidelines promulgated by the facility or by regulatory agencies. In these cases, therapists who want to enhance engagement have two options.

Therapists may choose to look for moments in the standard interview in which they can insert elements of the engagement session—for example, while inquiring about previous treatment episodes, the therapist could ask what the client did and did not find helpful in each of those experiences. Alternatively, the therapist may conduct the initial visit in the standard way and then initiate an engagement session at the follow-up meeting. In these cases, the client is likely to have already articulated key elements of her story, and the admitting diagnosis may have been discussed. Rather than repeating this material, the therapist can begin by summarizing what has already been discussed and then either ask for elaboration (if this seems likely to deepen the encounter) or move on to the next phase of the session.

Using the Engagement Session Prior to Other Forms of Treatment

Although developed as a prelude to IPT-B, the engagement session seems easily transferable to other contexts. Many of the issues the session is intended to address are found frequently in the treatment of persons with anxiety, substance use, and other disorders. O'Mahen and colleagues (2013) successfully added an engagement session to a CBT intervention for depressed perinatal women, and we think it likely that therapists can adapt the intervention for use prior to other treatment modalities as well. The goal of helping clients to see how the help they want can be provided by a given treatment extends to multiple treatment approaches.

Conclusions

We view the engagement session with promise. At face value, the MI, ethnographic interviewing, and psychoeducational strategies work well together to address common barriers to treatment. Anecdotally, women who have completed the session have consistently expressed the sense that it had helped them to clarify their treatment needs and goals and facilitated their participation in treatment. We have also trained numerous therapists from a variety of disciplines in both research and community settings to conduct the intervention, with good results. The engagement session is worthy of further investigation to determine the extent to which the addition of an MI-based integrative engagement intervention can help to address the pressing problem of limited treatment engagement and participation among depressed individuals.

References

American Psychiatric Association. (1994). *Diagnostic and statistical manual of mental disorders* (4th ed.). Washington, DC: Author.

Attkisson, C. C., & Greenfield, T. K. (2004). The UCSF Client Satisfaction Scales: 1. The Client Satisfaction Questionnaire–8. In M. Maruish (Ed.), *The use of psychological testing for treatment planning and outcome assessment* (3rd ed., pp. 799–812). Hillsdale, NJ: Earlbaum.

Daley, D. C., Salloum, I. M., Zuckoff, A., Kirisci, L., & Thase, M. E. (1998). Increasing treatment compliance among outpatients with comorbid depression and cocaine dependence: Results of a pilot study. *American Journal of Psychiatry, 155,* 1611–1613.

Daley, D. C., & Zuckoff, A. (1998). Improving compliance with the initial outpatient session among discharged inpatient dual diagnosis patients. *Social Work, 43,* 470–473.

Daley, D. C., & Zuckoff, A. (1999). A motivational approach to improving compliance. In D. C. Daley & A. Zuckoff, *Improving treatment compliance: Counseling and systems strategies for substance abuse and dual disorders* (pp. 105–123). Center City, MN: Hazelden.

Flynn, H. A., Blow, F. C., & Marcus, S. M. (2006). Rates and predictors of depression treatment among pregnant women in hospital-affiliated obstetrics practices. *General Hospital Psychiatry, 28,* 289–295.

Garcia, J. A., & Weisz, J. R. (2002). When youth mental health care stops: Therapeutic relationship problems and other reasons for ending youth outpatient treatment. *Journal of Consulting and Clinical Psychology, 70,* 439–443.

Grote, N. K., Bledsoe, S. E., Swartz, H. A., & Frank, E. (2004). Feasibility of providing culturally relevant, brief interpersonal psychotherapy for antenatal depression in an obstetrics clinic: A pilot study. *Research on Social Work Practice, 14,* 397–407.

Grote, N. K., Swartz, H. A., Geibel, S., Zuckoff, A., Houck, P. R., & Frank, E. (2009). A randomized trial of culturally relevant, brief interpersonal psychotherapy for perinatal depression. *Psychiatric Services, 60,* 313–331.

Grote, N. K., Swartz, H. A., & Zuckoff, A. (2008). Enhancing interpersonal psychotherapy for mothers and expectant mothers on low incomes: Additions and adaptations. *Journal of Contemporary Psychotherapy, 38,* 23–33.

Grote, N. K., Zuckoff, A., Swartz, H. A., Bledsoe, S. E., & Geibel, S. L. (2007). Engaging women who are depressed and economically disadvantaged in mental health treatment. *Social Work, 52,* 295–308.

Hettema, J., Steele, J., & Miller, W. R. (2005). Motivational interviewing. *Annual Review of Clinical Psychology, 1,* 91–111.

Kroenke, K., Spitzer, R. L., & Williams, J. B. (2001). The PHQ-9: Validity of a brief depression severity measure. *Journal of General Internal Medicine, 16,* 606–613.

Levy, L. B., & O'Hara, M. W. (2010). Psychotherapeutic interventions for depressed, low-income women: A review of the literature. *Clinical Psychology Review, 30,* 934–950.

Lorant, V., Deliège, D., Eaton, W., Robert, A., Philippot, P., & Ansseau, M. (2003). Socioeconomic inequalities in depression: A meta-analysis. *American Journal of Epidemiology, 157,* 98–112.

Lundahl, B. W., Kunz, C., Brownell, C., Tollefson, D., & Burke, B. L. (2010). A meta-analysis of motivational interviewing: Twenty-five years of empirical studies. *Research on Social Work Practice, 20,* 137–160.

Mackenzie, C. S., Knox, V. J., Gekoski, W. L., & Macaulay, H. L. (2004). An adaptation and extension of the Attitudes Toward Seeking Professional Psychological Help Scale. *Journal of Applied Social Psychology, 34,* 2410–2435.

Marcus, S. M., Flynn, H. A., Blow, F. C., & Barry, K. L. (2003). Depressive symptoms among pregnant women screened in obstetrics settings. *Journal of Womens Health, 12,* 373–380.

McCarthy, K. S., Iacoviello, B., Barrett, M., Rynn, M., Gallop, R., & Barber, J. P. (2005, June). *Treatment preferences impact the development of the therapeutic alliance.* Paper presented at the annual meeting of the Society for Psychotherapy Research, Montreal, Canada.

McKay, M. M., & Bannon, W. M. (2004). Engaging families in child mental health services. *Child and Adolescent Psychiatric Clinics of North America, 13,* 905–921.

Miller, W. R., & Rollnick, S. (2013). *Motivational interviewing: Helping people change* (3rd ed.). New York: Guilford Press.

Miranda, J., Azocar, F., Komaromy, M., & Golding, J. M. (1998). Unmet mental health needs of women in public-sector gynecologic clinics. *American Journal of Obstetrics and Gynecology, 17,* 212–217.

Miranda, J., Azocar, F., Organista, K. C., Dwyer, E., & Areane, P. (2003). Treatment of depression among impoverished primary care patients from ethnic minority groups. *Psychiatric Services, 54,* 219–225.

Miranda, J., Azocar, F., Organista, K. [C.], Muñoz, R., & Lieberman, A. (1996). Recruiting and retaining low-income Latinos in psychotherapy research. *Journal of Consulting and Clinical Psychology, 64,* 868–874.

Mojtabai, R., Olfson, M., Sampson, N. A., Jin, R., Druss, B., Wang, P. S., et al. (2011). Barriers to mental health treatment: Results from the National Comorbidity Survey Replication. *Psychological Medicine, 41,* 1751–1761.

O'Mahen, H., Himle, J. A., Fedock, G., Henshaw, E., & Flynn, H. (2013). A pilot randomized controlled trial of cognitive behavioral therapy for perinatal depression adapted for women with low incomes. *Depression and Anxiety, 30,* 679–687.

Pollard, C. A. (2006). Treatment readiness, ambivalence, and resistance. In M. M. Antony, C. Purdon, & L. J. Summerfeldt (Eds.), *Psychological treatment of obsessive compulsive disorder: Fundamentals and beyond* (pp. 61–78). Washington, DC: APA Books.

Rush, A. J., Trivedi, M. H., Ibrahim, H. M., Carmody, T. J., Arnow, B., Klein, D. N., et al. (2003). The 16–Item Quick Inventory of Depressive Symptomatology (QIDS), clinician rating (QIDS-C), and self-report (QIDS-SR): A psychometric evaluation in patients with chronic major depression. *Biological Psychiatry, 54,* 573–583.

Schensul, S. L., Schensul, J. J., & LeCompte, M. D. (1999). *Essential ethnographic methods: Observations, interviews, and questionnaires.* Walnut Creek, CA: AltaMira Press.

Scholle, S. H., Hasket, R. F., Hanusa, B. H., Pincus, H. A., & Kupfer, D. J. (2003). Addressing depression in obstetrics/gynecology practice. *General Hospital Psychiatry, 25,* 83–90.

Swartz, H. A., Frank, E., Shear, M. K., Thase, M. E., Fleming, M. A. D., & Scott, J. (2004). A pilot study of brief interpersonal psychotherapy for depression in women. *Psychiatric Services, 55,* 448–450.

Swartz, H. A., Frank, E., Zuckoff, A., Cyranowski, J. M., Houck, P. R., Cheng, Y., et al. (2008). Brief interpersonal psychotherapy for depressed mothers whose children are receiving psychiatric treatment. *American Journal of Psychiatry, 165,* 1155–1162.

Swartz, H. A., Grote, N. K., & Graham, P. (2014). Brief interpersonal psychotherapy (IPT-B): Overview and review of the evidence. *American Journal of Psychotherapy, 68,* 443–462.

Swartz, H. A., Shear, M. K., Wren, F. J., Greeno, C., Sales, E., Sullivan, B. K., et al. (2005). Depression and anxiety among mothers who bring their children to a pediatric mental health clinic. *Psychiatric Services, 56,* 1077–1083.

Swartz, H. A., Zuckoff, A., Frank, E., Spielvogle, H. N., Shear, M. K., Fleming, M. A. D., et al. (2006). An open-label trial of enhanced brief interpersonal psychotherapy in depressed mothers whose children are receiving psychiatric treatment. *Depression and Anxiety, 23,* 398–404.

Swartz, H. A., Zuckoff, A., Grote, N. K., Spielvogle, H., Bledsoe, S. E., Shear, M. K., et al. (2007). Engaging depressed patients in psychotherapy: Integrating techniques from motivational interviewing and ethnographic interviewing to improve treatment participation. *Professional Psychology: Research and Practice, 38,* 430–439.

Walitzer, K. S., Derman, K. H., & Connors, G. J. (1999). Strategies for preparing clients for treatment—a review. *Behavior Modification, 23,* 129–151.

Zerler, H. Motivational interviewing and suicidality. In H. Arkowitz, H. A. Westra, W. R. Miller, & S. Rollnick (Eds.), *Motivational interviewing in the treatment of psychological problems* (pp. 173–193). New York: Guilford Press.

Zuckoff, A., & Daley, D. C. (2001). Engagement and adherence issues in treating persons with non-psychosis dual disorders. *Psychiatric Rehabilitation Skills, 5,* 131–162.

Zuckoff, A., & Hettema, J. E. (2007, November). Motivational interviewing to enhance engagement and adherence to treatment: A conceptual and empirical review. In H. B. Simpson (chair), *Using motivational interviewing to enhance CBT adherence.* Paper presented at the 41st annual convention of the Association for Behavioral and Cognitive Therapies, Philadelphia, PA.

Zweben, A., & Zuckoff, A. (2002). Motivational interviewing and treatment adherence. In W. R. Miller & S. Rollnick, *Motivational interviewing: Preparing people for change* (2nd ed., pp. 299–319). New York: Guilford Press.

CHAPTER 7

• • • • • •

Motivational Interviewing and the Treatment of Depression

Sylvie Naar
Heather Flynn

Advances in the understanding of depression drive the need for innovations in intervention delivery. Major depressive disorder (MDD), for example, is still poorly detected and treated in the United States, and randomized controlled trials of treatment effectiveness show that many persons do not adhere to treatment or recover from their disorder (Santaguida et al., 2012). This chapter begins with a rationale for the use of motivational interviewing (MI) in the treatment of depression. We review MI as a brief stand-alone intervention for depression as well as MI integrated with other treatments such as cognitive-behavioral therapy (CBT) with behavioral activation (BA) and interpersonal psychotherapy (IPT). Whereas Chapter 6 (by Zuckoff, Swartz, & Grote) focused on MI as a *pretreatment* to engage individuals in treatment for their depression, this chapter shifts the focus to MI during the course of the depression treatment. We begin where the empirical evidence is strongest: MI for the treatment of depressive symptoms in the context of other medical conditions and medical settings, such as primary and chronic care. We also include coverage of MI for perinatal depression in light of preliminary evidence for the value of MI in this area. We then describe clinical issues related to the integration of MI with prominent psychotherapies for depression and conclude with recommendations for future treatment research.

Clinical Problems and Usual Treatment

There is an urgent need to explore novel treatments and adaptations, given that depression continues to be among the leading causes of disability in the United States and worldwide (Ferrari et al., 2013). Despite the availability of treatments such as antidepressant medications and psychotherapy, and costly investments in clinical research, the prevalence and burdens of depression have not improved in the United States. The majority of adults in the United States with depression do not receive evidence-based depression care (Rost, Smith, & Dickson, 2004; Shim, Baltrus, Ye, & Rust, 2011; Young, Klap, Sherbourne, & Well, 2001). Women in the postpartum period are particularly at risk, with a prevalence of 22% the year after birth and treatment rates of only 14% as compared to 26% in the general population (Wisner et al., 2013).

According to DSM-5, depressive disorders is a category that includes a number of diagnoses in addition to major depressive disorder: premenstrual dysphoric disorder, persistent depressive disorder, substance/medication-induced depressive disorder, and unspecified depressive disorders. All share the common feature of sad, empty, or irritable mood along with behavioral, somatic, and cognitive changes that significantly affect the ability to function. This chapter focuses on the critical need for innovation in the treatment of MDD and depression in other contexts.

Rationale for Using MI in the Treatment of Depression

Arkowitz and Burke (2008) suggested that MI "fits the symptoms" of depression. Symptoms and features of depression such as motivational deficits, ambivalence about change, and problematic decision making are specific MI foci. Watkins et al. (2011) note that, in addition to addressing ambivalence, MI focuses on supporting self-efficacy and reinforcing optimism, which may be key to reducing symptoms of depression. As elaborated upon below, there are myriad behaviors that worsen mood, exacerbate depression severity, or prolong course (such as interpersonal stress) that may be targets of MI, which is aimed at positive behavior change. In this way, MI may be used as a stand-alone treatment to address the symptoms of depression, particularly in populations and settings where depression is less severe, less chronic, or secondary to another physical condition.

MI may also be combined or integrated with existing evidence-based psychotherapies. For example, although it is clear that CBT has been shown to be largely effective for depression, aggregated response and remission rates can be improved upon (Cuijpers et al., 2013; Hollon, Thase, & Markowitz, 2002). Remission and response rates for IPT are comparable to those of CBT (Hollon et al., 2002). MI can be conceptually and practically integrated throughout CBT and IPT whenever motivational issues arise, thereby perhaps enhancing CBT outcomes. Adherence to psychotherapy is vital to treatment response, and MI directly addresses ambivalence about change and treatment. CBT and IPT do not formally address ambivalence; rather, the primary focus is on assisting clients with specific changes and skills. In that sense, MI can add a specific and strategic focus for building treatment motivation and adherence and for specific behavioral changes or decisions. MI also has an explicit focus on client–clinician relationship factors that may directly affect therapy outcome. For example, expressing empathy, a core MI skill, has been linked to CBT outcome in treatment studies (Burns & Nolen-Hoeksema, 1991, 1992; Miller, Taylor, & West, 1980). Therefore, MI has the potential to increase the efficacy of existing therapies.

Clinical Applications and Relevant Research

Brief MI to Address Depressive Symptoms

MI delivered in four sessions or less is considered a brief treatment for depression as an alternative to a low-intensity CBT approach (Hides, Carroll, Lubman, & Baker, 2010), or as part of a stepped-care approach in primary care (Robinson, Triana, & Olson, 2013). Much of the research to date has focused on depressive symptoms in individuals with physical health concerns. Naar-King and colleagues (Naar-King et al., 2009; Naar-King, Parsons, Murphy, Kolmodin, & Harris, 2010) adapted motivational enhancement therapy (MET) for young adults living with HIV. MET is a manualized four-session MI-based intervention originally developed to target alcohol use (Project MATCH Research Group, 1997). It differs from MI in that it includes a feedback component informing the client about where the severity of his or her problem falls as compared to others with the same problem. The Healthy Choices Intervention targeted general health behaviors, medication adherence, substance use, and sexual risk. It consisted of four 60-minute sessions, focusing on the two most problematic behaviors from the baseline assessment. Session 1 began with an overview of the approach, emphasizing how the intervention focuses on the client's readiness to change rather than pressuring an individual to change. The practitioner elicited the client's view of his or her choice of the first of the two behaviors and utilized OARS (Open Questions, Affirmations, Reflections, Summaries) to increase treatment engagement and elicit and reinforce change talk. Then the practitioner reviewed the structured personalized feedback from the baseline assessment and initiated a discussion of the consequences of these behaviors. The remainder of the session focused on increasing the client's commitment to change and completing a written plan for change including goals and potential barriers. For clients who were not ready to change behaviors, goals included preliminary steps such as thinking about change, talking to someone about change, or simply attending the next session.

The second session occurred the following week and followed a similar format focusing on the second behavior. In the third session (during Week 6), the practitioner and the client reviewed progress, renewed motivation, and affirmed commitment. The practitioner and the client examined the client's current importance of and confidence to change as well as a decisional balance activity for both behaviors (eliciting pros and cons). The session ended with a review and revision of the client's goal statement and change plan, integrating both behaviors into a single change plan. It is important to note that in more recent updates of MI, the use of a decisional balance activity is no longer recommended as a routine strategy for all clients but rather as a possible strategy for individuals less motivated to change who are exhibiting high levels of sustain talk (Naar-King & Suarez, 2011). The fourth session focused on termination and included a final review and revision of the client's goals and change plan. Particular emphasis was placed on assessing the client's self-efficacy for maintaining his or her goals for the two behaviors. In addition to improvements in health outcomes (Naar-King et al., 2009) and risk behaviors (Chen, Murphy, Naar-King, & Parsons, 2011; Murphy, Chen, Naar-King, Parsons, & for the Adolescent Trials Network, 2012), youth receiving Healthy Choices reported significantly greater improvements in self-report of self-efficacy and depressed mood as compared to youth receiving standard care alone in a randomized clinical trial (Naar-King et al., 2010).

Two additional randomized clinical trials support the use of MI to improve depressed mood in patients with physical health conditions. In a randomized controlled trial, Bombardier et al. (2009) found that MI delivered by phone focusing on improving functional recovery after traumatic brain injury (TBI) significantly improved multiple measures of self-report of depressive symptoms as compared to usual care. The intervention did not focus directly on depression but rather on increasing adherence to TBI treatment. However, the sessions incorporated several components of depression treatment such as exploration of client concerns, increasing engagement with rewarding activities, problem-solving skills, and goal setting. In a randomized controlled trial with patients following acute stroke, Watkins et al. (2011) reported that an MI intervention not only improved depressed mood but also improved mortality rates. Patients in the intervention group received up to four sessions of MI using agenda setting to focus on the patient's goals for recovery, compared to a usual care control group.

Collaborative care models, often referred to as depression care management, involve the incorporation of several intervention components into primary care practices and are aimed at improving the detection and treatment of depression. Such components typically include screening for depression in primary care, supports for the physician to treat depression such as interface and/or consultation with a care manager (such as social worker) or psychiatrist, as well as systematic monitoring of depression treatment adherence and response. Depression care management interventions that integrate MI have been shown to enhance the efficacy of depression treatment care management outcomes in adult primary care settings. In a large-scale randomized controlled trial, Rost and colleagues (Rost, Nutting, Smith, Werner, & Duan, 2001) trained nurses in a low-cost and exportable MI-based protocol for the treatment of depression. The intervention significantly increased the odds of engaging in and adhering to evidence-based treatment for depression including pharmacotherapy or psychotherapy over a 6-month period as compared to standard primary care (Rost et al., 2001). Improvements in clinical and cost outcomes were observed after 2 years (Dickinson et al., 2005). Therefore, MI may be integrated with depression intervention programs in primary care in order to directly affect motivational factors that impact treatment engagement and outcomes.

Integration of MI with depression interventions for women around the time of childbearing (perinatal depression) may be particularly effective in addressing the critical problem of undertreatment (i.e., no treatment or inadequate treatment) in this population. The problem of undertreated depression during pregnancy (especially among low-income and underserved women) is a critical public health issue because it constitutes a costly and burdensome risk to obstetrical and birth outcomes, such as premature labor and delivery, problematic birth weight, increased fetal activity, and infant neurobehavioral problems (Dieter et al., 2001; Field, Diego, & Hernandez-Reif, 2006; Hoffman & Hatch, 2000). Infants of mothers with prenatal depression may also manifest sleep, feeding, and temperament problems, all of which have been linked to later developmental, behavioral, and psychiatric risk (Armitage et al., 2009; Righetti-Veltema, Conne-Perréard, Bousquet, & Manzano, 2002) Moreover, the strongest risk for postpartum depression exists when prenatal depression is not adequately treated (Beck, Gable, Sakala, & Declercq, 2011).

A few recent studies illustrate the need for treatment engagement, highlighting the importance of addressing motivational factors by using client-centered counseling approaches (Flynn, Henshaw, O'Mahen, & Forman, 2010; Henshaw et al., 2011; O'Mahen & Flynn, 2008). A recent qualitative study showed that eliciting women's preferences and values along with providing a menu of options for treatment were paramount in increasing the likelihood of treatment follow-through (Henshaw et al., 2011). In a pilot study aimed at improving perinatal treatment engagement and outcomes, O'Mahen and colleagues (O'Mahen, Himle, Fedock, Henshaw, & Flynn, 2013) found that a CBT intervention modified to include MI components was feasible and effective for low-income women with MDD.

Integrating MI with Psychotherapy for Depression

In addition to the direct targeting of symptoms, several existing evidence-based depression treatments are ideally suited to integration with MI with the goal of improving overall treatment response rates. Antidepressant medications are the most commonly used treatment for MDD worldwide; however, initiation and adherence are known to be suboptimal, limiting their impact on the overall illness burden (American Psychiatric Association, 2010). The use of MI for medication adherence is covered by Balán, Moyers, and Lewis-Fernández (Chapter 9, this volume). The two most commonly studied psychotherapeutic treatments for depression are cognitive-behavioral therapy (CBT) and interpersonal psychotherapy (IPT). Both CBT and IPT are usually time-limited (e.g., up to 20 sessions) and aimed at remission of target symptoms.

There are now multiple studies suggesting that MI in combination with more intensive treatments like CBT is effective and perhaps more effective than a single treatment alone (see Burke, 2011, and Moyers & Houck, 2011, for reviews), though most studies targeted substance abuse and not depression. To our knowledge, there have been no studies combining MI and IPT. Burke (2011) notes that MI may work best to build motivation for change, whereas treatments like CBT provide the skills to take action for change.

MI and CBT

Westra and Arkowitz (2011) discuss several ways that MI can be combined with CBT. MI may be a delivered as a prelude to CBT (see Zuckoff, Swartz, & Grote, Chapter 6, this volume) or as an adjunct when ambivalence arises during CBT. Alternatively, MI can serve as an integrative framework in which other interventions such as CBT can be delivered. Specific MI skills that may be used include reflecting, asking open-ended questions, affirming, summarizing, and informing/advising (see Miller & Arkowitz, Chapter 1, this volume). The basic CBT model emphasizes the interplay among events, thoughts, behavior, and mood. Key elements of CBT include a problem-oriented focus, individualized case formulations, cognitive restructuring, skills training, and behavioral activation (Wright, Basco, & Thase, 2006). Next we will discuss the main elements of CBT and how each can be done in MI-style while using the MI-3 framework (Miller & Rollnick, 2013).

PROBLEM-ORIENTED FOCUS

Both MI and CBT share a problem-oriented focus in which a specific goal or target behavior is the focus of the therapeutic interaction. However, to promote the engaging process when integrating MI with CBT, the target behavior is not identified as a "problem" per se, as that is counter to a client-centered perspective. Rather, depression is seen as resulting in behaviors that the client perceives as interfering with functioning. In this way, the practitioner avoids words like "problem" or "disorder" and instead reflects the client's language regarding the target behaviors, emotions, or goals.

CASE FORMULATION AND TREATMENT PLANNING

In CBT, the case formulation addresses the connections between thoughts, emotions/moods, and behaviors. Case formulation guides the course of treatment by prioritizing goals and planning the choice and timing of interventions as well as predicting possible problems. This process often begins with an assessment, or functional analysis. During the functional analysis, the practitioner assesses thought and behavior patterns by helping the client identify antecedents or triggers for depression and the positive and negative consequences of depressive symptoms. In CBT, this typically proceeds in a question-and-answer format. As is consistent with the engaging and focusing processes of MI (Miller & Rollnick, 2013), integrated CBT-MI would involve use of MI skills (open-ended questions, reflections, summaries) throughout the case formulation. The assessment might begin with permission to ask more open-ended questions: "If it's OK with you, I want to find out more about your mood patterns. Some things that get in the way of reducing depression might be certain people, certain places, the time of day— things like that. What types of things get in the way for you?" In this example, aspects of the CBT case formulation, such as hypothesis testing, can be done in an MI style.

Following the assessment and case formulation, the client and practitioner collaboratively set goals and plan for treatment, consistent with the focusing and planning processes of MI. Agenda setting can be as simple as offering the choice of what to discuss first: "Would you prefer to talk first about mood, activity level, or what's going on with your family?" A more comprehensive approach involves eliciting the client's view of his or her situation and then placing these ideas in the context of collaborative goals for treatment: "So, we have talked about several things that make you feel like you are not reaching your full potential. Now let's talk about which of these targets will give you the biggest bang for your buck." If the client is not able to set an agenda or develop treatment goals independently, presenting a menu of options provides direction while simultaneously supporting autonomy consistent with the spirit of MI.

SKILLS TRAINING AND COGNITIVE RESTRUCTURING

The skills training and cognitive restructuring components of CBT involve identifying and modifying automatic thoughts and schemas and then learning and practicing skills to change these thoughts and develop new coping patterns. Ensuring the engaging process is critical during this process, for when the practitioner must take an expert role during this teaching phase, the therapeutic alliance may suffer. Without ensuring collaboration and evoking motivation, clients may passively accept the practitioner's suggestions and yet not fully commit to learning the skill. Several communication strategies can ensure that the MI processes are maintained throughout the restructuring and skills training components of treatment. A primary strategy for maintaining engagement is to ask for permission before engaging in any therapeutic task.

As the therapist begins to undertake the more expert-driven teaching elements of CBT, the elicit–provide–elicit strategy (E–P–E strategy) can serve to maintain an MI style when providing information or feedback (Rollnick & Prout, 2008). First, the practitioner elicits what the client is thinking about the information or skill. Then the practitioner reflects back the client's statements while adding additional information (again, emphasizing respect and choice), "So, you can see how managing your thoughts might help you be less depressed, and if you are ready we can consider some intervention strategies to address these thoughts—starting with recording when they happen and what they feel like." Finally, the practitioner elicits the client's view of the information, advice, or new skill. In this way, the practitioner avoids the "expert trap" and maintains relational components of MI even in the context of offering new information or advice.

The E–P–E strategy is particularly powerful when discussing the rationale for such treatment components as skills training. Often in CBT, the practitioner provides the rationale. Consistent with the evoking process of MI, the client rather than the therapist expresses the reasons to engage in session activities. In this example, the practitioner also uses E–P–E to evoke and reinforce change talk about engaging in treatment tasks. Here's an example of this process:

PRACTITIONER: I am wondering what you think it means to do a careful assessment and record your triggers for feeling sad. [Elicit]

CLIENT: Well, I guess it's like when am I most likely to feel sad.

PRACTITIONER: Right, we want to know when as in the timing [Reflect] but also what situations and maybe what thoughts and feelings you have when you miss [Provide]. So, why do you think it would be important to carefully look at how all that fits together? [Elicit]

CLIENT: I guess because then you can help me figure out what to do.

PRACTITIONER: You are hoping we can figure out how to manage these triggers [Reflect]. When we know the different things that trigger feeling depressed, we can come up with specific plans for situations—like when you're fighting with your husband, or thoughts and feelings, like when you feel like you are no good. If you record what situations or activities make you feel good, this can also help us to schedule more pleasurable activities down the road. [Provide] What do you think about these reasons for recording situations, thoughts, and feelings in the next week? [Elicit]

CLIENT: Makes sense.

Cognitive restructuring and skills training typically involve homework assignments such as tracking thoughts or practicing coping skills. Homework assignments are a recommended component of virtually all CBT manuals, and homework completion has been associated with improved outcomes (Carroll, Nich, & Ball, 2005). The E–P–E approach builds motivation for homework completion by ensuring that the client agrees with the purpose of the assignments and how they are related to his or her goals. When homework is missed, a pros and cons activity may help address sustain talk. Here, the practitioner first elicits the client's reasons for avoiding homework in an attempt to understand the barriers and reduce discord between the client and practitioner. Next, the practitioner elicits the "pros" of completing the assignment. If sustain talk around homework continues to emerge, an MI approach suggests "rolling" with it by allowing the client to consider alternatives and to reconsider whether the skill is important to his or her personal plan for change. Rulers may be tailored to evoke motivation for the specific skill or homework assignment. For example, "On a scale from 1 to 10, how would you rate the importance of keeping a thought record at home this week?" Following this question with "Why did you say a 5 and not a lower number?" may help to build motivation for homework.

BEHAVIORAL ACTIVATION

The behavioral component of CBT is commonly referred to as behavioral activation (BA), which has emerged as a "stand-alone" treatment for depression as well (Coffman, Martell, Dimidjian, Gallop, & Hollon, 2007; Dimidjian et al., 2006). BA includes functional analyses of triggers for mood and symptom followed by interventions aimed at gradually increasing the patient's engagement in experiences, behaviors, and activities that boost positive mood and improve symptoms. A major clinical challenge to the effective use of BA is patient ambivalence. MI can be helpful in this respect.

MI was developed specifically for targeting behavior change. There are a number of specific behaviors that are commonly targeted in BA, such as increasing engagement in pleasant events, exercising, changing negative interpersonal behaviors, and reducing avoidance behaviors (i.e., avoidance of behaviors that would improve mood) and rumination. Each of these behavior change goals may be met with client ambivalence and resistance. It is here that MI may be most useful in potentially decreasing ambivalence and increasing engagement in treatment.

CLIENT: I had a really bad day yesterday again. I woke up in a bad mood, and it got worse throughout the day.

PRACTITIONER: You've learned a lot about things that worsen your mood and make it better from your mood tracking work. What would have made it better?

CLIENT: Well, definitely if I had gone for a walk and listened to music—but I was just not feeling like it.

PRACTITIONER: You know it would have helped, but it's getting over that hump that you'd like to work on?

CLIENT: Yes, that's really the problem. It's not that I don't know what to do, it's making myself do it.

PRACTITIONER: We can focus on that aspect of it now—would that be helpful?

CLIENT: Yes, I think it would.

MI and IPT

IPT emphasizes the link between depression and interpersonal relationships and functioning. Within the IPT framework, depressed patients are often lacking varied aspects of social support, owing either to interpersonal conflict, losses, or other life changes. Integration of MI, therefore, has the potential to enhance the effectiveness of IPT by improving adherence to specific IPT behavior change targets as well as by facilitating explicit exploration of relationship problems. No published studies have specifically evaluated the efficacy of MI–IPT integration throughout the course of IPT treatment. However, MI has been used successfully as an IPT treatment engagement strategy for low-income women (see Zuckoff, Swartz, & Grote, Chapter 6, this volume).

Components of MI spirit such as expression of empathy and collaboration have been shown to enhance client–practitioner engagement in psychotherapy (Burns & Nolen-Hoeksema, 1992; Castonguay, Goldfried, Wiser, Gaue, & Hayes, 1996). Given that a key focus of IPT is on improving interpersonal connection, functioning, and support, the practitioner's use of skills to promote MI spirit serve as a therapeutic model for the IPT client. In fact, it may be useful for therapists specifically to teach clients some of the basic skills of MI as a way of relating to others. The example below illustrates one way in which integration of MI spirit may be explicitly used to help the client understand, articulate, and then communicate with significant others:

CLIENT: The problem is that I have no one else like you I can talk to about this stuff.

PRACTITIONER: You have plenty of people in your life, but there is a certain need for support you get here and nowhere else.

CLIENT: Yes, I don't know if it's possible, they don't listen the way you do.

PRACTITIONER: What is it exactly about the way you feel interacting with me that you don't feel with others?

CLIENT: Well, I don't feel like you are trying to push me in any one direction, but you listen and then ask me what I want to do. So, I don't feel defensive.

PRACTITIONER: That's something you need, is for someone to listen and then help you figure out what to do rather than tell you or dictate to you?

CLIENT: Exactly.

PRACTITIONER: Yes, it's not something people do naturally, especially when they care about you and get into "fix it" mode—so, we have to actually clearly ask for that sometimes. How would you feel about asking specifically for that from someone?

CLIENT: I feel like my mom is probably the best person to try with.

As with CBT, ambivalence is commonly encountered in IPT. Here, again, MI can be useful to resolve ambivalence about specific behaviors and decisions. For example, in IPT, depressed mood and other symptoms may be linked to deficient or unsatisfactory social support. One target of treatment, therefore, is changing the ways in which patients communicate their needs for support to others.

PRACTITIONER: In the last session you mentioned that you planned to talk to your husband about helping watch the kids for an hour at night while you take some time for yourself. How did that go?

CLIENT: Well, I never actually got around to talking to him about that.

PRACTITIONER: You had some mixed feelings about whether or not this was the right time.

CLIENT: Yes, every time we had a few minutes I chickened out.

PRACTITIONER: You're not sure exactly what to say?

CLIENT: Yes, and I am sort of afraid of his reaction—like what if he gets angry or says "no"?

PRACTITIONER: It seems that you know that it's critical to your mental health to have that downtime for yourself, and you'd like to get more comfortable and confident with asking. How confident are you on a scale of 1–10, with 10 being very confident in your ability to ask him for this?

CLIENT: I'd say about a 6.

PRACTITIONER: Why a 6 and not a 0?

CLIENT: Well, I'm pretty good at being assertive in a friendly way at work, and I have been able to ask him some things before that actually went well.

PRACTITIONER: You definitely have the skills to do this.

CLIENT: Yes, I guess so; I think I just need to be ready for any reaction and figure out how I will handle that.

PRACTITIONER: That makes sense—would it be OK if we practiced some scenarios here to help you prepare?

CLIENT: Yes, I think that would take away some of the anxiety.

MI and Relapse Prevention

As noted above, relapse rates for depression are high. The primary model of relapse prevention comes from the addictions literature (Marlatt & George, 1984), with a focus on changing cognitions around how the client views lapses and helping the client to understand the difference between lapses and relapse (Curry, Marlatt, & Gordon, 1987). If setbacks or lapses are viewed as irreparable failures by the client, relapse is more likely to occur. However, if lapses are viewed more as learning experiences, it is more likely that relapses will be reduced and perhaps even eliminated. Furthermore, the engaging process of MI suggests avoiding the terms "lapse" and "relapse" and instead expressing empathy about the difficulties of maintaining changes, as well as supporting autonomy and choice with regard to maintaining behavior change (Miller, Forcehimes, & Zweben, 2011). In the following sections, we prefer to use terms like "slips" and "maintenance" instead of "lapse" and "relapse prevention."

Increasing the Importance of Behavior Change

One way to evoke motivation and address a slip (formerly lapse) is to revisit the importance of maintaining the behavior changes. This can be done using an *importance ruler*. The practitioner asks the person to rate the level of commitment to the specified goal on a 10-point scale. After reflecting on the response, the practitioner asks why the person picked that number and not a lower number to elicit the person's own reasons for the importance of maintenance. The specificity of the language is important here. Whereas change talk earlier in treatment may address desire, ability, reasons, need, and commitment to making initial changes, change talk about maintenance could emphasize arguments in favor of maintaining changes (e.g., "It is important for me to *stay* active because I don't want to go back to spending so much time in bed; I like the way I am feeling since I started treatment, and I want it to stay that way"). Change talk about maintenance may also include desire, ability, reasons, needs, and commitment to the maintenance phase of treatment (e.g., "I know I need to keep coming to sessions even though I am feeling better, because I don't want to start all over again").

Increasing Confidence

Self-efficacy is considered a key predictor of maintenance success. However, few maintenance interventions specify exactly how a practitioner might support self-efficacy (Beshai, Dobson, Bockting, & Quigley, 2011; Herz et al., 2000; Lam & Wong, 2005; Marlatt & Donovan, 2005; Minami et al., 2008; Nigg, Borrelli, Maddock, & Dishman, 2008).

MI has specific strategies for supporting self-efficacy. One is the use of affirmations ("You are very persistent in your goals") as opposed to praise ("I think it's great that you are so persistent"). There are several types of questions a practitioner may ask to support self-efficacy, including asking about past change successes or asking about successfully accomplished goals from earlier treatment sessions and discussing how to use these to maintain change. Indeed, open-ended questions can be useful in eliciting self-affirmations. For example: "How have you achieved these changes in the past" or "How does it feel having committed energy and effort to this behavior and achieved change?"

When a client does not easily identify personal strengths, particularly in relation to maintenance, an exploration of what others (friends, family) say about strengths may be fruitful. An affirmation card sort activity may also help to identify these strengths. The client can endorse qualities he or she possesses from a list of strengths and then answer questions about how these qualities are currently evident in his or her life, both in relation to past successes and the maintenance of behavior change. For example: "You mentioned you've always been a strong person. How might being a strong person help you maintain the changes you have made in overcoming depression?" It is also critical for the practitioner to directly convey hope and optimism regarding the client's ability to maintain changes. This does not have to be a blanket belief in change but rather can be linked to certain constraints. For example, "I believe you can get back on track (after a slip-up) when you get the help from your family." Research suggests that practitioner optimism is a common factor evident in positive therapeutic outcomes (Lambert & Barley, 2001).

Another way to increase self-efficacy is to use a confidence ruler—similar to the rulers described earlier but instead asking about confidence in maintaining a specific behavior or using a particular skill. An important point about self-efficacy has been emphasized by Polivy and Herman (2002), who define the "false hope syndrome" as "unrealistic expectations about the likely speed, amount, ease, and consequences of self-change attempts" (p. 677). Overconfidence and setting unrealistic goals often undermine successful change. In fact, the Polivy and Herman review suggests that self-efficacy at the end of treatment is more predictive of success than that at the onset of treatment. They note that confidence that is earned is more likely to be associated with future success than is confidence that has not been earned. Furthermore, realistic and flexible goal setting will also help avoid the false hope syndrome. These strategies demonstrate how MI can increase the importance accorded, and confidence in maintaining changes, and decrease the high rates of relapse in depression treatment.

Conclusions and Future Directions

MI has clear potential for enhancing depression treatment outcomes, both in terms of addressing depressive symptoms directly in brief MI and integrating MI with other psychotherapies. While several studies support the use of brief MI to reduce depressed mood in populations with physical health conditions, studies targeting depressed mood in other populations within primary care (e.g., subclinical depression in the context of nonchronically ill persons and adolescent populations) are lacking. Also lacking are studies of the efficacy of MI with people with primary depression who do not necessarily have any significant health problems.

There are a few studies addressing the integration of MI and CBT for depressed people with health-related concerns. Results of these studies have demonstrated the potential of this approach, but additional research is needed specifically to test whether integrating MI with depression-specific psychotherapies as compared to depression treatment alone significantly improves depression and quality of life outcomes. Such studies should be done with samples large and diverse enough to understand whether particular characteristics of patients (such as demographic or illness characteristics) influence (moderate) the effects of the treatment on outcomes.

There is little literature available on how to successfully implement integration of MI and other psychotherapies into "real-world" settings.

For example, little is known about the training length and format needed for community clinicians in order to produce effective results. Also, little is known about the sustainability of MI in the context of routine clinical services in community settings. Moyers and Houck (2011) contend that combining MI with other psychotherapies often requires the practitioner to make decisions when the two treatments have competing goals or priorities. Studies of decision rules are necessary to provide guidance on how practitioners should proceed at different choice points.

We know little about the use of traditional MI fidelity measures to code interactions when MI is integrated with other treatments, and further research is necessary on fidelity measures for combined treatments. We have some preliminary data on a supervisor rating scale for MI fidelity within sessions where practitioners are expected to integrate MI and CBT for a family-based treatment. In a small pilot study, supervisors rated counselors on MI components by using a four-point rating scale. The preliminary results from Rasch measurement models (Chapman, Sheidow, Henggeler, Halliday-Boykins, & Cunningham, 2008) are promising: the components formed a single dimension, the four-point rating scale performed as intended, the components assessed the full range of counselors and families, and the components could differentiate about five levels of MI fidelity in the sample. The final measure is presented in Table 7.1.

Finally, an innovative approach to depression treatment emerging in recent years is physical activity. Both cross-sectional and longitudinal studies in several countries over the past 20 years consistently show a link between exercise and improved mood (Otto & Smits, 2011), and a meta-analysis of 70 intervention studies showed that exercise resulted in improvements in depressed mood in nonpsychiatric populations (Conn, 2010). Several studies have shown that physical activity interventions are at least as effective in improving depressed mood in both clinical and nonclinical samples as is treatment through antidepressants or psychotherapy (Blumenthal et al., 2007; Stathopoulou, Powers, Berry, Smits, & Otto, 2006). Despite its multiple benefits, the majority of adults in the United States and other developed countries do not engage in sufficient physical activity to substantially improve their mental and physical health (Lee et al., 2012). It is likely that undertaking an exercise regimen is even more difficult for those with depression. MI has the potential of increasing motivation to exercise so that it becomes even more effective. There is a growing literature on the use of MI to promote physical activity (Martins & McNeil, 2009), and future studies are warranted to address the use of MI in encouraging physical activity to improve depression.

TABLE 7.1. Measures of MI Fidelity in CBT Sessions

Item	Definition
1. The counselor cultivates empathy and compassion with the client.	The counselor understands or makes an effort to grasp the client's perspectives and feelings and conveys that understanding to the client.
2. The counselor fosters collaboration with the client.	The counselor negotiates with the client and avoids an authoritarian stance. A metaphor for collaboration is dancing instead of wrestling.
3. The counselor supports the autonomy of the client.	The counselor emphasizes the client's freedom of choice and conveys an understanding that the critical variables for change are within the client and cannot be imposed by others.
4. The counselor works to evoke the client's ideas and motivations for change.	The counselor conveys an understanding that motivation for change, and the ability to move toward that change, reside mostly within the client and therefore focuses efforts on eliciting and expanding it within the therapeutic interaction.
5. The counselor balances the client's agenda with focusing on the target behaviors.	The counselor maintains appropriate focus on a specific target behavior or concerns directly tied to it while still addressing the client's concerns.
6. The counselor demonstrates reflective listening skills.	The frequency of reflective statements is kept in balance with questions.
7. The counselor uses reflections strategically.	The quality of the reflections is always considered—low-quality reflections are inaccurate, lengthy, or unclear. High-quality reflections are used to express empathy, develop discrepancy, reinforce change talk, reduce resistance, and in general strategically increase motivation.
8. The counselor reinforces strengths and positive behavior change.	The counselor affirms personal qualities or efforts made by the client that promote productive change or that the client might harness in future change efforts.

(continued)

TABLE 7.1. (*continued*)

9. The counselor uses summaries effectively.	Summaries are used to pull together points from two or more prior client statements. At least two different ideas must be conveyed, as opposed to two reflections of the same idea. Summaries are a way to express active listening and reflect back to the client the "story." Summaries are also used to structure the session as well as to guide clients in the direction of change.
10. The counselor asks questions in an open-ended way.	An open-ended question is one that allows a wide range of possible answers. Closed-ended questions may be answered with a one-word response. Multiple-choice questions are considered open, particularly with clients who struggle with open and more abstract questions.
11. The counselor solicits feedback from the client.	The counselor asks the client for his or her response to information, recommendations, feedback, and the like. This is analogous to the ask–tell–ask or elicit–provide–elicit strategy in Motivational Interviewing.
12. The counselor addresses THE client's ambivalence.	The counselor responds to ambivalence either reflectively or strategically. Ambivalence may emerge as statements against change either directly about the target behaviors, about engaging in the treatment program, or discord in the relationship. Clients who are ambivalent may mix statements against change (sustain talk) with statements for change. Sometimes ambivalence is indicated more indirectly— lack of homework completion, minimal communication in the session, or statements such as "I guess so" or "I will do that if you want me to" indicating acquiescence or only half-hearted agreement with the plan for change.

MI was never intended to be a comprehensive psychotherapy (Miller & Rollnick, 2009). Yet, studies suggest that MI alone can improve mood (Bombardier et al., 2009; Naar-King et al., 2010; Watkins et al., 2011) and provide a strong foundation to address therapeutic alliance and motivational concerns in other interventions.

References

American Psychiatric Association. (2010). *Practice guideline for the treatment of patients with major depressive disorder* (3rd ed.). Washington, DC: American Psychiatric Press.

Arkowitz, H., & Burke, B. L. (2008). Motivational interviewing as an integrative framework for the treatment of depression. *Motivational interviewing in the treatment of psychological problems* (pp. 145–172). New York: Guilford Press.

Armitage, R., Flynn, H., Hoffmann, R., Vazquez, D., Lopez, J., & Marcus, S. (2009). Early developmental changes in sleep in infants: The impact of maternal depression. *Sleep, 32*(5), 693–696.

Beck, C. T., Gable, R. K., Sakala, C., & Declercq, E. R. (2011). Posttraumatic stress disorder in new mothers: Results from a two-stage U.S. national survey. *Birth, 38*(3), 216–227.

Beshai, S., Dobson, K. S., Bockting, C. L., & Quigley, L. (2011). Relapse and recurrence prevention in depression: Current research and future prospects. *Clinical Psychology Review, 31*(8), 1349–1360.

Blumenthal, J. A., Babyak, M. A., Doraiswamy, P. M., Watkins, L., Hoffman, B. M., Barbour, K. A., et al. (2007). Exercise and pharmacotherapy in the treatment of major depressive disorder. *Psychosomatic Medicine, 69*(7), 587–596.

Bombardier, C. H., Bell, K. R., Temkin, N. R., Fann, J. R., Hoffman, J., & Dikmen, S. (2009). The efficacy of a scheduled telephone intervention for ameliorating depressive symptoms during the first year after traumatic brain injury. *Journal of Head Trauma Rehabilitation, 24*(4), 230–238.

Burke, B. L. (2011). What can motivational interviewing do for you? *Cognitive and Behavioral Practice, 18*(1), 74–81.

Burns, D. D., & Nolen-Hoeksema, S. (1991). Coping styles, homework compliance, and the effectiveness of cognitive-behavioral therapy. *Journal of Consulting and Clinical Psychology, 59*(2), 305–311.

Burns, D. D., & Nolen-Hoeksema, S. (1992). Therapeutic empathy and recovery from depression in cognitive-behavioral therapy: A structural equation model. *Journal of Consulting and Clinical Psychology, 60*(3), 441–449.

Carroll, K. M., Nich, C., & Ball, S. A. (2005). Practice makes progress?: Homework assignments and outcome in treatment of cocaine dependence. *Journal of Consulting and Clinical Psychology, 73*(4), 749.

Castonguay, L. G., Goldfried, M. R., Wiser, S., Raue, P. J., & Hayes, A. M. (1996). Predicting the effect of cognitive therapy for depression: A study of unique and common factors. *Journal of Consulting and Clinical Psychology, 64*, 497–504.

Chapman, J. E., Sheidow, A. J., Henggeler, S. W., Halliday-Boykins, C. A., & Cunningham, P. B. (2008). Developing a measure of therapist adherence to contingency management: An application of the Many-Facet Rasch Model. *Journal of Child and Adolescent Substance Abuse, 17*(3), 47–68.

Chen, X., Murphy, D. A., Naar-King, S., & Parsons, J. T. (2011). A clinic-based motivational intervention improves condom use among subgroups of youth living with HIV: A multicenter randomized controlled trial. *Journal of Adolescent Health, 49*(2), 193–198.

Coffman, S. J., Martell, C. R., Dimidjian, S., Gallop, R., & Hollon, S. D. (2007). Extreme nonresponse in cognitive therapy: Can behavioral activation succeed where cognitive therapy fails? *Journal of Consulting and Clinical Psychology, 75*(4), 531–541.

Conn, V. S. (2010). Depressive symptom outcomes of physical activity interventions: Meta-analysis findings. *Annals of Behavioral Medicine, 39*(2), 128–138.

Cuijpers, P., Berking, M., Andersson, G., Quigley, L., Kleiboer, A., & Dobson, K. S. (2013). A meta-analysis of cognitive-behavioural therapy for adult depression, alone and in comparison with other treatments. *Canadian Journal of Psychiatry, 58*(7), 376–385.

Curry, S., Marlatt, G. A., & Gordon, J. R. (1987). Abstinence violation effect: Validation of an attributional construct with smoking cessation. *Journal of Consulting and Clinical Psychology, 55*(2), 145–149.

Dickinson, L. M., Rost, K., Nutting, P. A., Elliott, C. E., Keeley, R. D., & Pincus, H. (2005). RCT of a care manager intervention for major depression in primary care: 2–year costs for patients with physical vs psychological complaints. *Annals of Family Medicine, 3*(1), 15–22.

Dieter, N., Field, T., Hernandez-Reif, M., Jones, N. A., Lecanuet, J., Salman, F., et al. (2001). Maternal depression and increased fetal activity. *Journal of Obstetrics and Gynecology, 21*(5), 468–473.

Dimidjian, S., Hollon, S. D., Dobson, K. S., Schmaling, K. B., Kohlenberg, R. J., Addis, M. E., et al. (2006). Randomized trial of behavioral activation, cognitive therapy, and antidepressant medication in the acute treatment of adults with major depression. *Journal of Consulting and Clinical Psychology, 74*(4), 658–670.

Ferrari, A. J., Charlson, F. J., Norman, R. E., Patten, S. B., Freedman, G., Murray, C. J., et al. (2013). Burden of depressive disorders by country, sex, age, and year: Findings from the global burden of disease study 2010. *PLoS Medicine, 10*(11), e1001547.

Field, T., Diego, M., & Hernandez-Reif, M. (2006). Prenatal depression effects on the fetus and newborn: A review. *Infant Behavior and Development, 29*(3), 445–455.

Flynn, H. A., Henshaw, E., O'Mahen, H., & Forman, J. (2010). Patient perspectives on improving the depression referral processes in obstetrics settings: A qualitative study. *General Hospital Psychiatry, 32*(1), 9–16.

Henshaw, E. J., Flynn, H. A., Himle, J. A., O'Mahen, H. A., Forman, J., & Fedock, G. (2011). Patient preferences for clinician interactional style in treatment of perinatal depression. *Qualitative Health Research, 21*(7), 936–951.

Herz, M. I., Lamberti, J. S., Mintz, J., Scott, R., O'Dell, S. P., McCartan, L., et al. (2000). A program for relapse prevention in schizophrenia: a controlled study. *Archives of General Psychiatry, 57*(3), 277–283.

Hides, L., Carroll, S. P., Lubman, D. I., & Baker, A. (2010). Brief motivational interviewing for depression and anxiety. In J. Bennett-Levy, D. Richards,

P. Farrand, & H. Christensen (Eds.), *Oxford guide to low intensity CBT interventions* (pp. 177–185). Oxford, UK: Oxford University Press.

Hoffman, S., & Hatch, M. C. (2000). Depressive symptomatology during pregnancy: Evidence for an association with decreased fetal growth in pregnancies of lower social class women. *Health Psychology, 19*(6), 535–543.

Hollon, S. D., Thase, M. E., & Markowitz, J. C. (2002). Treatment and prevention of depression. *Psychological Science in the Public Interest, 3*(2), 39–77.

Lam, D., & Wong, G. (2005). Prodromes, coping strategies and psychological interventions in bipolar disorders. *Clinical Psychology Review, 25*(8), 1028–1042.

Lambert, M. J., & Barley, D. E. (2001). Research summary on the therapeutic relationship and psychotherapy outcome. *Psychotherapy: Theory, Research, Practice, Training, 38*(4), 357–361.

Lee, I-M., Shiroma, E. J., Lobelo, F., Puska, P., Blair, S. N., & Katzmarzyk, P. T. (2012). Effect of physical inactivity on major non-communicable diseases worldwide: An analysis of burden of disease and life expectancy. *The Lancet, 380*(9838), 219–229.

Marlatt, G. A., & Donovan, D. M. (2005). *Relapse prevention: Maintenance strategies in the treatment of addictive behaviors.* New York: Guilford Press.

Marlatt, G. A., & George, W. H. (1984). Relapse prevention: Introduction and overview of the model. *British Journal of Addiction, 79*(3), 261–273.

Martins, R. K., & McNeil, D. W. (2009). Review of motivational interviewing in promoting health behaviors. *Clinical Psychology Review, 29*(4), 283–293.

Miller, W. R., Forcehimes, A. A., & Zweben, A. (2011). *Treating addiction: A guide for professionals.* New York: Guilford Press.

Miller, W. R., & Rollnick, S. (2009). Ten things that motivational interviewing is not. *Behavioural and Cognitive Psychotherapy, 37*(2), 129–140.

Miller, W. R., & Rollnick, S. (2013). *Motivational interviewing: Helping people change* (3rd ed.). New York: Guilford Press.

Miller, W. R., Taylor, C. A., & West, J. C. (1980). Focused versus broad-spectrum behavior therapy for problem drinkers. *Journal of Consulting and Clinical Psychology, 48*(5), 590–601.

Minami, T., Wampold, B. E., Serlin, R. C., Hamilton, E. G., Brown, G. S. J., & Kircher, J. C. (2008). Benchmarking the effectiveness of psychotherapy treatment for adult depression in a managed care environment: A preliminary study. *Journal of Consulting and Clinical Psychology, 76*(1), 116–124.

Moyers, T. B., & Houck, J. (2011). Combining motivational interviewing with cognitive-behavioral treatments for substance abuse: Lessons from the COMBINE research project. *Cognitive and Behavioral Practice, 18*(1), 38–45.

Murphy, D. A., Chen, X., Naar-King, S., Parsons, J. T., & the Adolescent Trials Network. (2012). Alcohol and marijuana use outcomes in the Healthy

Choices motivational interviewing intervention for HIV-positive youth. *AIDS Patient Care and STDs, 26*(2), 95–100.

Naar-King, S., Parsons, J. T., Murphy, D., Kolmodin, K., & Harris, D. R. (2010). A multisite randomized trial of a motivational intervention targeting multiple risks in youth living with HIV: Initial effects on motivation, self-efficacy, and depression. *Journal of Adolescent Health, 46*(5), 422–428.

Naar-King, S., Parsons, J. T., Murphy, D. A., Chen, X., Harris, D. R., & Belzer, M. E. (2009). Improving health outcomes for youth living with the human immunodeficiency virus: A multisite randomized trial of a motivational intervention targeting multiple risk behaviors. *Archives of Pediatrics and Adolescent Medicine, 163*(12), 1092–1098.

Naar-King, S., & Suarez, M. (2011). *Motivational interviewing with adolescents and young adults.* New York: Guilford Press.

Nigg, C. R., Borrelli, B., Maddock, J., & Dishman, R. K. (2008). A theory of physical activity maintenance. *Applied Psychology, 57*(4), 544–560.

O'Mahen, H., Himle, J. A., Fedock, G., Henshaw, E., & Flynn, H. (2013). A pilot randomized controlled trial of cognitive behavioral therapy for perinatal depression adapted for women with low incomes. *Depression and Anxiety, 30*(7), 679–687.

O'Mahen, H. A., & Flynn, H. A. (2008). Preferences and perceived barriers to treatment for depression during the perinatal period. *Journal of Women's Health, 17*(8), 1301–1309.

Otto, M. W., & Smits, J. A. (2011). *Exercise for mood and anxiety: Proven strategies for overcoming depression and enhancing well-being.* New York: Oxford University Press.

Polivy, J., & Herman, C. P. (2002). If at first you don't succeed: False hopes of self-change. *American Psychologist, 57*(9), 677–689.

Project MATCH Research Group (1997). Project MATCH secondary a priori hypotheses. *Addiction, 92,* 1671–1698.

Righetti-Veltema, M., Conne-Perréard, E., Bousquet, A., & Manzano, J. (2002). Postpartum depression and mother–infant relationship at 3 months old. *Journal of Affective Disorders, 70*(3), 291–306.

Robinson, W., Triana, A., & Olson, M. (2013). Treatment of depression in primary care: A motivational interviewing, stepped-care approach. *Consultant, 53*(7), 495–499.

Rollnick, S., & Prout, H. (2008). Behavior change counselling. *Nutrition and Health,* 130–138.

Rost, K., Nutting, P., Smith, J., Werner, J., & Duan, N. (2001). Improving depression outcomes in community primary care practice. *Journal of General Internal Medicine, 16*(3), 143–149.

Rost, K. M., Smith, J. L., & Dickinson, L. M. (2004). The effect of improving primary care depression management on employee absenteeism and productivity: A randomized trial. *Medical Care, 42,* 1202–1210.

Santaguida, P. L., MacQueen, G., Keshavarz, H., Levine, M., Beyene, J., & Raina, P. (2012). *Treatment for depression after unsatisfactory response to SSRIs. AHRQ Comparative Effectiveness Reviews.* Rockville, MD: Agency for Healthcare Research and Quality (US).

Shim, R. S., Baltrus, P., Ye, J., & Rust, G. (2011). Prevalence, treatment and control of depressive symptoms in the United States. *Journal of the American Board of Family Medicine, 24,* 33–38.

Stathopoulou, G., Powers, M. B., Berry, A. C., Smits, J. A., & Otto, M. W. (2006). Exercise interventions for mental health: A quantitative and qualitative review. *Clinical Psychology: Science and Practice, 13*(2), 179–193.

Watkins, C. L., Wathan, J. V., Leathley, M. J., Auton, M. F., Deans, C. F., Dickinson, H. A., et al. (2011). The 12–month effects of early motivational interviewing after acute stroke: A randomized controlled trial. *Stroke, 42*(7), 1956–1961.

Westra, H. A., & Arkowitz, H. (2011). Introduction. *Cognitive and Behavioral Practice, 18*(1), 1–4.

Wisner, W. L., Sit, D. K. Y., McShea, M. C., Rizzo, D. M., Zoertich, R. A., & Hughes, C. L. (2013). Onset timing, thoughts of self-harm, and diagnosis of post partum women with screen-positive depression findings. *JAMA Psychiatry, 79,* 490–498.

Wright, J. H., Basco, M. R., & Thase, M. E. (2006). *Learning cognitive-behavior therapy: An illustrated guide.* Arlington, VA: American Psychiatric Press.

Young, A. S., Klap, R., Sherbourne, C., & Wells, K. B. (2001). The quality of care for depressive and anxiety disorders in the United States. *Archives of General Psychiatry, 58*(1), 55–61.

CHAPTER 8

• • • • • •

Motivational Interviewing to Address Suicidal Ideation

Peter C. Britton

In 2015, some 40,600 people died by suicide in the United States (Centers for Disease Control and Prevention, 2015), making suicide the 10th leading cause of death overall and the 4th leading cause of years of potential life lost before age 65. Studies indicate that over 90% of individuals who die by suicide struggle with a diagnosable psychiatric disorder (Cavanagh, Carson, Sharpe, & Lawrie, 2003; Yoshimasu, Kiyohara, & Kazuhisa, 2008). These individuals often seek care for psychological and other problems shortly before their death, and an estimated 20% of decedents make contact with mental health care services during the month before suicide and 45% make contact with primary care (Luoma, Martin, & Pearson, 2002). Clinicians working in these settings must have access to empirically supported treatments they can use with patients whom they believe are at elevated risk. Although a number of interventions have been shown to reduce risk for suicide attempts in high-risk patients (Tarrier, Taylor, & Gooding, 2008), there is a paucity of empirically supported brief treatments and none has used a motivational approach.

Usual Treatments

Suicide researchers frequently use suicide attempts as a proxy for suicide, because they are more common and are robust predictors of suicide

193

(Harris & Barraclough, 1997; Owens, Horrocks, & House, 2002). To date, four behavioral interventions have been shown to reduce risk for suicide attempts in high-risk populations. Dialectical behavior therapy (DBT), a 1-year treatment using individual and group modalities, has been shown to reduce suicide attempts in women with borderline personality disorder (Linehan et al., 2006). Cognitive therapy (CT) for suicide prevention, a 10-session treatment, has been shown to reduce reattempts in attempters when combined with case management (Brown, Newman, Charlesworth, Crits-Christoph, & Beck, 2004). Brief cognitive-behavioral therapy (B-CBT) for suicide prevention is a 12-session treatment that has been shown to reduce attempts in a military population with recent attempts or suicidal ideation with intent (Rudd et al., 2014). Problem solving therapy, a five-session treatment conducted on inpatient units and/or in the home after discharge, has also been shown to reduce reattempts in attempters (Salkovskis, Atha, & Storer, 1990). The obvious benefit of DBT, CT for suicide prevention, B-CBT for suicide prevention, and problem solving is that they have been shown to reduce risk for suicide attempts where other approaches have failed and should therefore be integrated into practice wherever possible. Because they utilize a cognitive-behavioral framework, these treatments use a modality that is familiar to many practitioners.

The Clinical Problem

These treatments do, however, have limitations. The majority of these interventions are costly, as DBT requires yearlong individual and group treatment, CT for suicide prevention uses case management to ensure basic needs are met, B-CBT was effective in the military (which provides one's living quarters, food, and an income), and the efficacious problem solving treatment required in-home sessions after discharge from inpatient units. Many providers do not have the resources, and insurance companies and health care systems may not cover the costs required, to provide these treatments; moreover, it is unclear whether these approaches are efficacious without their costly components. DBT, CT, and B-CBT for suicide prevention also require 10 or more sessions and are inappropriate for settings that treat large numbers of individuals at acute risk such as emergency departments and acute psychiatric inpatient units. With the exception of B-CBT, the treatments were found to reduce risk for reattempts and may or may not reduce risk for suicide.

This distinction is important for a number of reasons. Suicide attempts and suicide are different behaviors, as most attempts are overdoses whereas most suicides are by firearms (Desai, Dausey, & Rosenheck, 2008; Kellermann et al., 1992; Wiebe, 2003). Although reducing risk for suicide attempts in high-risk suicide attempters is critical, these cited studies may have limited generalizability, as they exclude the estimated 50% or more of individuals who die by suicide on the first attempt (Isometsa & Lonnqvist, 1998). The majority of participants in three of the studies (involving DBT, CT, and problem solving) were also female, and it is unclear whether the findings generalize to males, who have higher rates of suicide in the United States (Centers for Disease Control and Prevention, 2014).

Treatments that are briefer than 10 sessions, require fewer resources, are generalizable, and are appropriate for practitioners in most settings must therefore be developed and tested. It is important to note that there is precedence for the success of such approaches. In a study of hospitalized depressed or suicidal patients who refused follow-up treatment, having an attending clinician send 24 caring letters over 5 years was shown to reduce suicide risk for up to 2 years (Motto & Bostrom, 2001), and a similar intervention was found to reduce risk for nonfatal self-poisoning (Carter, Clover, Whyte, Dawson, & D'Este, 2007; Carter, Clover, Whyte, Dawson, & D'Este, 2005), indicating that simple interventions can be surprisingly efficacious. Brief interventions can also be used as adjuncts to more intensive treatments such as DBT, CT for suicide prevention, B-CBT, and in-person or telephone follow-ups. A 1-hour educational intervention (about suicide risk, protection, and treatment) paired with nine follow-up telephone calls or home visits was shown to reduce risk for suicide over 18 months in patients in emergency care across five low- to middle-income countries (Fleischmann et al., 2008).

Rationale for Using Motivational Interviewing for Suicidal Ideation (MI-SI)

Suicidality Conceptualized as a Motivational Issue

One of the reasons that motivational interviewing (MI) has been proposed as a brief one- to three-session suicide prevention intervention is that suicide can be conceptualized as a motivational issue (Britton, Patrick, & Williams, 2011; Britton, Williams, & Conner, 2008; Zerler, 2008, 2009). In 1977, Kovacs and Beck (1977, p. 361) described the suicidal act "as the outcome of the internal subjective struggle between the wish to live and the wish to die, rather than the consequence of a single unidirectional motivation." Research generally supports the "internal struggle" hypothesis, showing that outpatients who wanted to live as much or more than they want to die made less severe attempts (Kovacs & Beck, 1977) and are less likely to die by suicide (Brown, Steer, Henriques, & Beck, 2005). Increasing the motivation to live in patients who are thinking about suicide may reduce their risk for continuing to think about and engage in suicidal behavior (Britton et al., 2008) and likely increases their likelihood of engaging in mental health and/or substance abuse treatment to resolve their problems (Britton et al., 2011).

The Theory of MI and Suicide Prevention

The theory of MI can be used to model how it might be used to help patients regain the motivation to live (Miller & Rose, 2009). Process outcome research suggests that MI works through interpersonal and technical pathways. Interpersonally, MI provides patients with a therapeutic relationship that fosters openness and supports growth and development, known as the MI spirit. At the same time, there is a desired outcome, and clinicians use their MI skills to actively elicit and reinforce change talk (indicating that the patient is thinking about making changes) and commitment talk (indicating that the patient will be making changes) while simultaneously reducing counterchange talk (usually called "sustain talk"), all of which are predictive of posttreatment change (Moyers, Martin, Houck, Christopher, & Tonigan, 2009; Moyers et al., 2007). A similar model can be applied to suicidal patients (see Figure 8.1). In MI-SI, clinicians seek to provide patients with a caring listener who is supportive of growth and adaptation. Such a relationship is hypothesized to directly reduce the client's risk of thinking about and engaging in suicidal behavior (i.e., both attempts and actual suicide). Clinicians also use MI skills to evoke talk associated with living and reduce talk associated with death and suicide. Increased exploration of living and reduced discussion about suicide is hypothesized to decrease the client's risk of thinking about or engaging in suicidal behavior after the session is over. As noted previously (Miller & Rose, 2009), it is unlikely that merely talking about living will decrease a person's risk for suicide, but when it is genuine and meaningful, such talk may be reflective of the resolution of the internal struggle between the wish to live and the wish to die.

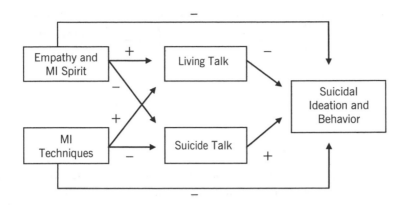

FIGURE 8.1. Hypothesized MI-SI process model.

Clinical Applications and Considerations

MI-SI as a Component of Treatment

Individuals who are at risk for suicide are a heterogeneous population that often has complex and chronic problems, and it is unlikely that one to three sessions of any treatment will be sufficient. MI-SI may therefore be most effective as an adjunct to more intensive treatment, as people who are motivated to live might also be motivated to engage in life-sustaining and enhancing activities such as treatment. This may be particularly critical with suicidal patients, for whom it is better to err on the side of too much care rather than too little. An MI session cannot replace a structured risk assessment that can be used to identify critical risk factors for suicide that need to be addressed, such as a suicide attempt history (Harris & Barraclough, 1997; Owens et al., 2002) or access to firearms (Hemenway & Miller, 2002; Miller, Azrael, & Hemenway, 2002; Miller & Hemenway, 1999). Patients are also likely to require additional treatment to adequately address their risk, such as coping skills training, problem solving therapy, or substance abuse treatment. In the sequence of treatment with suicidal patients (see Figure 8.2), MI-SI is therefore best conceptualized as a component of treatment that follows a structured suicide risk assessment and is followed by additional treatment to directly address the patient's risk or problems that may be contributing to it. Although some treatments such as coping skills, problem solving, or reducing substance use can be implemented using an MI-based approach, such components would have to be added after basic MI-SI.

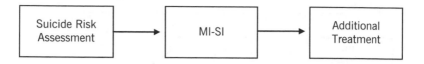

FIGURE 8.2. MI-SI in the sequence of treatment.

The MI Spirit and Suicidality

Care must also be taken when applying the MI spirit to suicidal patients. The concept of the MI spirit was developed by Miller and Rollnick (1991) and further refined in 2013 (Miller & Rollnick, 2013) to describe the relational characteristics that are needed to create an interpersonal environment that is supportive of change and growth.

Miller and Rollnick's (2013) most recent model of MI spirit includes partnership, acceptance, compassion, and evocation. When using MI, clinicians strive to develop a good collaborative *partnership* with the patient, *accept* the patient as a fellow human being with his or her own perspective, have an attitude of *compassion* in which the welfare and needs of the other are actively promoted, and *evoke* the person's strengths and resources rather than deficits. When using MI with suicidal patients, clinicians should aspire to interact according to these beliefs or values. However, they must do so thoughtfully in a manner that does not increase risk. All suicidal patients are ultimately autonomous, as the rates of suicide attempts and suicides after signing no-harm contracts and during and after hospitalization attest (Appleby et al., 1999; Goldacre, Seagroatt, & Hawton, 1993; Meehan et al., 2006; Qin & Nordentoft, 2005; Rudd, Mandrusiak, & Joiner, 2006). Denying patients autonomy can have a negative impact on treatment outcome, as power struggles focused on establishing autonomy can sometimes exacerbate risk for suicidal behavior (Filiberti et al., 2001; Hendin, Haas, Maltsberger, Koestner, & Szanto, 2006). Although it is important to respect suicidal patients' autonomy, there are inherent differences in substance abuse behaviors and suicidal behaviors that require consideration. There is little risk in supporting the autonomy of substance abusers, as relapses can be expected, are rarely fatal, and may increase the patient's motivation to address his or her substance use (Anglin, Hser, & Grella, 1997; Miller, Walters, & Bennett, 2001). There is obviously greater risk in supporting the autonomy of suicidal patients, as attempts often result in serious injury and can end in death. When using MI with suicidal patients, clinicians may therefore feel that they are in a bind between supporting their patient's autonomy and providing adequate protection.

This bind, however, exists for all clinicians working with suicidal patients and requires an informed and thoughtful approach to autonomy support. When exploring patients' motivation for and plans to make life worth living, clinicians can support patients' autonomy in much the same way they do with substance abusers. However, when patients are actively thinking about suicide, clinicians must reserve and exercise the right to protect patients when they are at imminent risk to themselves or others, whether they are using MI or any other intervention. Like all clinicians, MI clinicians should share with patients the limits of confidentiality and the need to take protective action if the person is deemed a danger to self or others, but should do so in way that is respectful of the individual's autonomy. From an MI perspective, it may be helpful for clinicians to clarify that their preference is not to hospitalize patients or keep them hospitalized but, rather, to help them identify their reasons for living and collaboratively develop a plan to keep them safe. It may also be helpful to emphasize the desire to help patients develop a plan to make life worth living so that hospitalization is not needed. Although arguments about autonomy tend to be rare in our experience, they are to be avoided whenever possible, as there is little to be gained. When pressed, clinicians can acknowledge that patients are ultimately autonomous and will eventually leave the clinician's office or the hospital, as both are true and unlikely to increase risk. However, clinicians should avoid supporting the patient's "right" to suicide, as the patient may mistakenly believe the clinician condones the option.

The Technical Component of MI and Suicidality

In the context of a supportive relationship based on the MI spirit, clinicians use MI skills strategically to promote living talk and reduce suicide talk, which is hypothesized to be predictive of increased engagement in life-sustaining and enhancing behavior and reduced suicide-related behavior (see Figure 8.1). Similar to MI clinicians working with individuals with substance abuse problems, clinicians use *open questions* to elicit their patients' perspective, *reflections* to share their understanding of patients' thoughts and feelings about living, *affirmations* to reinforce patients' motivation to live and to encourage engagement in life-sustaining and -enhancing activities, and *summaries* to integrate patients' thoughts, feelings, and actions into a coherent and life-affirming narrative. However, recent advances in MI theory and research and our clinical experience have significantly impacted our strategic approach to applying MI to suicidal patients.

In early applications (Britton et al., 2008, 2011), clinicians were instructed to start the intervention by asking patients why they were thinking about suicide. The idea was based on use of the decisional balance, a structured exploration of the pros and cons of changing and not changing, to resolve ambivalence about changing (Miller & Rollnick, 2002); findings suggested that when sustain talk about suicide transitioned to change talk about living, positive changes occurred (Bertholet, Faouzi, Gmel, Gaume, & Daeppen, 2010). However, the model for using MI with suicidal patients posits that evoking living talk should reduce risk for suicidal behavior whereas evoking suicide talk should increase the risk for suicidal behavior, which would suggest that the decisional balance could be ineffective and even harmful (Miller & Rose, in press). In fact, the most recent version of MI (Miller & Rollnick, 2013) views the use of decisional balance for effecting change as inappropriate. Instead, the focus is on eliciting and reinforcing change talk. Clinical experience also supports this latter view. Discussing reasons for suicide often unnecessarily returns patients to the thought patterns and overwhelming emotions that characterize the suicidal state. Because the intervention is only one to two sessions long, time spent in exploring patients' suicidality would replace time spent in exploring motivations to live. Clinicians using MI with suicidal patients should avoid deliberately evoking suicidal thoughts and should instead provide patients with an opportunity to talk about their reasons for living, hopes, wishes, and dreams. This can be accomplished by empathically tailoring the opening question to the patient.

If the patient is thinking about suicide, the clinician can ask:

> "I know you are in a lot of pain and have been thinking about suicide. I'm wondering why you thought it was important to talk to me instead of making an attempt?"

If the patient made an attempt and admitted him- or herself to the Emergency Department or hospital, the clinician can ask:

> "I know that you are here because you made a suicide attempt and called 911. Obviously you've been in a lot of pain, and there are reasons that you have been thinking about suicide. What I'm curious about is why did you call 911?"

It can be challenging to come up with an opening question when a patient makes a potentially lethal suicide attempt and did not die or someone else contacted emergency services, but there are questions that clinicians can ask:

> "You made a very serious attempt and came very close to dying. Obviously, you were in a lot of pain before you made the attempt. I'm wondering how were you able to keep fighting to live for so long before you made the attempt?"

If clinicians believe that the patient is not engaged, want to understand the patient better, think the patient is not ready to discuss reasons for living, or the starting question fails to elicit reasons to live, it may be helpful to inquire about patients' personal values and beliefs, abilities or strengths, accomplishments, or a time in their life when things were going well and they felt that life was worth living. Such information provides clinicians with the positive side of suicidal patients' ambivalence, which clinicians can reinforce, and can serve as the first step to exploring the motivation to live.

The model also raises questions about how clinicians should respond when patients engage in suicide talk, as is bound to happen. Following MI theory and research as well as the MI mantra to "let your patient be your guide," clinicians should respond to suicide talk in an empathic patient-centered manner that does not evoke more suicide talk. Responses that reflect patients' suicide talk in the context of their motivations to live and provide an opportunity for positive or at least neutral responses can be particularly helpful. For example, if a patient says "I still think about suicide," the clinician can:

- Reframe: "You could use some help with the problems that make you think about suicide."
- Agree with a twist: "You still think about suicide sometimes and are still trying to find another way out."
- Use double-sided reflections: "On the one hand, you still think about suicide sometimes, and, on the other hand, you know that killing yourself may really hurt your children."

Clinical Illustration

MI is conceptualized as consisting of four phases: (1) engaging, (2) focusing, (3) evoking, and (4) planning (Miller & Rollnick, 2013). The phases are conceptualized as successive and yet recursive, such that each phase builds on the preceding one, but progress is expected to require the ability to transition between phases when needed. For example, patients have to engage in the process before a focus can be decided, but clinicians may have to ask questions to facilitate engagement. The phases are therefore more similar to compass directions—which allow for the flexibility to travel in other directions to avoid lakes and mountains—than they are to a map, which is used to plan the necessary detours.

To illustrate MI-SI, we will examine the case of a veteran who is at increased risk for suicide. The illustration is divided by phases, starting with a discussion examining the critical topics to consider when working with suicidal patients and ending with a clinical interchange that exemplifies the phase. To respect the patient's confidentiality, the one portrayed is deliberately a composite of many patients that have been seen. Throughout the interchange we identify the MI skill that is being used, whether it is a *reflection, open-ended question, affirmation*, or *summary* or another action, such as giving information or structuring when appropriate.

Engaging

Clinicians should start the session by trying to engage the patient in the treatment process. Although the importance of engaging patients who are thinking about suicide in treatment seems obvious, there are many pressures that can interfere, such as the fear of having a patient die by suicide, the reflexive use of no-harm contracts and hospitalization, as well as patient characteristics such as a challenging interpersonal style or fear of hospitalization. When suicidal patients never engage or disengage, clinicians lose the opportunity to help them rediscover their reasons for living and find the motivation they need to resolve their problems. To engage patients, clinicians should help them feel as comfortable as possible and provide them with a sense of what the process may look like and ask them what they think about it. It may be helpful for clinicians to share their perspective on working with suicidal patients, such as the limits of confidentiality, as well as their desire to help patients avoid hospitalization by helping them rediscover their motivation to live and develop a plan to resolve their problems. As mentioned earlier, asking patients about their values, beliefs, strengths, accomplishments, and desires can also facilitate engaging. Here is an example of an interview emphasizing the engagement phase of MI:

CLINICIAN: So, we just finished a risk assessment, and it looks like you have been thinking about suicide and even have a plan to overdose, although you said you are not sure whether you are going to do it or not.

VETERAN: Yeah, I've been thinking about it . . . I just don't know.

CLINICIAN: It's kind of hard to talk about. [Reflection]

VETERAN: It's really hard to talk about; I don't want you to send me to the hospital!

CLINICIAN: Would it be OK for me to give you some information on how I look at this? [Asking permission]

VETERAN: Yeah, go ahead.

CLINICIAN: Suicide is obviously a very serious issue. Just like any other therapist you are going to work with, I have a responsibility to take steps to protect you or other people if I think you are a threat to yourself or others. Although I think hospitalization is helpful in some situations, I don't think it is the right decision for everyone, so my goal is not to hospitalize you. What I'd really like to do is to work with you to figure out what has prevented you from making an attempt and what would give you the best chance of getting through this difficult time. [Giving information] How does that sound? [Open question]

VETERAN: That makes sense. I think suicide is something that people just think of when they hit bottom. I've hit bottom lots of times, and I've been down there so long that I can't imagine finding my way out.

CLINICIAN: And that's why we're talking, because it sounds like there's a part of you that wants to make it out of that hole alive. [Reflection]

VETERAN: Yeah, I never thought of it that way, but I guess there's something in me that's not ready to die.

Focusing

After engagement, the next step is to agree to focus on rediscovering the motivation to live. This can be easy when the focus of treatment is determined by the context. For instance, when a patient calls a suicide crisis line, both the patient and the responder understand that the discussion is most likely going to address suicide. However, in other settings such as outpatient mental health, patients frequently have a number of problems, and the focus may have to be negotiated. If there is disagreement, the clinician's approach to determining the focus can have a substantial impact on the treatment process. In such cases clinicians can take a directive, following, or guiding approach. When taking a directive approach, the clinician decides the focus of treatment without asking for the patient's input. With suicidal patients, prematurely deciding to focus on their motivation to live may make them feel their pain is being ignored and cause them to disengage, resulting in a step backward. When taking a following approach, clinicians allow patients to determine the focus, which may prevent clinicians who are working with suicidal patients from ever discussing suicide versus living. A guiding approach is halfway between a directive approach and a following approach. When guiding, clinicians try to understand each patient's perspective but introduce potentially important topics such as the motivation to live, and bring patients back to those topics when they stray. Such a flexible approach enables clinicians to keep clients engaged in the process of exploring sensitive topics such as their reasons for living despite their pain and suicidal thoughts. Here is an example of an interview emphasizing the focusing phase of MI:

VETERAN: Yeah, I never thought of it that way, but I guess there's something in me that's not ready to die.

CLINICIAN: You're obviously in a lot of pain. From the assessment I know that you're feeling depressed, your PTSD symptoms have returned, and you've been drinking a lot to manage them. Your relationship with your wife is also strained, and you've been feeling disconnected and lonely. And yet, there is also that other side, that side of you that's not ready to die. [Reflection]

VETERAN: I don't know what it is, but it has kept me from doing anything, you know, permanent.

CLINICIAN: There's a sense that these feelings you have now may not be permanent, they may not last forever. [Reflection]

VETERAN: It doesn't feel that way right now, but that's basically it. Something has to change, because I can't keep going into this dark hole. Every time I fall back down I feel more hopeless, like it's just a matter of time before I'm in the hole for good.

CLINICIAN: Something really does need to change, and I really want to talk about that. However, I'm also very curious about that part of you that keeps trying to climb out of that hole. [Affirmation, structuring statement] Can we explore that first? [Asking permission]

VETERAN: I know it's there, but I don't know what it is.

Evoking

In the evocation phase, clinicians elicit, listen for, and reinforce reasons for living. They try to identify living talk expressing the *desire* (e.g., "I don't really want to die"), *ability* (e.g., "I can make my life worth living"), *reasons* (e.g., "I need to live for my kids"), and *need* to live (e.g., "I need to live"). To reinforce each patient's desire, ability, reasons, and need to live, and make these more personal, clinicians acknowledge them, affirm them, and explore them in detail. Patients' reasons for living typically consist of such common things as the belief that they can cope with their problems and will survive, as responsible to family members, or have child related concerns, moral or religious beliefs, a fear of attempt-related pain or of death, or a fear of others' disapproval of their suicide (Linehan, Goodstein, Nielsen, & Chiles, 1983). However, there may also be unexpected reasons that do not fall into common categories, such as the desire to explore the world or the realization that little things in life such as dew on the grass have beauty and meaning. Such verbalizations are thought to signal that the patient is considering living and believed to be preparatory. They often precede stronger statements expressing *commitment* (e.g., "I am not going to kill myself"), *activation* (e.g., "I am going to give treatment a try"), and *taking steps* to resolving problems (e.g., "I have already gotten rid of my firearms"). Some patients may have difficulty expressing their motivation to live, and sometimes the clinician's goal is simply to encourage the patient to begin thinking about living. Clinicians can ask patients about their core beliefs and values and explore their congruence with living and discrepancy with suicide and what life was like when it was worth living, what a life worth living would look like, and what might have to change to make life worth living. At the conclusion of this phase, clinicians should ask patients for a commitment to living, as it may be helpful for patients to hear themselves say it out loud. Here is an example of an interview emphasizing the evoking phase of MI:

VETERAN: I know it's there, but I don't know what it is.

CLINICIAN: Why did you come in to see me today instead of making an attempt? [Open question]

VETERAN: I honestly didn't want to kill myself today. I woke up and was a little disappointed I did—but I didn't really think about trying to kill myself. I mean, I don't really want to die, but sometimes I think it's the only thing I can do to stop feeling so bad.

CLINICIAN: Although you haven't been able to find another way out, you don't really want to kill yourself, at least not all the time. On some days you want to live more than you want to die. [Reflection]

VETERAN: But on the bad days I forget that I don't want to die. Anyway, I know that I need help.

CLINICIAN: It takes a lot of courage to admit you need help. [Affirmation] So, what does it look like when your life is going well? What makes it worth living? [Open question]

VETERAN: When I was doing well, my relationship with my wife was good, we had a lot of fun together. She said I was strong and dependable, but that was before my PTSD got bad and I started drinking to deal with it. Now she can't get away fast enough.

CLINICIAN: You value your relationships with your wife and family. [Reflection]

VETERAN: That's what's so hard. I feel like my kids and definitely my wife would be better off without me, but they tell me it's not true.

CLINICIAN: Tell me about your kids. [Open question]

VETERAN: My kids are great. My son is a doctor, and he has two kids, and my daughter is a journalist and is always traveling.

CLINICIAN: You're really proud of them. [Affirmation]

VETERAN: I am very proud.

CLINICIAN: And they would be upset if you killed yourself. [Reflection]

VETERAN: They would be devastated, for a while at least. I don't want to hurt them anymore, but I don't know what to do.

CLINICIAN: So, one of the reasons you're still living is that on some level you know your suicide would hurt your family, and that's not the kind of husband, father, or grandfather you want to be. You also said that when you get along with them life is more enjoyable. [Reflection]

VETERAN: It's great when we are getting along! I feel like I'm worth something, and I don't even think about suicide.

CLINICIAN: The good times with your family—they make life worth living. [Reflection] What are some other things that make life worth living? [Open question]

VETERAN: I've always loved the outdoors, hiking, hunting, fishing, and stuff like that. But it's been a while since I've done anything like that. When my PTSD hits I don't want to leave the house. I have nightmares and sleep in a different room than my wife. I'm always tired and grouchy . . . I'm hell to be around.

CLINICIAN: Your PTSD takes you away from your family and the activities you love. You really miss being in touch with nature, there's something special about it. [Reflection]

VETERAN: It's really like my spirituality. I love smelling the pine trees, feeling the air on my face.

CLINICIAN: Like those good moments with your family, you really feel alive when you can get out into nature. It's very personal for you. [Reflection]

VETERAN: I'm not religious and I don't go to church, but the woods are kind of like my church.

CLINICIAN: You need to get back in touch with your spiritual side. It gives you a sense of perspective—that there's something bigger than you. [reflection]

VETERAN: I feel alive and my problems don't feel like as big of a deal. It's a good feeling, and I need to find a way to get myself to do those things that I enjoy.

CLINICIAN: And that's one reason why you're here. [Reflection]

VETERAN: That . . . and the other day I thought about my first order. Every once in a while I think about boot camp, and I think about reciting my first order. Never leave your post until you have orders to do so.

CLINICIAN: That's really stuck with you. You're not the type of soldier who leaves his post. [Reflection]

VETERAN: I was a good soldier, and that was important to me. I took pride in serving and felt I was doing something important. I have to find a way to stay at my post.

CLINICIAN: You said that your service gave you a sense of meaning— that you were serving a purpose. [Reflection] I'm wondering, what kind of purpose you can find going forward? [Open question]

VETERAN: I don't know. If I get through this, I want to do something valuable like help other veterans. I don't even care if I get paid, but I want to show other veterans that they aren't alone and that we can all stand by each other.

CLINICIAN: You have to stand by your post, but there's nothing that says you have to do it alone. One purpose you can find for yourself is to help other veterans who are having some of the same struggles that you are having. [Reflection]

VETERAN: I can help them, and they can help me.

CLINICIAN: So, you have reasons for living. Your wife and your kids are important to you, and when you get along with them, life has meaning and is even fun. Nature has always been important to you spiritually, and you find meaning and peace when you are in the woods. And when you think about creating meaning going forward, you think about helping other veterans—doing something you feel is important and that you can be proud of. So, after thinking about these reasons for living, how committed are you to living? [Open question]

VETERAN: I'm committed. I don't want to kill myself, but I can't go on living this way.

Planning

When patients have fully explored their motivation for living, verbalized a commitment to living, or already taken steps toward making life worth living, it may be time to introduce the possibility of making a plan. Clinicians can assess patients' readiness by summarizing the patient's living or commitment talk and asking an open question such as "What do you think you could do to make life worth living?" The process of planning may require a variety of strategies. Some patients have no ideas, and plans need to be developed from scratch; other patients have numerous ideas and have to make choices or set priorities; still others know exactly what they want to do and how to do it. Activities should match patients' needs and may include brainstorming, weighing the pros and cons of various options, troubleshooting concerns or barriers, identifying the steps that need to be taken, developing alternative plans in case the primary plan is unsuccessful or more difficult than expected, and eliciting and reinforcing the patient's motivation to engage in the plan. Clinician may ask if putting the plan in writing would be helpful, as it could provide patients with a resource they can refer to after they leave and that clinicians can refer to in later sessions. Clinicians may also want to inquire about enlisting the help of others so that patients have some assistance in following through on their plan. Like verbally committing themselves to living, it may also be helpful to ask for a patient's commitment to following through with the plan so that the patients hear themselves agree to do it. If continued contact is possible, clinicians should also ask permission to inquire about the patient's progress at a later date so that they can reinforce any changes the patient makes, troubleshoot any barriers, and revise the plan if necessary. Here is an example of an interview emphasizing the planning phase of MI:

VETERAN: I'm committed. I don't want to kill myself, but I can't go on living this way.

CLINICIAN: You are committed to living, but something needs to change. [Reflection] What steps can you take to make sure your life is worth living? [Open question]

VETERAN: I've been taking my medication and coming to therapy, but they don't seem to be working as well as they could.

CLINICIAN: You're feeling that your treatment needs some adjustments. [Reflection]

VETERAN: My PTSD symptoms have been really bad lately. I'm not sure why, but I haven't been able to sleep because of the nightmares, and I've been jumpy and irritable all the time. I've been really mean lately, so my family can't stand to be around m—and I don't blame them.

CLINICIAN: Could we talk about some options that I know about? [Asking permission]

VETERAN: Definitely.

CLINICIAN: Well, I'm aware that they have recently made some advancements in the use of medication to treat nightmares. I'm a psychologist, so I can't prescribe medication, but there are psychiatrists in the VA who are familiar with the medications who you can talk to. It also sounds like you may want to discuss other medication adjustments as well. [Giving information]

VETERAN: That would be great if there is something that could help with the nightmares. My wife stopped sleeping with me years ago because I would thrash and accidentally hit her.

CLINICIAN: It also sounds like what we've been doing hasn't been helping you with your PTSD symptoms. We have some specialists in empirically supported treatments for PTSD, and that means they are trained in treatments that have been scientifically shown to reduce PTSD symptoms in veterans. [Giving information]

VETERAN: That would be great too. I've been thinking about suicide— that's how bad things have gotten—so I'll try anything. Can't you help me with that treatment?

CLINICIAN: I know enough about them to talk about how they work, but I don't have the training and expertise that some of my colleagues do. [Giving information] I'd like you to be able to get the best treatment you can get. [Affirmation]

VETERAN: OK, let's do it!

CLINICIAN: You said you were drinking. What are your thoughts about your substance use? [Open question]

VETERAN: I've got to go back to AA. It's worked for me before, and I just have to get back to the steps.

CLINICIAN: You've been successful in changing your drinking in the past and already know what you have to do about your drinking. [Affirmation] What else do you think will be helpful? [Open question]

VETERAN: I have to get out of the house and figure out a way to spend more time in nature, and I really want to help other veterans—so, I have to figure out how I can do that. But it's so easy to come up with reasons not to do it—I'm tired, I'm depressed, it's cold out, I don't know how to make sure I do it.

CLINICIAN: So, it's important to figure out a way to hold you accountable so that you actually spend some time in the woods. [Reflection]

VETERAN: I think if I scheduled a time to hike with my wife or go fishing with a friend, I would be more likely to do it.

CLINICIAN: Involving others in your plans is one way of making sure you do it, and it's also a way of building your relationships with your wife and your friends. [Affirmation]

VETERAN: They've wanted to help, asking what they can do, and I've just been telling them to go away and leave me alone because they don't understand. I don't want to hurt them anymore—but I can't be alone all the time either, I just feel worse.

CLINICIAN: And spending time with them in nature, where you feel more peaceful and spiritual, is one way you can be around them without being angry. [Reflection]

VETERAN: My wife and I used to love to go hiking and camping. It's something we always shared, but we had kids and were working and just got away from it. It would be nice to build that back into our relationship.

CLINICIAN: That's something your wife might enjoy too. It may also help her figure out how she can be there for you. [Reflection]

VETERAN: It will get me some exercise, too. I've been gaining a lot of weight lately, and my doctor has been getting on my case.

CLINICIAN: There may be some health benefits as well. [Reflection]

VETERANS:: But I don't know how to get into helping veterans. Do you know how I can do that?

CLINICIAN: How did you get the idea? [Open question]

VETERAN: I was in the VA and saw one of those peer specialists and was thinking that I'd like to do that. He said I could look at USA jobs and submit an application.

CLINICIAN: What do you think about that? [Open question]

VETERAN: I haven't gotten around to it but I'm going to do it.

CLINICIAN: Sounds like you're already taking steps. [Affirmation] I'll also look into it and see if I can come up with any additional information. [Giving information] Anything else you think might be helpful? [Open question]

VETERAN: No, I think that's a good place to start.

CLINICIAN: Would you be willing to write down what you are committed to doing on this piece of paper? Sometime people find it helpful to write down their plan so they can return to it when they aren't sure what to do or don't feel like they are making progress. It's totally up to you though. [Asking permission, giving information]

VETERANS:: Sure (*writing*). I'm going to go to a psychiatrist to see if the nightmare medication will work for me and to see if other medications can help me. I'll see a therapist who has special training in PTSD so I can work on my symptoms. I'm going to go back to AA. I'm going to schedule trips into nature with my wife and friend once a week. I'm also going to find a VA peer specialist to see if there is any way that I can volunteer to help other veterans.

CLINICIAN: It sounds like you are committed to living and working on this plan. [Reflection]

VETERAN: I am. I don't want to die, I just couldn't figure out what I needed to do. It's good to have a plan.

CLINICIAN: So, you are committed to living. You are not ready to leave your post, and you want to be there with your family and especially your wife. You also don't want to leave the other veterans behind, the ones you may be able to help. Your plan is to make sure you are getting the best treatment you can by asking a psychiatrist about medication for your nightmare and to see if there are any other medications that might help. You are going to see a psychologist to focus on your PTSD symptoms so that your symptoms don't interfere with your life as much, and you are going to go back to AA to address your drinking. You also feel like life is worth living when you are in nature and smelling the pine trees and feeling the wind on your face. Once a week you are going to go on a hike or go fishing with your wife or a friend. That will allow you to get in touch with your spirituality and may even help repair your relationships. You also want to look into volunteering to help other veterans. Your military service gave you a sense of meaning, and maybe you can continue to find meaning by helping other veterans. [Summarizing]

VETERAN: If I can be there for other veterans—help them get through what I've been struggling with—then going through this will be worth something.

CLINICIAN: You've done a lot of work today! [Affirmation] Why don't you start putting your plan into place, and we'll review it in a couple of weeks and see how it is going and if anything needs to be tweaked. [Structuring]

Current Research and Preliminary Findings

The primary limitation of MI-SI is that there is currently no evidence that it is an efficacious intervention for suicidal patients. Clinicians should therefore familiarize themselves with and use treatments that have already been found to be efficacious. However, research on MI-SI is in progress.

Colleagues and I (Britton, Connor, & Maisto, 2012). have conducted an open trial to test the acceptability of MI-SI for psychiatrically hospitalized veterans with suicidal ideation, estimate its pre–posteffect size on the severity of suicidal ideation, and examine the rate of treatment engagement after discharge. Inpatients were eligible if they were veterans who were 18 or over, able to understand the description of the study and the informed consent process, eligible to receive VHA health care at the local Veterans Affairs Medical Center or outpatient facilities so they could return for follow-up assessments, clinically cleared to participate (e.g., not aggressive or violent with staff or other patients), had thoughts of suicide, and were not currently psychotic, manic, or demented. The presence of current suicidal ideation was determined with a score over 2 on Beck's Scale for Suicidal Ideation (SSI) (Beck, Kovacs, & Weissman, 1979), which prospectively predicts death by suicide (Brown, Beck, Steer, & Grisham, 2000). Participants received a screening assessment, baseline assessment, one to two MI-SI sessions (depending on their length of stay), a posttreatment assessment, and a 60-day follow-up assessment.

Thirteen veterans were enrolled, 9 (70%) completed both MI-SI sessions and the posttreatment assessment, and 11 (85%) completed the follow-up assessment. Participants who received MI-SI found it acceptable. The mean (SD) CSQ-8 (Client Satisfaction Questionnaire, adapted to assess satisfaction with therapy) score was 3.58 (.40), indicating participants were "3 = mostly satisfied" to "4 = very satisfied" with the intervention. Participants also experienced reductions in the severity of their suicidal ideation with a large pre–post effect size that ranged from 1.66 (using baseline observations carried forward [BOCF] for missing data) to 1.95 (using list-wise deletion [LWD] for participants with missing data). BOCF can underestimate effects, as baseline scores are used to replace missing data (tending to ensure that no change is observed). Conversely, LWD can overestimate effects because patients who are doing poorly are more likely to miss follow-up assessments and as a consequence are deleted from the dataset. Together these two measures may provide a very rough estimate of what the range for the actual effect may be. Additionally, 54% (BOCD) to 64% (LWD) of scores fell below the high-risk threshold of lower than 3 on the SSI at follow-up. All participants attended one mental health or substance abuse treatment session after discharge (indicating initiation of outpatient treatment), and 8 (73%) of the 11 participants with follow-up data completed two or more sessions in each of the 2 months after discharge, indicating engagement in treatment. One patient who was engaged with treatment made a suicide attempt that was interrupted by police after he called 911 for help. These preliminary findings suggest that MI-SI has potential and that a more rigorous trial is needed.

Potential Problems

Not all MI-SI therapy sessions proceed as well as clinicians hope. Some patients have difficulty identifying any motivation to live even after clinicians inquire about their personal values and beliefs, abilities or strengths, accomplishments, or times in their lives when they were happy. With these patients, clinicians can attempt to reframe their problems from a change perspective and ask what would have to change for life to be worth living and what would have to change for that to happen. Patients who are intent on suicide may also require a few days of hospitalization before they are willing to explore their motivation to live. Additionally, some patients may be in so much emotional and/or physical pain that a brief intervention will do little to help them resolve their suicidality. With these patients it may be more helpful to focus on eliciting a commitment to a treatment or treatments that have already been found to be efficacious or to explore the possibility that a yet untried treatment may be helpful. Although it may seem callous to state, clinicians can at least help patients realize that they have to be alive for treatment to work and they should therefore refrain from making an attempt until they have exhausted all of the treatments that may be helpful (Jobes, 2010; Linehan, 1993; Wenzel, Brown, & Beck, 2009).

Conclusions

There is a real scarcity of brief interventions that can be used to reduce high-risk patients' suicide risk and none that takes a motivational approach. Individuals who are motivated to live may be more likely to engage in potentially life-saving activities such as treatment than those who are not motivated to live. The goal of MI-SI is therefore to elicit and reinforce the motivation to live and engage in life-sustaining and life-enhancing activities. Clinicians using MI-SI with patients who are at risk for suicide must take certain precautions. They should not use MI-SI as a stand-alone treatment but as a component of treatment, following a structured risk assessment and followed by additional empirically supported treatments. They should support patients' autonomy whenever possible but be open about their need to take protective action when a patient is determined to be a risk to him- or herself and scrupulously avoid supporting the "right" to suicide. After engaging with the patient, clinicians should start to explore each patient's motivations to live with an empathic question that is cstom-tailored to the patient's experience. When they hear living talk, clinicians should ask for more detail, reflect patients' motivations to live, affirm their reasons for living, and construct summaries that support the living side of the internal struggle. Clinicians should avoid evoking patients' motivations for thinking about suicide as doing so may unnecessarily return them to the suicidal state. When they hear suicide talk, clinicians should reflect it in an empathic way that does not evoke additional suicide talk. After the patient expresses a commitment to living, clinicians should explore the possibility of making a plan to ensure that life remains worth living. Although MI-SI shows promise, rigorous efficacy studies are needed.

Acknowledgments

I would like to thank Kenneth R. Conner, PsyD, MPH, and Stephen A. Maisto, PhD, ABPP, for their support and their invaluable intellectual contributions to the work discussed in this chapter. This work was supported, in part, by a grant from Department of Veterans Affairs, Clinical Science Research and Development (No. IK2CX000641).

References

Anglin, M. D., Hser, Y., & Grella, C. E. (1997). Drug addiction and treatment careers among clients in the drug abuse treatment outcome study (DATOS). *Psychology of Addictive Behaviors, 11*(4), 308–323.

Appleby, L., Shaw, J., Amos, T., McDonnell, R., Harris, C., McCann, K., et al. (1999). Suicide within 12 months of contact with mental health services: National clinical survey. *British Medical Journal, 318*(7193), 1235–1239.

Beck, A. T., Kovacs, M., & Weissman, A. (1979). Assessment of suicidal intention: The scale for suicide ideation. *Journal of Consulting and Clinical Psychology, 47*(2), 343–352.

Bertholet, N., Faouzi, M., Gmel, G., Gaume, J., & Daeppen, J. B. (2010). Change talk sequence during brief motivational intervention, towards or away from drinking. *Addiction, 105*(12), 2106–2112.

Britton, P. C., Connor, K. R., & Maisto, S. A. (2012). An open trial of motivational interviewing to address suicidal ideation with hospitalized veterans. *Journal of Clinical Psychology, 68,* 961–971.

Britton, P. C., Patrick, H., & Williams, G. C. (2011). Motivational interviewing, self-determination theory, and cognitive behavioral therapy to prevent suicidal behavior. *Journal of Cognitive Behavioral Practice, 18*(1), 16–27.

Britton, P. C., Williams, G. C., & Conner, K. R. (2008). Self-determination theory, motivational interviewing, and the treatment of clients with acute suicidal ideation. *Journal of Clinical Psychology, 64*(1), 52–66.

Brown, G. K., Beck, A. T., Steer, R. A., & Grisham, J. R. (2000). Risk factors for suicide in psychiatric outpatients: A 20–year prospective study. *Journal of Consulting and Clinical Psychology, 68*(3), 371–377.

Brown, G. K., Newman, C. F., Charlesworth, S. E., Crits-Christoph, P., & Beck, A. T. (2004). An open clinical trial of cognitive therapy for borderline personality disorder. *Journal of Personality Disorders, 18*(3), 257–271.

Brown, G. K., Steer, R. A., Henriques, G. R., & Beck, A. T. (2005). The internal struggle between the wish to die and the wish to live: A risk factor for suicide. *The American Journal of Psychiatry, 162*(10), 1977–1979.

Carter, G. L., Clover, K., Whyte, I. M., Dawson, A. H., & D'Este, C. (2005). Postcards from the EDge project: Randomised controlled trial of an intervention using postcards to reduce repetition of hospital treated deliberate self poisoning. *BMJ: British Medical Journal, 331*(7520), 805–809.

Carter, G. L., Clover, K., Whyte, I. M., Dawson, A. H., & D'Este, C. (2007). Postcards from the EDge: 24–month outcomes of a randomised controlled trial for hospital-treated self-poisoning. *British Journal of Psychiatry, 191,* 548–553.

Cavanagh, J. T. O., Carson, A. J., Sharpe, M., & Lawrie, S. M. (2003).

Psychological autopsy studies of suicide: A systematic review. *Psychological Medicine, 33*(3), 395–405.

Centers for Disease Control and Prevention. (2014). *Wisqars injury mortality reports 2003–2010.* Available at *www.cdc.gov/injury/wisqars.*

Desai, R. A., Dausey, D., & Rosenheck, R. A. (2008). Suicide among discharged psychiatric inpatients in the department of veterans affairs. *Military Medicine, 173*(8), 721–728.

Filiberti, A., Ripamonti, C., Totis, A., Ventafridda, V., Conno, F., Contiero, P., et al. (2001). Characteristics of terminal cancer patients who committed suicide during a home palliative care program. *Journal of Pain and Symptom Management, 22*(1), 544–553.

Fleischmann, A., Bertolote, J. M., Wasserman, D., De Leo, D., Bolhari, J., Botega, N. J., et al. (2008). Effectiveness of brief intervention and contact for suicide attempters: A randomized controlled trial in five countries. *Bulletin of the World Health Organization, 86*(9), 703–709.

Goldacre, M., Seagroatt, V., & Hawton, K. (1993). Suicide after discharge from psychiatric inpatient care. *Lancet, 342*(8866), 283–286.

Harris, E. C., & Barraclough, B. (1997). Suicide as an outcome for mental disorders: A meta-analysis. *British Journal of Psychiatry, 170*(3), 205–228.

Hemenway, D., & Miller, M. (2002). Association of rates of household handgun ownership, lifetime major depression, and serious suicidal thoughts with rates of suicide across U.S. census regions. *Injury Prevention, 8*(4), 313–316.

Hendin, H., Haas, A. P., Maltsberger, J. T., Koestner, B., & Szanto, K. (2006). Problems in psychotherapy with suicidal patients. *American Journal of Psychiatry, 163*(1), 67–72.

Isometsa, E. T., & Lonnqvist, J. K. (1998). Suicide attempts preceding completed suicide. *British Journal of Psychiatry, 173*, 531–535.

Jobes, D. A. (2010). *Managing suicidal risk: A collaborative approach.* New York: Guilford Press.

Kellermann, A. L., Rivara, F. P., Somes, G., Reay, D. T., Francisco, J., Banton, J. G., et al. (1992). Suicide in the home in relation to gun ownership. *New England Journal of Medicine, 327*(7), 467–472.

Kovacs, M., & Beck, A. T. (1977). The wish to die and the wish to live in attempted suicides. *Journal of Clinical Psychology, 33*(2), 361–365.

Linehan, M. M. (1993). *Cognitive-behavioral treatment of borderline personality disorder.* New York: Guilford Press.

Linehan, M. M., Comtois, K. A., Murray, A. M., Brown, M. Z., Gallop, R. J., Heard, H. L., et al. (2006). Two-year randomized controlled trial and follow-up of dialectical behavior therapy vs therapy by experts for suicidal behaviors and borderline personality disorder. *Archives of General Psychiatry, 63*(7), 757–766.

Linehan, M. M., Goodstein, J. L., Nielsen, S. L., & Chiles, J. A. (1983). Reasons for staying alive when you are thinking of killing yourself: The reasons for living inventory. *Journal of Consulting and Clinical Psychology, 51*(2), 276–286.

Luoma, J. B., Martin, C. E., & Pearson, J. L. (2002). Contact with mental health and primary care providers before suicide: A review of the evidence. *American Journal of Psychiatry, 159*(6), 909–916.

Meehan, J., Kapur, N., Hunt, I. M., Turnbull, P., Robinson, J., Bickley, H., et al. (2006). Suicide in mental health in-patients and within 3 months of discharge: National clinical survey. *British Journal of Psychiatry, 188,* 129–134.

Miller, M., Azrael, D., & Hemenway, D. (2002). Household firearm ownership and suicide rates in the United States. *Epidemiology, 13*(5), 517–524.

Miller, M., & Hemenway, D. (1999). The relationship between firearms and suicide: A review of the literature. *Aggression and Violent Behavior, 4*(1), 59–75.

Miller, W. R., & Rollnick, S. (1991). *Motivational interviewing: Preparing people to change addictive behavior.* New York: Guilford Press.

Miller, W. R., & Rollnick, S. (2002). *Motivational interviewing: Preparing people for change* (2nd ed.). New York: Guilford Press.

Miller, W. R., & Rollnick, S. (2013). *Motivational interviewing: Helping people change* (3rd ed.). New York: Guilford Press.

Miller, W. R., & Rose, G. S. (2009). Toward a theory of motivational interviewing. *American Psychologist, 64*(6), 527–537.

Miller, W. R., & Rose, G. S. (2015). Motivational interviewing and decisional balance: Contrasting responses to client ambivalence. *Behavioral and Cognitive Psychotherapy, 43*(2), 129–141.

Miller, W. R., Walters, S. T., & Bennett, M. E. (2001). How effective is alcoholism treatment in the United States? *Journal of Studies on Alcohol, 62*(2), 211–220.

Motto, J. A., & Bostrom, A. G. (2001). A randomized controlled trial of postcrisis suicide prevention. *Psychiatric Services, 52*(6), 828–833.

Moyers, T. B., Martin, T., Christopher, P. J., Houck, J. M., Tonigan, J. S., & Amrhein, P. C. (2007). Client language as a mediator of motivational interviewing efficacy: Where is the evidence? *Alcoholism: Clinical and Experimental Research, 31*(Suppl. 3), 40S–47S.

Moyers, T. B., Martin, T., Houck, J. M., Christopher, P. J., & Tonigan, J. S. (2009). From in-session behaviors to drinking outcomes: A causal chain for motivational interviewing. *Journal of Consulting and Clinical Psychology, 77*(6), 1113–1124.

Owens, D., Horrocks, J., & House, A. (2002). Fatal and non-fatal repetition of self-harm: Systematic review. *British Journal of Psychiatry, 181,* 193–199.

Qin, P., & Nordentoft, M. (2005). Suicide risk in relation to psychiatric hospitalization: Evidence based on longitudinal registers. *Archives of General Psychiatry, 62*(4), 427–432.

Rudd, M. D., Bryan, C. J., Wertenberger, E., Delano, K., Wilkinson, E., Breitbach, J., et al. (2014, November). *Brief cognitive behavioral therapy for suicidal military personnel: Results of a two-year randomized controlled trial.* Paper presented at the annual meeting of the Association for Behavioral and Cognitive Therapies, Philadelphia, PA.

Rudd, M. D., Mandrusiak, M., & Joiner, T. E. J. (2006). The case against no-suicide contracts: The commitment to treatment statement as a practice alternative. *Journal of Clinical Psychology, 62*(2), 243–251.

Salkovskis, P. M., Atha, C., & Storer, D. (1990). Cognitive-behavioural problem solving in the treatment of patients who repeatedly attempt suicide: A controlled trial. *British Journal of Psychiatry, 157*, 871–876.

Tarrier, N., Taylor, K., & Gooding, P. (2008). Cognitive-behavioral interventions to reduce suicide behavior: A systematic review and meta-analysis. *Behavior Modification, 32*(1), 77–108.

Wenzel, A., Brown, G. K., & Beck, A. T. (2009). Cognitive therapy for suicidal patients with substance dependence disorders. In A. Wenzel, G. K. Brown, & A. T. Beck (Eds.), *Cognitive therapy for suicidal patients: Scientific and clinical applications* (pp. 283–310). Washington, DC: American Psychological Association.

Wiebe, D. J. (2003). Homicide and suicide risks associated with firearms in the home: A national case-control study. *Annals of Emergency Medicine, 41*(6), 771–782.

Yoshimasu, K., Kiyohara, C., & Kazuhisa, M. (2008). Suicidal risk factors and completed suicide: Meta-analyses based on psychological autopsy studies. *Environmental Health and Preventive Medicine, 13*(5), 243–256.

Zerler, H. (2008). Motivational interviewing and suicidality. In H. Arkowitz, H. A. Westra, W. R. Miller, & S. Rollnick (Eds.), *Motivational interviewing in the treatment of psychological problems* (pp. 173–193). New York: Guilford Press.

Zerler, H. (2009). Motivational interviewing in the assessment and management of suicidality. *Journal of Clinical Psychology, 65*(11), 1207–1217.

CHAPTER 9

• • • • • •

Motivational Pharmacotherapy

Combining Motivational Interviewing and Antidepressant Therapy to Improve Treatment Outcomes

Iván C. Balán
Theresa B. Moyers
Roberto Lewis-Fernández

This chapter describes motivational pharmacotherapy (MPT), which was developed by integrating motivational interviewing (MI; Miller & Rollnick, 2013) with psychopharmacotherapy to complete the tasks of antidepressant therapy in an MI-consistent manner. Typical psychopharmacotherapy sessions tend to be brief, focusing on illness history, current symptoms, medication information, and dosing. Although the psychiatrist's demeanor can certainly be warm and pleasant, the interaction is usually dominated by close-ended questions that allow the psychiatrist to quickly assess the patient's current state and to offer treatment. Although treatment adherence is recognized as critical to the effectiveness of pharmacotherapy, it is usually discussed in a simple, didactic, exhortative manner, with a curious lack of emphasis on how to guide the patient to achieve the desired change (i.e., take the medicine).

Clients coming for a psychopharmacotherapy evaluation often experience ambivalence about taking antidepressants. On the one hand, they want to overcome their depression and its impact on their life; on the other, they are concerned about possible side effects, addiction, and cultural taboos about taking psychiatric medication (Vargas et al., in press). In integrating MI into psychopharmacotherapy, our aim was to create an intervention that respected this ambivalence and that, once the ambivalence was overcome, motivated clients to take their medication consistently. Furthermore, we sought to establish a client-centered interaction throughout the treatment to help patients express any concerns or doubts about their care and to encourage them to find solutions together with their psychiatrists, rather than unilaterally deciding to discontinue treatment, thus prolonging their depression.

Consistent with the four processes in MI (engagement, focus, evocation, and planning), MPT is conducted with the spirit of MI, taking time to engage and understand the client in order to provide a sturdy relationship on which to ground the treatment. The focusing process is brief, as patients entering MPT are there specifically to discuss antidepressant therapy. Next, we identify opportunities for evoking change talk during the session. This is often achieved by shaping fact-gathering questions into evocative questions and eliciting from patients the potential benefits of taking antidepressants rather than simply informing them.

Lastly, and very importantly, we want to ensure that treatment planning, such as the decisions to take the medication, change the dose, or switch to a different antidepressant, is made collaboratively. This entails a shift in the traditional roles of pharmacotherapy, where the psychiatrist is the expert and the client accepts the recommendations of the psychiatrist. Instead, we sought to create in both clients and clinicians the acknowledgment of mutual expertise: the psychiatrist's in the medication and the client's in his or her adherence plans, concerns, and bodily reactions to the antidepressant. With this reconceptualization of the relationship, decisions about medication dosing and changes are made jointly, not just by asking the client if the psychiatrist's decision was acceptable but by the psychiatrist sharing treatment options, including their pros and cons, so that the client and psychiatrist can together choose among them.

The Clinical Problem and Relevant Research

Treatment nonadherence represents a major challenge in the pharmacotherapy of psychiatric disorders, whether nonadherence is defined as clients not taking medications as prescribed, missing scheduled appointments, or terminating treatment prematurely. Reviews of full or partial *medication nonadherence* typically show median rates of > 40%

in schizophrenia and bipolar disorder and > 50% in major depressive disorder (MDD) across various treatment durations (Bulloch & Patten, 2010; Velligan et al., 2006, 2010). *Treatment retention* among individuals with MDD, for example, is very low, with 30% of clients on average discontinuing antidepressant therapy after 1 month and 45–60% after 3 months (Velligan et al., 2010), much earlier than recommended by treatment guidelines (American Psychiatric Association Work Group on Major Depressive Disorder, 2010). All aspects of nonadherence typically show worse rates among underserved racial/ethnic groups as compared to non-Latino whites (Harman, Edlund, & Fortney, 2004; Lanouette, Folsom, Sciolla, & Jeste, 2009; Schraufnagel, Wagner, Miranda, & Roy-Byrne, 2006; Warden et al., 2007).

Factors contributing to nonadherence include attitudes and expectations about antidepressant therapy, side effects, poor client–provider relationship, and few perceived benefits or improvement, as well as structural barriers such as cost and availability of treatment (Cabassa, Lester, & Zayas, 2007; Interian et al., 2010; Lanouette et al., 2009; Lingam & Scott, 2002; Mitchell & Selmes, 2007). Although many of these factors can be overcome through better client–provider communication, education about antidepressant therapy, and changes in dosing or medication, most clients who discontinue their antidepressant do so without consulting their provider (Demyttenaere et al., 2001; Maddox, Levi, & Thompson, 1994).

Nonadherence presents a major target for intervention in psychopharmacotherapy because antidepressants are frequently effective when taken properly. For example, the cumulative remission rate in the STAR*D trial, a major study of comparative effectiveness in pharmacotherapy, was 67% if all clients stayed in treatment over a sequence of four treatment steps. Yet, the percentage of clients exiting the protocol after each step was substantial: 20.9% after Step 1, 29.7% after Step 2, and 42.3% after Step 3 (Rush et al., 2006). Irregular medication adherence and early discontinuation among clients with antidepressants are associated with increased recurrence, leading to shorter well intervals, higher severity, lower treatment responsiveness, worsening disability, rehospitalization, and higher health care costs (Edwards, 1998; Melfi et al., 1998; Roy-Byrne, Post, Uhde, Porcu, & Davis, 1986). Since truly innovative psychotropics are still years in the future, a substantial public health benefit could be derived in the meantime from maximizing adherence to existing treatments, including medications.

Considerable attention has been paid, therefore, to interventions that enhance adherence in psychopharmacotherapy. A major barrier to their implementation is that simple adherence interventions are minimally effective and more effective interventions are not simple. Standard psychoeducation, a typically didactic approach in which clients receive treatment information (e.g., duration, side effects), improves adherence only slightly or for a limited period (Zygmunt, Olfson, Boyer, & Mechanic, 2002). More complex approaches, such as adjunctive case management, intensive behavioral interventions, or Assertive Community Treatment teams, are more effective but require substantial investment in ancillary staff, time, and cost, which can limit their implementation, especially in small clinical practices (Haynes, Ackloo, Sahota, McDonald, & Yao, 2008; Kreyenbuhl, Nossell, & Dixon, 2009; Zygmunt et al., 2002). Furthermore, high-resource interventions are unlikely to eliminate racial/ ethnic disparities in care since minority groups usually receive treatment in settings with the highest resource constraints. Moreover, such adherence interventions have rarely been tested with underserved racial/ethnic populations, raising questions about their cross-cultural effectiveness. The need for sustainable, culturally validated, and cost-effective approaches to enhancing adherence in psychopharmacotherapy remains acute.

Curiously, one potentially cost-effective approach to improving adherence that has received only limited attention relies on rethinking the way that psychopharmacotherapy itself is conducted. Adherence-promotion techniques could be integrated throughout the process of care rather than supplementing standard pharmacotherapy with additional interventions by adjunctive personnel. To be widely implementable, however, the intervention would need to avoid complicating or prolonging the medication session beyond what is feasible in a busy pharmacotherapy practice. Thus MI, which has shown efficacy in improving treatment adherence in brief interventions, may be particularly applicable.

Rationale for Using MI in This Context

MI has been effective in enhancing treatment adherence in multiple health conditions, even during brief medical visits (Burke, Arkowitz, & Menchola, 2003; Hettema, Steele, & Miller, 2005; Rubak, Sandbaek, Lauritzen, & Christensen, 2005). In mental health, it has been combined with cognitive-behavioral therapy (CBT) to increase treatment initiation and adherence for various psychiatric problems (Arkowitz, Miller, Rollnick, & Westra, 2008; Arkowitz & Westra, 2009; Westra & Arkowitz, 2011). In psychopharmacotherapy, however, the application of MI remains limited. To date, it has been applied as a stand-alone intervention or in combination with CBT to deliver adjunctive psychotherapy to promote pharmacotherapy adherence in clients with MDD (Interian, Martínez, Iglesias Rios, Krejci, & Guarnaccia, 2010; Interian, Lewis-Fernández, Gara, & Escobar, 2013) and psychotic disorders (Compliance Therapy; Kemp, Kirov, Everitt, Hayward, & David, 1998). These have shown initial efficacy, although replications of compliance therapy have failed to reproduce the original results (Drymalski & Campbell, 2009).

Clinical Applications

This chapter is based on two studies of MPT conducted at the Hispanic Treatment Program of the New York State Psychiatric Institute, an outpatient psychiatry research clinic in a primarily Latino neighborhood in New York City. Participants in both studies were informed that the treatment consisted of antidepressant medication and would be free of charge. During the first study, the intervention was developed and pilot tested in an open trial of 50 Latino outpatients with MDD treated for 12 weeks (Lewis-Fernández et al., 2013). The second study was a randomized clinical trial, which was just completed, comparing MPT to standard pharmacotherapy for MDD. This study was designed to more closely mimic treatment in a typical outpatient setting. Participants were followed for 36 weeks, with visits scheduled first weekly, then biweekly, then monthly for the duration of the study. Participants were not discontinued from the study for missing sessions or for not taking the antidepressant, and they could use the treatment sessions to discuss their ambivalence about antidepressant therapy. Available antidepressants included SSRIs, SNRIs, bupropion, mirtazapine, and nortriptyline; dosing changes and medication switches followed an algorithm designed to mimic standard practice (Crismon et al., 1999); and medications were free of charge. Participants were not offered psychotherapy at the clinic, including from their psychiatrist during sessions; however, those interested were offered referrals for concomitant psychotherapy elsewhere. The case material we present here comes from the treatment of participants in the randomized clinical trial, with verbatim transcriptions translated from the original Spanish.

Development of MPT

We now describe the specific manner in which MI was integrated with standard antidepressant therapy to develop MPT. Our goal is to convey a summary of the intervention training manual that may be useful to clinicians, including case illustrations. First, however, we discuss the cultural and clinical issues that were considered in tailoring the intervention to our study population, namely, low-income, mostly Spanish-monolingual, U.S. Latino outpatients with MDD.

From the outset, we considered what adaptations might be needed to make MPT most efficacious with depressed Latinos. The ease of use across cultures has often been attributed to MI's focus on evocation, reflection, and empathy, which may help bridge cultural differences across clients and providers. Its emphasis on self-efficacy and a strengths-based perspective guides the clinician to evoke solutions to problems from the client instead of recommending solutions, which might otherwise highlight cultural incongruities between clients and clinicians. Furthermore, MI's focus on empathy facilitates the clarification of unexpected culturally specific meanings and their negotiation between client and clinician in order to arrive at a mutual goal. At the same time, however, this emphasis on client-originated solutions, which requires a high level of activity and engagement, could be difficult for depressed clients, whose low mood interferes with energy, motivation, and concentration. Our adaptation of MPT to depressed Latino clients forced us to mediate between these two requirements.

In terms of cultural adaptation, we embedded into MPT what Resnicow, Baranowski, Ahluwalia, and Braithwaite (1999) term "surface-" and "deep-structure" cultural elements. Surface-structure adaptations involved matching intervention materials to the target population, such as conducting the intervention in the preferred language of the client (whether Spanish or English), using the clients' terms when describing depression—such as the Latino idiom for mental distress, "nervios" (nerves; Guarnaccia, Lewis-Fernández, & Rivera, 2003)—and wording session materials in a manner easily understandable to clients with limited health literacy. Conversely, deep-structure adaptations "require an understanding of the cultural, social, historical, environmental, and psychological forces that influence the target health behavior in the proposed target population" (Resnicow et al., 1999, p. 12) and it is these adaptations which are proposed to determine the efficacy of an intervention.

Various deep-structure elements were also embedded in MPT. The content of the handouts used during the sessions (i.e., the list of potential reasons for nonadherence) was derived from the treating psychiatrists' clinical expertise and from the results of our formative qualitative study on treatment adherence and retention among depressed Latino clients

(Lewis-Fernández, 2003). These materials reflect the concerns about antidepressant therapy expressed by Latino clients through their cultural lens. Another deep-structure adaptation involved presenting antidepressant therapy in a manner compatible with many Latino clients' concerns about "medications for *nervios*," (i.e., whether the medication will cause addiction, as only people who are "crazy" take medication for *nervios*) while at the same time complying with approved treatment guidelines for MDD. For instance, we emphasized that minimally effective doses were being prescribed for a minimally effective period in order to reduce the risk of side effects and/or overreliance on medication; we discussed the pros and cons of brief drug holidays (e.g., on some weekends) in responding to clients' impressions that interrupting the medication occasionally encouraged the body to kick-start its own recovery; we encouraged clients' self-coping as a way of achieving the cultural value of *poner de su parte* (doing one's share), thereby decreasing the need for the antidepressant; and we agreed with the hope that someday medication would no longer be needed while also discouraging premature discontinuation (Vargas et al., in press).

Other deep-structure elements incorporated into MPT involved the cultural norms relating to psychiatrist–client interactions. For example, we were concerned that the culturally expected power differential between psychiatrists and clients might lead the latter to limit their expressions of concern or disagreement in order to avoid being "disrespectful" (Laria & Lewis-Fernández, 2006). This deference, in the context of treatment difficulties, often leads clients to discontinue therapy rather than discuss the difficulties with the psychiatrist in order to seek out a mutual solution. As such, the psychiatrist must often work to preempt treatment discontinuation without the benefit of obvious signs of resistance, such as sustain talk or discord, that typically alert a clinician to the possibility that a client is at odds with his or her treatment or the provider. To address this shortcoming, clinicians' elicitation of clients' concerns or obstacles in MPT was typically prefaced by statements such as "Many people have expressed concerns to me about . . . " or by offering handouts about common obstacles to adherence or retention, in order to help normalize and facilitate discussion of these topics.

We also worried that the psychiatrists' collaborative approach, which deemphasizes an expert role, might diminish their standing in the eyes of clients who, from a cultural perspective, expect psychiatrists to provide authoritative answers and recommendations related to their treatment. In MPT, this was dealt with by demarcating the areas of expertise held by both clinicians and clients. When the issue of a client's expectations of the psychiatrist as an "expert" arose—(e.g., "Well, you're the doctor, what do you think I should do?"), psychiatrists would refer to their *mutual* expertise—the clinician as an expert in psychiatric treatment and the client as an expert in his or her personalized health knowledge, expectations, and care-related behavior. The expertise of the psychiatrist was thereby preserved, and the client's position was elevated to that of a true collaborator in the treatment. Using these approaches, we found clients to be verbal and engaged. Nonetheless, the impact of culturally prescribed roles and the expectations of physicians and clients are likely to vary across groups and should be kept in mind when using this intervention with other populations.

In adapting MPT to the clinical requirements of depressed clients, we looked for ways to assist clients in being active during sessions. For example, while one might effectively elicit concerns, values, or obstacles to treatment through dialogue with a client, we found more structured and preprepared materials typical of MI interventions (i.e., lists, bubble sheets, confidence rulers, card sorts—described in later sections) very useful in engaging these clients. Of particular concern was how to foster self-efficacy in clients whose depression might impede it. The confidence-building exercises in the Week 1 session were specifically added for this reason. These exercises, discussed in more detail below, included eliciting from the client a story of success in achieving a goal that appeared unattainable. If clients were unable to come up with an example on their own, the psychiatrist suggested one of several challenges commonly experienced by Latino immigrants (e.g., attaining their goal of reaching the United States). We found that these adaptations were sufficient to promote client participation in the MPT sessions.

Overview of MPT

Typical MPT sessions follow a standard format, which is depicted in Table 9.1. The psychiatrist begins each visit by welcoming the client, affirming the commitment to treatment evidenced by his or her attendance, and suggesting a brief structure for the session. Using open-ended questions, the psychiatrist then inquires about changes the client might have noted in his or her condition, including side effects. Improvements are highlighted through the use of reflections and explored in order to evoke more change talk; lack of improvement or deterioration is reflected empathically and assessed, using open-ended questions and reflections. Medication adherence is also explored and successful adherence highlighted and affirmed, even if suboptimal, in order to help build

TABLE 9.1. Outline of Motivational Pharmacotherapy Sessions

1. Welcome the patient to session.
   a. Affirm the patient's commitment to getting better.
   b. Explain the structure for session.

2. Discuss the patient's state/symptoms.
   a. Assess symptoms/side effects, primarily using open-ended questions and reflections.
   b. Improvements in state are reflected and explored to elicit more change talk.

3. Assess treatment adherence.
   a. Focus on adherence successes to build self-efficacy.
   b. Collaboratively identify ways of overcoming obstacles to adherence.

4. Use MI techniques to elicit change talk and commitment language (early sessions).
   a. Goals and values card sort (Week 0).
   b. Confidence ruler and story of overcoming obstacles (Week 1).

5. Elicit and resolve obstacles to treatment (midtreatment).
   a. Obstacles to adherence bubble sheet (Week 4).
   b. Thoughts about early termination from treatment (Week 8).

6. Review medication dosage and treatment plan.
   a. Collaboratively reach decisions about treatment.

self-efficacy in relation to treatment adherence. The client is then typically asked to describe what steps or supports enabled him or her to adhere to the treatment (e.g., "I put the pills where I can't miss them every morning," "My husband helps me to remember"). Then, obstacles to adherence are elicited and followed by a discussion of strategies to overcome them. To foster self-efficacy, clients are first asked for their own strategies before any additional solutions are proposed by the clinician. Sessions end with a review of the treatment regimen and a joint decision about any treatment changes that might be warranted. The exact order of the steps varies somewhat according to clients' priorities during the session. Below, we provide a transcript that illustrates the opening exchanges of a typical Week 2 session.

PSYCHIATRIST: I am glad to see you, this is the third time we meet like this—which is great! Now we have the opportunity to continue talking about the treatment, how things are going with the medication, what you think about the medication, any obstacle that might have come up in relation to taking the medication, and seeing how we might overcome those obstacles. How does that sound?

CLIENT: That's fine.

PSYCHIATRIST: Tell me, how have you been since we last saw each other?

CLIENT: Really, until now, everything has been going pretty well. I have been feeling better, and it looks like the medicine is helping me a lot, with more energy, and it's helping me be more motivated than before.

PSYCHIATRIST: Really? What do you notice?

CLIENT: It's helping me a lot, actually, with things that I had not been able to do before. I am taking computer classes and classes for my GED so that I can take the exam . . . I want to do more with my life. Before, I hadn't been able to do that. I tried a few times, but because of the same problem [depression] I couldn't motivate myself to do it, but now, I feel more motivated.

PSYCHIATRIST: Good! So the motivation has increased so much that you have even taken this step. What helped you make this decision?

CLIENT: I had always wanted to. I had tried to do the GED course before but never got to do it because by the time the date arrived I would feel depressed and would want to stay home, not care about anything, it would really affect me—but now I am feeling good.

PSYCHIATRIST: Good! And what has helped you continue with your treatment?

CLIENT: The improvement I see, I am getting better—until now the treatment hasn't affected me in the least . . .

PSYCHIATRIST: You haven't noticed *any* problem with the treatment.

CLIENT: No, no problems.

PSYCHIATRIST: Good, that's great. You notice more energy, more concentration, you were telling me . . .

CLIENT: More concentration, like I see things more realistically now, I see things more positively than how I saw them before—things or problems that were really insignificant, and I gave them such importance. Now I see the situation a different way and even laugh about how I would give such importance to things that don't deserve it.

PSYCHIATRIST: Wow! Now you have a much broader perspective . . .

CLIENT: The way I think about things now is very different from how I used to think before.

PSYCHIATRIST: How has it changed?

CLIENT: I see things in a more grounded way—more realistically—is what I have noticed. I see things more naturally, I see that some things really aren't important.

PSYCHIATRIST: Wow, those are some pretty important changes!

CLIENT: It's as if they had taken everything off me, all the negative things. I hope it continues . . .

PSYCHIATRIST: The negative things are gone . . . is what you are saying . . .

CLIENT: Yes, I don't have them anymore.

PSYCHIATRIST: Good, good.

CLIENT: And another thing I have really noticed is that the fears I had have disappeared, I mean, I don't feel those fears anymore.

PSYCHIATRIST: That sounds great! So, how has it been for you taking your medication regularly?

CLIENT: I am taking it at the same time, always. I started thinking, what is a good time to take the medication? What time do I go to sleep? At what time do I get hungry? And I think it's a good time for me to take the medication.

PSYCHIATRIST: You have established a routine for yourself. Do you have any concerns or questions about the pills, any obstacle that interferes with you taking it?

CLIENT: No.

PSYCHIATRIST: None.

CLIENT: No.

PSYCHIATRIST: Well, if at any point any questions arise . . .

CLIENT: Yes, if I see anything or have any questions about the treatment, I will let you know right away.

PSYCHIATRIST: Perfect.

Throughout, the psychiatrist conducting MPT works collaboratively with the client to identify and overcome any obstacles to treatment adherence and retention that may arise. The main methods used to achieve these goals are open-ended questions, affirmations, reflections, and summaries. Close-ended questions and didactic exhortations are generally avoided as much as possible because they tend to disrupt the client's momentum by turning attention to the clinician as the center of the session, either as the expert in charge of gathering the information in order to reach a conclusion or as the primary holder of motivation for why treatment is needed. Of course, some clinical situations require the psychiatrist to move away from the specific task of building motivation in order to address a critical issue such as suicidal or homicidal ideation or to assess for potentially dangerous side effects (e.g., rash). At these times, the psychiatrist follows a technique of "bracketing," specifically stating the need to explore in more detail what the client is reporting before proceeding with the rest of the session. The clinician then conducts the necessary assessment and "closes" the bracketed period by acknowledging the client for the valuable information provided. When it becomes necessary to adjust or switch medication over the course of treatment, the clinician works collaboratively with the client to reach decisions about changes in medication dosage or type. After obtaining permission from the client to offer options or suggestions, the clinician presents the client with several alternatives to address the situation (i.e., wait another week to see if there will be greater improvement, increase the dose, or switch to another medication). In effect, the psychiatrists share with the clients their own thinking about possible next steps and invite the clients to suggest their own treatment modifications. The scenario below is a particularly interesting example of this approach, as it depicts a patient who, when offered treatment options, opts for a more aggressive approach than the psychiatrist.

The client comes to the Week 4 visit complaining about troublesome headaches over the past 2 weeks. So far, he has had minimal improvement in his depressive symptoms and attributes the headaches to a side effect of the increase in sertraline dose to 75mg 2 weeks earlier. Below, the clinician and the client discuss possible steps to deal with the headaches. Although the client does not express ambivalence about continuing in treatment, this combination of minimal improvement and bothersome side effects suggests high risk of treatment discontinuation. In such situations, psychiatrists tend to favor a more cautious approach to treatment in order to minimize discomfort from side effects and the potential for early treatment discontinuation.

PSYCHIATRIST: So, you have been at 75 mg these 2 weeks and we have various alternatives, and I would like to discuss them with you to see what you think. One idea is to keep the medication at 75 mg another 2 weeks, see how things go, and see if, even though you are having the headaches, they are decreasing. The other is that we can reduce the medicine to 50 mg, and the other alternative is that we raise the medication a little bit to 100 mg, which would be two 50-mg tablets. Remember that I am the expert in medications but you are the expert in your body, and you are the one who is feeling these things and you decide if you are willing to tolerate more or less of what you are feeling. What are you thinking? What are your ideas about this?

CLIENT: Well, yesterday and today I took the medication, and the headache is a little . . .

PSYCHIATRIST: It's disappearing, it's less now.

CLIENT: . . . like if the pill, the body is adapting.

PSYCHIATRIST: It has adapted a bit better. So, how does that affect your decision—would you like to keep it at 75 mg or raise it a little bit? What would you like?

CLIENT: I would like you to raise it to 100 mg. I think that's better.

PSYCHIATRIST: Yes, we can do that. Remember, if anything happens during the week, give me a call, and I would be happy to help you deal with it. And if you see that you cannot tolerate the 100 mg, drop it to 75 mg. As you said you observed at the beginning, there are some side effects and after some time they diminish. So, what do you think? We do that then?

CLIENT: Yes, of course.

PSYCHIATRIST: Fine, then let's raise it to 100 mg. And we can wait and see what happens over the next 2 weeks, although—remember—if you need to, call me before our next appointment.

The format of these "typical" MPT sessions is augmented in Weeks 0, 1, 4, and 8 with a more structured series of processes and tasks to yield four "enhanced" sessions. These additional techniques address key reasons for nonadherence in antidepressant trials (Demyttenaere, 1997, 1998; Pekarik, 1992) and were placed early in the treatment process in order to build and maintain the client's motivation to begin a course of antidepressant medication. The timing of these "enhanced" sessions also allowed us to target adherence concerns and behavior prior to the biggest wave of discontinuation from mental health treatment, which comes after the first or second session in the general population, with Latino ethnicity particularly associated with nonretention after three or more visits (Olfson et al., 2009). The enhanced sessions are described in more detail below.

Week 0: Building Motivation to Change and Addressing Obstacles to Change

The specific objective of this session is for the client to decide to begin antidepressant therapy. This first session begins by affirming the client's attendance and briefly presenting what the session entails, ending with a question to the client about what he or she thought of the plan for the session. After exploring how the depression has been affecting the client's life, the psychiatrist inquires about any concerns the client has about taking antidepressants. If the client is hesitant to report any, the psychiatrist presents those typically expressed by other clients in order to normalize having concerns and facilitate their expression during the session. The specific concerns suggested by the clinician were drawn from previous research with depressed Latinos at our clinic and include "Antidepressants are addictive," "Taking medicines harms the body," and "Taking medication means the person is crazy" (Vargas et al., in press). Also helpful in eliciting concerns is beginning the inquiry indirectly by asking about what the client has heard from others about antidepressants, with this serving as an effort to reduce the client's anxiety about challenging the psychiatrist early on. Framing this question about "medicines for *nervios* [nerves]" instead of "antidepressants" is particularly useful for clients who are less familiar with biomedical terminology. To prevent the discussion of concerns from overwhelming the session, a list of concerns is generated at the beginning of the session but addressed later, just prior to discussing whether the client will begin treatment.

At this point, the focus of the session shifts to building an awareness of the importance of entering treatment. The approach used is to explore important values in a client's life and how these values have been affected by the depression (Miller & Rollnick, 2013). These value explorations can be a powerful way to accentuate the discrepancy between the client's current state and how he or she wishes to be (Grube, Rankin, Greenstein, & Kearney, 1977; Rokeach, 1973; Schwartz & Inbar-Saban, 1988). Values "card sorts" have often been used in MI to facilitate the exploration of values and elicit change talk (Graeber, Moyers, Griffith, Guajardo, & Tonigan, 2003; Miller, C'de Baca, Matthews, & Wilbourne, 2001; Moyers & Martino, 2006). In MPT, clients are handed a deck of 24 cards with a single value listed on each card (including two blank cards enabling the client to identify personal values not included in the deck) and asked to select the three most important values. The actual values were derived from our clinical experience with

Latino clients and included a range of life areas, such as "Being a good mother," "Not losing hope," "Supporting my family in my country," "Working," and "Devotion to God." The psychiatrist evokes an account of the importance of these values and selectively reflects statements to accentuate their importance in the client's life prior to the onset of the depression. Once the chosen values are explored, the clinician summarizes the discussion and asks how the depression has affected the client's ability to live by and pursue those values. The desired discrepancy is created as the client experiences the gap between his or her current condition and where he or she would like to be. For example:

> "I see that for you there are numerous things that are important to you related to your family, to being calm, to being happy and not losing hope, and with going to church and raising your children in a Christian way. How has your depression affected those things—the caring for your children, not losing hope, those things?"

Having set the stage by accentuating the sense of discrepancy for the client and identifying the depression as its source, the psychiatrist then follows up with a key question about the client's plans to cope with the situation. This question usually is: "So, what do you make of all this?" or "So, what do you think you need to do now?" Since the values exercise has typically built the importance of overcoming the depression and the client is attending the first session of a treatment based on antidepressants, responses to this question often focus on *needing* (an example of change talk) to do something about the depression, including a comment about "giving this medicine a chance." The psychiatrist then responds to these statements with reflections in order to highlight and magnify the client's decision to change (e.g., "You really are fed up with the problems the depression is causing for you, and you are willing to try a new way of coping with it").

Once some motivation to enter treatment begins to emerge, the psychiatrist addresses the concerns about antidepressant therapy expressed earlier in the session. Consistent with an MI style, the psychiatrist uses an elicit (concerns about treatment)–provide (information about treatment)–elicit (reaction from client) approach in order to personalize information or recommendations to address a client's specific concerns and to maintain a collaborative relationship. This approach also avoids giving information that is already known. When necessary, the psychiatrist also asks permission to offer information about MDD, antidepressants, and how other clients have dealt with similar concerns. Once this step is completed, the focus shifts to providing the client with information about his or her own antidepressant therapy (i.e., choice of medication, dosing, frequency, speed of effect). In order to retain engagement in this discussion, after every two to three points the psychiatrist asks the client for feedback and whether he or she wants more information. Clients are also handed an information sheet with frequently asked questions about antidepressants and given the option of reviewing these on their own after the session. The interactions and decisions about treatment are framed collaboratively, with the psychiatrist explicitly stating that it is the client's decision whether to begin treatment and that decisions as to changes in dosing or medications will be made jointly. Clients who express their willingness to start antidepressant therapy are given the study medication; those who remain ambivalent are asked to return to the next appointment to continue discussing treatment options. The session ends with a general prophylactic statement about clients who, at times, decide not to continue with treatment after leaving the session. Even if the client discontinues the medication, he or she is asked to return for the next appointment in order to discuss what led to this decision.

Week 1: Building Confidence to Adhere to Treatment

The second session focuses on building confidence and self-efficacy toward treatment retention and medication adherence. It also continues to address a second goal in MI, reducing obstacles to change, and introduces a third goal, maintaining motivation to change.

Following the standard opening previously described, the focus shifts to two exercises. The first, a confidence ruler (Rollnick, Butler, & Mason, 1999), asks clients about adherence: "On a scale of 0 to 10, where 0 is not confident at all and 10 is very confident, how confident are you that you could take this medication daily?" The follow-up question, "Why is it a [client's number] and not a 0?," elicits from the client statements of self-confidence and commitment to the treatment (i.e., "Because I have gotten through worse," "Because I take my other medications every day," "Because I know that once I set my mind to something I do it"). Only then does the psychiatrist ask the client what it would take to move him or her from the chosen number up a couple of numbers. This is often helpful in identifying other obstacles to medication adherence that can be subsequently addressed.

The second confidence-building exercise asks the client about a success story, but with a twist. Clients are asked to recall a challenge they were unsure of accomplishing at first but which turned out well because of their perseverance. Clients unable to provide an example are asked about situations common to this client population, such as obstacles encountered in the process of migration or challenges in raising their children with limited resources in often dangerous inner-city environments. Throughout the story, psychiatrists selectively reflect statements of self-confidence and determination and explore what clients did when they lost hope of achieving their goal. The purpose of the exercise is to help clients recognize their perseverance in the face of challenges, which can easily be overlooked amid one's depression. The exercise ends with the psychiatrist linking the client's perseverance in that successful past situation with the expected positive effect of persevering in treatment in order to overcome his or her depression. The rest of the session follows the typical format of MPT sessions.

Week 4: Maintaining Commitment and Addressing Obstacles to Treatment Adherence

The goal of this session is to maintain motivation to change by reviewing the client's progress and reinforcing his or her commitment to change. The session also focuses on exploring and overcoming obstacles to treatment adherence.

Only one additional procedure is added to the typical MPT format in this session. During the discussion of medication adherence, the client is presented with a list of 21 obstacles, written in individual bubbles, which were culled from our formative work with depressed Latinos (Lewis-Fernández, 2003). Using a list normalizes the presence of obstacles by indicating that others have faced similar difficulties. This procedure helps the client express the obstacles affecting him or her and work collaboratively with the psychiatrist to overcome them and remain in treatment. Items include "I don't want people to think I am crazy," "I forget to take the pills," "They have too many side effects," and a blank bubble for other unlisted concerns that are then identified. The obstacles identified are then problem-solved collaboratively, first by evoking solutions from the client and then by supplementing these solutions if necessary through the elicit–provide–elicit approach. Clients who do not report any obstacles are affirmed for their commitment to treatment and invited to raise future obstacles as needed during subsequent sessions.

Week 8: Maintaining Commitment and Addressing Obstacles to Treatment Completion

The final enhanced session focuses on reinforcing the client's commitment to change by celebrating his or her achievements and success at tackling obstacles to treatment adherence and retention. These goals are achieved through two exercises.

First, the psychiatrist again checks in with the client about possible obstacles to continuing in treatment, using a list of 14 obstacles that are prominent during the middle stages of treatment, typically after the onset of improvement. We compiled the list from our formative work with this population, with such obstacles including: "I don't want to be addicted to the pills," "I feel better already," "Stopping the pills would tell me if I still need them," as well as a blank statement ("_____") to be filled in by the client for concerns not specifically listed. The client is then asked about his or her thoughts regarding premature termination to address any concerns that might interfere with the guideline-concordant duration of care for that client. As in Week 4, clients who do not express concerns are invited to raise them anytime in the future as needed. Although evoking potential obstacles to treatment continuation with clients who are adherent appears inconsistent with MI, we wanted to facilitate and normalize this type of discussion so that, if thoughts of discontinuing treatment arose in the future, the clients would feel comfortable raising them on their own before taking action.

The second exercise focuses on emphasizing the discrepancy between clients' current state and their baseline condition in order to reinforce commitment to the treatment and maintain motivation to change. Clients are asked about two things: (1) how things have changed since the onset of treatment and (2) how they currently view the future as compared to their baseline visit. In the ensuing conversation, the clinician selectively reflects and explores change talk in order to link the person's improvement with his or her participation in antidepressant therapy and thereby maximize adherence. The exercise ends with the psychiatrist's providing a summary of the changes the client has reported and offering affirmation for his or her sustained commitment to treatment.

Thoughts about premature termination are frequently reported during this MPT session, including but not exclusively in response to the list of potential concerns presented at the beginning of the session. Often these thoughts are related to the onset of initial improvement. Below, we illustrate how a psychiatrist negotiated a client's decision to terminate treatment prematurely at Week 20. MPT allowed the psychiatrist to disagree with the client's decision while also reinforcing the latter's role in decision making. Through an MI-consistent approach, the client and the clinician were able to reach a joint solution that reduced the client's ambivalence and allowed him to remain in treatment.

After achieving substantial improvement on 25 mg of sertraline during the first weeks of treatment, a client's baseline symptoms of depression and anxiety reemerged between Weeks 8 and 16. The client and the psychiatrist decided to increase the dose to 50 mg during their Week 16 visit, to consolidate treatment gains. The client then returned for his session in Week 20 reporting headaches, nausea, heart palpitations, and diarrhea for 4–5 days after taking the increased dose. He had reduced the dosage on his own to 25 mg, but (given the improvement in symptoms he had already sustained) the client concluded that his body was rejecting the medication and discontinued sertraline 5 days before the Week 20 visit, insisting he could not take this medication or any of the other antidepressants in the study. He was attending the session to inform the psychiatrist about what he had done. After exploring the client's decision and empathically reflecting the client's experience, the psychiatrist (in the transcript below) reaffirms the client's autonomy in deciding to take medication and moves to establish a plan:

PSYCHIATRIST: So, what would your plan be—what would be the next step?

CLIENT: You are the doctor, so you decide . . . and we had decided that I would take the medication for the next 9 months, but since I had to stop the medication—not because I wanted to but because my body was rejecting it—I would like to continue with the treatment for the 9 months and see how my body is doing without the medication during these 3 months. I don't know if you would be in agreement with that.

PSYCHIATRIST: So continuing to come, but evaluating the need for the medication; not necessarily taking it, but evaluating how you continue without it and seeing if there is a need for change.

CLIENT: If you want to, you can even give me the medications, though I wouldn't take it. And if there is a problem, I would have it there . . .

PSYCHIATRIST: To take.

CLIENT: Yes, to take if anything happens. But more than anything I would like you to do an evaluation of these 3 months to see what is my reaction to not taking the medication.

PSYCHIATRIST: What you propose is interesting. I understand that it's like an extended evaluation, like continuing to evaluate you without necessarily taking the pill, depending on what happens. I think it is fine. It's a process during which we evaluate jointly what needs to be done.

CLIENT: You are the specialist here, and you are the one that knows much more about these things.

PSYCHIATRIST: I think this is fine in principle. Let me tell you what I am thinking, and we can talk about it, OK? The positive aspect of what you are proposing is that we can evaluate your situation without you necessarily taking the pill. Nobody would be forcing you to take something that your body is telling you that it—at this specific time—shouldn't take. . . . The advantage to this is that we can continue to evaluate you without you having to take the medicine, and that might be the most advantageous thing for you, since your body is sending you a message.

CLIENT: Because in reality, if I have been with this treatment so long, I would like you to continue treating me in this manner and see what happens.

PSYCHIATRIST: Yes, I think that is perfectly fine. The concern that I have—and it's a concern that we can talk about and don't have to reach a decision about today—is that there is a risk that the depression might return more quickly if you take the medication for less time. That is, you have been taking the medication for a few months, and that is good, you have that treatment in your body, no one can take that from you, and it might be sufficient to protect you.

CLIENT: It's 6 months since I have been taking the medication, and I think that if I would have taken the medication for 9 months it would have been much better for me—but in this case it's not me who is making the decision.

PSYCHIATRIST: Yes, it's your body.

CLIENT: Yes, my body, and if I continue taking medication it can have consequences—be it headaches or vomiting—that could start.

PSYCHIATRIST: I understand. The only thing I might add is that possibility of a slightly higher risk that the depression might return. On the one hand, stopping the medication will not do anything to your body and, on the other hand, is the slightly higher risk that the depression might return. That is the balance that we have to consider. And, really my role is to provide you with information so we both have the information that is necessary to make a decision.

CLIENT: If it were for me . . . I am supposed to take the medication longer, and if it were possible, I would continue to do so. But in reality—maybe it sounds illogical—but really it's my body that is rejecting the medication.

PSYCHIATRIST: No, I hear that, that is very clear. How about if we do the following, because I like your plan. We are in agreement about you staying in treatment for 9 months, evaluating you and seeing you. What we would do during the visits is ask you how you are doing and, based on that, decide if it's worth trying to start the medication again or not. And we continue another month with that decision, and in the following visit we do the same and we continue that way. How does that sound?

CLIENT: Yes, yes.

PSYCHIATRIST: And if that is what happens for the next 3 months, fine— you don't restart it. If there is a change . . . we'll decide on a month-to-month basis. I can even give you some medication in case you decide you want to take some so you have them available—if not, no. Like you suggested, having them there just in case.

CLIENT: Yes, I actually brought back the pills I didn't take, so I can take those back with me. I don't like to take medication unless I have to, and right now I don't need them.

PSYCHIATRIST: And really, you are telling me that you are feeling really well right now . . .

CLIENT: Yes, I feel well—like I told you earlier, it's like I feel strong, positive, so I don't think I will need the medication right now. But, as you say, maybe in the future I might relapse.

PSYCHIATRIST: Well, but I think it is fine for us to continue talking about it and without any pressure that you should do one thing or another, we can do whatever we think will work.

CLIENT: No, I really want to keep coming here, and I am hoping that my decision to stop taking the medication will not change anything in the treatment.

PSYCHIATRIST: I agree, the idea is to continue with the treatment. Perfect. Let's do that.

Subsequently, the client asked the psychiatrist about how the antidepressant works in the body and how long the medication would remain in his system, questions that the psychiatrist answered. Although the psychiatrist took time to understand the client's experience and his ambivalence about continuing to take the medication, the whole session lasted only 19:58 minutes. The client returned for his session on Week 24 reporting that, 10 days after his previous session, he restarted the 25 mg of sertraline after the depressive symptoms reemerged. He continued to take the medication with sustained improvement and completed all 36 weeks of treatment.

MPT demonstrates how MI can be embedded into psychopharmacotherapy in order to address ambivalence about medication adherence in a manner that is feasible in clinical practice. This integration results in a substantially different approach to interacting with mental health clients during medication treatment. In our experience, MPT results in a client–clinician interaction that is more client-centered, collaborative, and personalized than standard psychopharmacotherapy. One major contribution of MI to pharmacotherapy is how it recasts the relationship between the clinician and the client as one of equal experts who explore together what course to follow. Whereas clinicians are experts in antidepressant therapy, clients are experts in their treatment expectations, subjective medication effects, barriers to treatment, and capacities to overcome these barriers. Within the MI framework, clients' expertise is even more crucial to the success of the therapy, since the decision whether to adhere to the treatment ultimately rests with them. Second, MI brings to pharmacotherapy its emphasis on basic counseling skills (i.e., open-ended questions, affirmations, reflections, and summaries) during the pharmacotherapy encounter. This contribution reshapes the interaction from one focused primarily on assessing and prescribing to one centered on understanding the client's experience with the treatment and responding accordingly. Such an approach fosters improved communication and engagement between clinician and client and also enables the clinician to more fully understand the obstacles to adherence that may arise as well as the personal strengths that the client brings to the therapy that can be used to overcome these obstacles.

Third, MI contributes to pharmacotherapy a strong focus on fostering in clients a desire to overcome their depression through antidepressant therapy as well as a belief in their ability to overcome barriers to achieve their desired goal. In MPT, the clinician becomes attuned to the stream of change talk in order to gauge and influence the momentum of the session. This is not a primary focus of standard pharmacotherapy sessions, where the emphasis is placed instead on illness history, current symptoms, side effects, adherence to dosing, and so on. By contrast, in MPT the psychiatrist tends to spend less time pursuing multiple details about symptom changes, for example, and more time managing the client's motivation, obstacles to adherence, and strategies to enhance it. This means the psychiatrist has to trust that, by inquiring generally about the client's condition, he or she will raise important symptoms, side effects, and concerns, and that only occasionally will a more detailed assessment be necessary. In many practitioners, this may raise concerns about missing some basic information, and the psychiatrists in our trial faced this worry during the development of MPT. Yet, it is important to balance this concern with the realization that by over-focusing on symptom elicitation the client may be lost to early termination. In effect, MPT does not consist of *adding* a series of MI techniques to what occurs in the standard pharmacotherapy sessions; instead, MPT requires that the pharmacotherapist *limit* some of the typical approaches used during these sessions and replace them with an interaction that is more consistent with MI. In so doing, the length of these sessions remains comparable to that of standard pharmacotherapy and compatible with routine psychiatric practice (Lewis-Fernández et al., 2013).

Research Findings

Findings from our pilot study showed that only 20% of the 50 first-generation Latino clients with MDD in the study discontinued treatment by Week 12, with a mean therapy duration of 74.2 out of 84 days. Clients' symptoms, psychosocial functioning, and quality of life improved significantly. After 12 weeks of treatment, 82% of clients were considered "responders" (defined as a ≥ 50% drop in depression symptoms) and 68% "remitters" (responders with a final symptom score in the normal range). Compared to published Latino proportions of nonretention (32–53%) and previous studies at our clinic with similar samples and medications using standard psychopharmacotherapy (36–46%), these findings suggest that MPT may be effective in reducing treatment nonretention among depressed Latino clients who seek antidepressant therapy. Data analysis of the randomized clinical trial comparing MPT to standard antidepressant therapy is now in progress.

Another MI-based approach to improving antidepressant adherence that is called motivational enhancement therapy for antidepressants (META) uses psychotherapists to deliver the intervention (Interian et al., 2010, 2013) rather than targeting the behavior of the prescribers themselves. META is a three 60-minute-session intervention that was developed through an iterative process that identified Latino cultural values and beliefs that could affect antidepressant adherence and incorporated these into the intervention (Interian et al., 2010). While empathizing with participants' concerns about antidepressant therapy, META also evokes their motivation to overcome the depression. Specific components include providing targeted antidepressant information, nonjudgmental sharing of adherence feedback, exploring previous episodes of nonadherence, anticipating and problem-solving potential barriers to future adherence, and sending a written adherence plan by mail.

In the pilot study assessing the efficacy of the intervention, participants were randomized to usual care (UC) or usual care plus META (Interian et al., 2013). Two META sessions were provided between the baseline and the 5-week assessments, with a booster session between the 5-week and 5-month assessments. Study participants received naturalistic psychopharmacologic/psychotherapeutic care from their usual providers, whose content was not altered for the study. META participants showed significantly higher antidepressant adherence than UC clients at 5 weeks (72.9% vs. 40.8%; $p < .01$) and 5 months (61.5% vs. 31.7%; $p < .01$). At 5 months, half of the META participants achieved symptom remission based on the Beck Depression Inventory–II, compared to only 20.8% of usual care participants. Thus, META appears to be another promising MI-based approach to improving antidepressant adherence.

Potential Problems

While MI approaches to improving retention and adherence in antidepressant therapy appear promising, study results to date also highlight that these interventions are not successful for all clients. Clearly there is a need to understand for whom MPT and META are most helpful, but we also need to understand for whom they are not and, potentially, for whom these approaches may be contraindicated.

A second challenge focuses on who would provide the intervention. The two interventions discussed offer different approaches, each with their pros and cons. A benefit of MPT is that it does not require visits with other mental health professionals since it is conducted by the prescriber him- or herself. This also allows the prescriber to continually assess the client's motivation to remain in treatment throughout the course of pharmacotherapy and immediately address concerns that might otherwise lead the client to premature discontinuation. However, the typical 2–3 days of training plus follow-up coaching that were used to develop expertise in MPT may not be feasible in all settings, especially in community mental health centers, where psychiatrists face substantial clinical responsibilities and resource limitations. It is possible that in some settings the use of adjunct providers to conduct the motivational intervention (as was done with META) may be more feasible. However, META has only been tested with doctoral-level psychologists, who are also frequently unavailable in low-resource settings. Research has shown that MI can be learned by providers with a wide range of formal training in psychotherapy and counseling. One possible future step for META is to test its feasibility and effectiveness among providers with less formal clinical training.

Lastly, the psychiatrists who provided MPT found it to be a significant shift in the way psychopharmacotherapy sessions are conducted. Not all clinicians will necessarily be comfortable with this approach, especially in terms of its emphasis on client autonomy. With depressed clients, we saw this discomfort manifested in two ways. First, it resulted in clinicians' providing less information than usual when prescribing medication, which occurs when clients answer "no" when asked by the provider whether they want additional information about the medication. Second, it more explicitly leaves the decision whether or not to take medication in the hands of the client. This challenge may be particularly difficult with certain client populations, such as those who are psychotic or suicidal, and may be perceived as colluding with a potentially very negative outcome. Psychiatrists also had to adapt to not assessing many specific symptoms at every visit and to trusting that open-ended questions would reveal the client's condition sufficiently to evoke critical information.

Conclusions

Both MPT and META appear to be promising interventions for improving adherence and retention in antidepressant therapy. Although the interventions vary in their structure and their provider, MI clearly informs them both, as can be seen in the greater focus on empathic attunement to the client's concerns about medications, the use of values to build motivation, and the personalized approach to providing information about antidepressants. This MI-consistent framework stands in sharp contrast to what is typically done to encourage clients to take antidepressants, where a prescriber, in an expert role, exhorts the client about the benefits of the medication to convince him or her to initiate treatment. Concerns and expectations about medication are often minimized as obstacles that can be easily overcome and should not be allowed to impede medication taking. While this approach may be sufficient for some clients considering antidepressants, MPT and META have the potential to improve treatment adherence, retention, and other clinical outcomes among a broader segment of clients prescribed antidepressants who might benefit from a more nuanced discussion that considers their concerns as well as the potential benefits of the medication.

A natural next step for META and MPT is to assess their effect on treatment adherence and retention in other clinical and cultural populations. MI has been used to augment engagement in psychotherapy and pharmacotherapy among clients with anxiety disorders and schizophrenia (Drymalski & Campbell, 2009; Graeber et al., 2003; Merlo et al., 2010; Simpson et al., 2010; Westra, Arkowitz, & Dozois, 2009), and these interventions may inform us as to how best to adapt MPT and META to these populations.

It is not surprising that both MPT and META proved amenable to cultural tailoring to first-generation Latinos, as MI is currently used throughout the world, and research has shown it to be effective across diverse cultures and social groups (Hettema et al., 2005). This experience suggests that META and MPT would be amenable to tailoring to other cultural groups. It is important to note that research applications of both interventions had the luxury of ethnic matching between clients and providers, something that is often not possible in community clinical settings. More research is needed on how MI processes may differ in culturally matched versus nonmatched interactions as well as on the added value of formal cultural tailoring of MI interventions to specific cultural groups.

Lastly, a study comparing MPT and META would also be very valuable, especially in identifying which clients might benefit the most from each of the approaches as well as to formally study the challenges of implementing the interventions in community clinical settings.

While the efficacy of MPT in improving treatment retention and adherence among depressed Latinos awaits the completion of the current randomized clinical trial, and META has only been studied in a pilot trial, our experience to date suggests that both MI-based interventions may be valuable tools in helping clients engage in pharmacotherapy. This would greatly facilitate their ability to participate in an efficacious treatment that is likely to result in symptomatic and functional improvement.

Acknowledgments

This project was directly supported by Research Grant Nos. R21 MH 066388 and R01 MH 077226 from the National Institute of Mental Health. Study medication (sertraline) and additional financial support were provided by Pfizer, Inc. The studies were supported in part by institutional funds from New York State Psychiatric Institute (to Roberto Lewis-Fernández). Portions of this chapter were previously published in Balán, I., Moyers, T., & Lewis-Fernández, R. (2013). Motivational pharmacotherapy: Combining motivational interviewing and antidepressant therapy to improve treatment adherence. *Psychiatry: Interpersonal and Biological Processes, 76*(3), 203–209. Copyright 2013 by Taylor & Francis. Reprinted by permission of Taylor & Francis and The Washington School of Psychiatry.

References

Alegría, M., Atkins, M., Farmer, E., Slaton, E., & Stelk, W. (2010). One size does not fit all: Taking diversity, culture, and context seriously. *Administration and Policy in Mental Health, 37*, 48–60.

American Psychiatric Association Work Group on Major Depressive Disorder. (2010). Practice guideline for the treatment of clients with major depressive disorder, 3rd edition. *American Journal of Psychiatry, 167*, S1–S118.

Arkowitz, H., Miller, W. R., Rollnick, S., & Westra, H. (2008). *Motivational interviewing in the treatment of psychological problems.* New York: Guilford Press.

Arkowitz, H., & Westra, H. A. (Eds.). (2009). Special issue on motivational interviewing and psychotherapy. *Journal of Clinical Psychology: In Session, 65*(11).

Bulloch, A. G. M., & Patten, S. B. (2010). Nonadherence with psychotropic medications in the general population. *Social Psychiatry and Psychiatric Epidemiology, 45*, 47–56.

Burke, B. L., Arkowitz, H., & Menchola, M. (2003). The efficacy of motivational interviewing: A meta-analysis of controlled clinical trials. *Journal of Consulting and Clinical Psychology, 71*, 843–861.

Cabassa, L. J., Lester, R., & Zayas, L. H. (2007). "It's like being in a labyrinth": Hispanic immigrants' perceptions of depression and attitudes toward treatments. *Journal of Immigrant Health, 9*, 1–16.

Crismon, M. L. Trivedi, M., Pigott, T. A., Rush, J. A., Hirschfeld, R. M. A., Kahn, D. A., et al. (1999). The Texas Medication Algorithm Project: Report on the Texas Consensus Conference Panel on medication treatment of major depressive disorder. *Journal of Clinical Psychiatry, 60*, 142–156.

Demyttenaere, K. (1997). Compliance during treatment with antidepressants. *Journal of Affective Disorders, 43*, 27–39.

Demyttenaere, K. (1998). Noncompliance with antidepressants: Who's to blame? *International Clinical Journal of Psychopharmacology, 13*(Suppl. 2), S19–S25.

Demyttenaere, K., Enzlin, P., Walthère, D., Boulanger, B., De Bie, J., De Troyer, W., et al. (2001). Compliance with antidepressants in a primary care setting. 1: Beyond lack of efficacy and adverse events. *Journal of Clinical Psychiatry, 62* (Suppl. 22), 30–33.

Drymalski, W. M., & Campbell, T. C. (2009). A review of motivational interviewing to enhance adherence to antipsychotic medication in patients with schizophrenia: Evidence and recommendations. *Journal of Mental Health, 18*, 6–15.

Edwards, J. (1998). Long term pharmacotherapy of depression. *British Medical Journal, 316*, 1180–1181.

Graeber, D. A., Moyers, T. B., Griffith, G., Guajardo, E., & Tonigan, S. (2003). A pilot study comparing motivational interviewing and an educational intervention in patients with schizophrenia and alcohol use disorders. *Community Mental Health Journal, 39*, 189–202.

Grube, J. W., Rankin, W. L., Greenstein, T. N., & Kearney, K. A. (1977). Behavior change following self-confrontation: A test of the value-mediation hypothesis. *Journal of Personality and Social Psychology, 35*, 212–216.

Guarnaccia, P. J., Lewis-Fernández, R., & Rivera, M. (2003). Toward a Puerto Rican popular nosology: *Nervios* and *ataques de nervios*. *Culture, Medicine and Psychiatry, 27*, 339–366.

Harman, J. S., Edlund, M. J., & Fortney, J. C. (2004). Disparities in the adequacy of depression treatment in the United States. *Psychiatric Services, 55*, 1379–1385.

Haynes, R. B., Ackloo, E., Sahota, N., McDonald, H. P., & Yao, X. (2008). Interventions for enhancing medication adherence. *Cochrane Database of Systematic Reviews, 2*, Art. No. CD000011.

Hettema, J., Steele, J., & Miller, W. R. (2005). Motivational interviewing. *Annual Review of Clinical Psychology, 1*, 91–111.

Interian, A., Ang, A., Gara, M. A., Link, B. G., Rodríguez, M. A., & Vega, W. A. (2010). Stigma and depression treatment utilization among Latinos: Utility of four stigma measures. *Psychiatric Services, 61*, 373–379.

Interian, A., Martínez, I., Iglesias Ríos, L., Krejci, J., & Guarnaccia, P. J. (2010). Adaptation of a motivational interviewing intervention to improve antidepressant adherence among Latinos. *Cultural Diversity and Ethnic Minority Psychology, 16*, 215–225.

Interian, A., Lewis-Fernández, R., Gara, M. A., & Escobar, J. I. (2013). A randomized, controlled trial of an intervention to improve antidepressant adherence among Latinos. *Depression and Anxiety, 30*, 688–696.

Kemp, R., Kirov, G., Everitt, B., Hayward, P, & David, A. (1998). Randomised controlled trial of compliance therapy: 18–month follow-up. *British Journal of Psychiatry, 172*, 413–419.

Kreyenbuhl, J., Nossell, I. R., & Dixon, L. B. (2009). Disengagement from mental health treatment among individuals with schizophrenia and strategies for facilitating connections to care: A review of the literature. *Schizophrenia Bulletin, 35*, 696–703.

Lanouette, N. M., Folsom, D. P., Sciolla, A., & Jeste, D. V. (2009). Psychotropic medication nonadherence among United States Latinos: A comprehensive literature review. *Psychiatric Services, 60*, 157–174.

Laria, A., & Lewis-Fernández, R. (2006). Issues in the assessment and treatment of Latino patients. In R. Lim (Ed.), *Clinical manual of cultural psychiatry:*

A handbook for working with diverse patients (pp. 119–173). Washington, DC: American Psychiatric Press.

Lewis-Fernández, R. (2003). *Role of cultural expectations of treatment in adherence research.* Presentation at the National Institute of Mental Health training conference "Beyond the Clinic Walls: Expanding Mental Health, Drug and Alcohol Services Research Outside the Specialty Care System" in Rockville, MD.

Lewis-Fernández, R., Balán, I., Patel, S., Moyers, T., Sanchez-Lacay, A., Alfonso, C., et al. (2013). Impact of motivational pharmacotherapy on treatment retention among depressed Latinos. *Psychiatry: Biological and Interpersonal Processes, 76*(3), 210–222.

Lingam, R., & Scott, J. (2002). Treatment nonadherence in affective disorders. *Acta Psychiatrica Scandinavica, 105,* 164–172.

Maddox, J., Levi, M., & Thompson, C. (1994) The compliance with antidepressants in general practice. *Journal of Psychopharmacology, 8,* 48–53.

Melfi, C. A., Chawla, A. J., Croghan, T. W., Hanna, M. P., Kennedy, S., & Sredl, K. (1998). The effects of adherence to antidepressant treatment guidelines on relapse and recurrence of depression. *Archives of General Psychiatry, 55,* 1128–1132.

Miller, W. R., C'de Baca, J., Matthews, D. B., & Wilbourne, P. L. (2001). Personal values card sort. Available at *http://casaa.unm.edu.*

Miller, W. R., & Rollnick, S. (2013). *Motivational interviewing: Helping people change* (3rd ed.). New York: Guilford Press.

Merlo, L. J., Storch, E. A., Lehmkuhl, H. D., Jacob, M. L., Murphy, T. K., Goodman, W. K., et al. (2010). Cognitive behavioral therapy plus motivational interviewing improves outcome for pediatric obsessive–compulsive disorder: A preliminary study. *Cognitive Behavior Therapy, 39,* 24–27.

Mitchell, A. J., & Selties, T. (2007). Why don't patients take their medicines?: Reasons and solutions in psychiatry. *Advances in Psychiatric Treatment, 13*(5), 336–346.

Moyers, T. B., & Martino, S. (2006). "What's important in my life": The Personal Goals and Values Card Sorting Task for individuals with schizophrenia. Available at *http://casaa.unm.edu.*

Olfson, M., Mojtabai, R., Sampson, N. A., Hwang, I. Druss, B., Wang, P. S., et al. (2009). Dropout from outpatient mental health care in the United States. *Psychiatric Services, 60,* 898–907.

Pekarik, G. (1992). Relationship of clients' reasons for dropping out of treatment to outcome and satisfaction. *Journal of Clinical Psychology, 48,* 91–98.

Resnicow, K., Baranowski, T., Ahluwalia, J. S., & Braithwaite, R. L. (1999). Cultural sensitivity in public health: Defined and demystified. *Ethnicity and Disease, 9,* 10–21.

Rokeach, M. (1973). *The nature of human values.* New York: Free Press.

Rollnick, S., Butler, C. C., & Mason, P. (1999). *Health behavior change: A guide for practiotioners.* Philadelphia: Elsevier.

Roy-Byrne, P., Post, R., Uhde, T., Porcu, T., & Davis, D. (1985). The longitudinal course of recurrent affective illness. *Acta Psychiatrica Scandinavica, 71*(Suppl. 317), 1–34.

Rubak, S., Sandbaek, A., Lauritzen, T., & Christensen, B. (2005). Motivational interviewing: A systematic review and meta-analysis. *British Journal of General Practice, 55,* 305–312.

Rush, A. J., Trivedi, M. H., Wisniewski, S. R., Nierenberg, A. A., Stewart, J. W., Warden, D., et al. (2006). Acute and longer-term outcomes in depressed outpatients requiring one or several treatment steps: A STAR*D report. *American Journal of Psychiatry, 163,* 1905–1917.

Schraufnagel, T. J., Wagner, A. W., Miranda, J., & Roy-Byrne, P. P. (2006). Treating minority patients with depression and anxiety: What does the evidence tell us? *General Hospital Psychiatry, 28,* 27–36.

Schwartz, S. H., & Inbar-Saban, N. (1988). Value self-confrontation as a method to aid in weight loss. *Journal of Personality and Social Psychology, 34,* 396–404.

Simpson, H. B., Zuckoff, A. M., Maher, M. J., Page, J. R., Franklin, M. E., Foa, E. B., et al. (2010). Challenges using motivational interviewing as an adjunct to exposure therapy for obsessive–compulsive disorder. *Behaviour Research and Therapy, 48,* 941–948.

Vargas, S., Cabassa L. J., Nicasio, A. V., De La Cruz, A. A., Jackson, E., Rosario, M., et al. (in press). Toward a cultural adaptation of pharmacotherapy: Latino views of depression and antidepressant therapy. *Transcultural Psychiatry.*

Velligan, D. I., Lam, Y. W. F., Glahn, D. C., Barrett, J. A., Maples, N. J., Ereshefsky, L., et al. (2006). Defining and assessing adherence to oral antipsychotics: A review of the literature. *Schizophrenia Bulletin, 32,* 724–742.

Velligan, D., Sajatovic, M., Valenstein, M., Riley, W. T., Safren, S., Lewis-Fernández, R., et al. (2010). Methodological challenges in psychiatric treatment adherence research. *Clinical Schizophrenia and Related Psychoses, 4,* 74–91.

Warden, D., Trivedi, M. H., Wisniewski, S. R., Davis, L., Nierenberg, A. A., Gaynes, B. N., et al. (2007). Predictors of attrition during initial (citalopram) treatment for depression: A STAR*D report. *American Journal of Psychiatry, 164,* 1189–1197.

Westra, H. A., & Arkowitz, H. (Eds.). (2011). Special issue on integrating motivational interviewing with cognitive behavioral therapy for a range of mental health problems. *Cognitive and Behavioral Practice, 18,* 1–81.

Westra, H. A., Arkowitz, H., & Dozois, D. J. A. (2009). Adding a motivational interviewing pretreatment to cognitive behavioral therapy for generalized anxiety disorder: A preliminary randomized controlled trial. *Journal of Anxiety Disorders, 23,* 1106–1117.

Zygmunt, A., Olfson, M., Boyer, C. A., & Mechanic, D. (2002). Interventions to improve medication adherence in schizophrenia. *American Journal of Psychiatry, 159,* 1653–1664.

CHAPTER 10

• • • • • •

Motivational Interviewing in Treating Addictions

William R. Miller

"Addiction" has long been a generic term applied to a wide range of excessive behaviors (Peele, 1985), and it is the title of one of the oldest scientific journals in this field. Addictions occur all along a continuum, though the term is sometimes associated only with the more severe end of the spectrum. Consistent with a public health model, the fifth edition of the *Diagnostic and Statistical Manual of Mental Disorders* (American Psychiatric Association, 2013) removed the prior distinction between "abuse" and "dependence" and recognized substance use disorders as continuously distributed. Alcohol use disorders, for example, vary along a continuum including risky use, harmful or problematic use, and dependence (Institute of Medicine, 1990; Miller & Muñoz, 2013). Alcohol, tobacco, and other drug use are increasingly recognized as public health issues that should be addressed in mainstream health care.

Addiction and Motivation

Motivational interviewing (MI) began as a tool for the treatment of alcohol problems (Miller, 1983) and quickly found applications in addressing other drug and gambling problems as well. Addiction is a prototypical focus for MI because it is fundamentally a problem of motivation. I do not mean this in a moralistic sense—that people who suffer with addictions somehow have insufficient or flawed motivations. Rather, I mean that the phenomena referred to as addictions involve powerful and often conflicting sources of reinforcement (Meyers & Smith, 1995; Miller, 2006). Some drugs of abuse directly activate central reward channels in the brain. Substance use is also strongly influenced by social reinforcement and modeling. Physiological dependence and withdrawal set up a pattern of negative reinforcement for continued use. The broader pattern of behavioral dependence involves progressive detachment from other natural sources of positive reinforcement in deference to drug use (Edwards & Gross, 1976). Real or imagined access to valued reinforcers (e.g., financial, social, sexual) can also be tied to alcohol and other drug use. Thus, any attempt to derail an addictive behavior competes with powerful incentives for continued use. This paradox of persistence is characteristic of substance use disorders, which are the focus of this chapter, as well as process addictions such as pathological gambling (see Hodgins, Swan, & Diskin, Chapter 11, this volume) and eating disorders (see Cassin & Geller, Chapter 14, this volume). All of these involve behavior that persists despite apparent harm or risk of harm, often accompanied by a subjective sense of compromised personal control (Baumeister, Heatherton, & Tice, 1994; Brown, 1998; Miller & Atencio, 2008).

Yet, despite impaired self-control in addiction, the vast majority of people who quit smoking, drinking, or using other drugs still do so without receiving any formal treatment. "Disease model" programs ultimately appeal to a personal decision to abstain one day at a time (AA World Services, 2001; Nowinski, 2003). Courts seldom find people not guilty by reason of alcohol/drug intoxication; more often it aggravates rather than mitigates an offense. Whatever the rhetoric, we generally tend to treat addictions as a matter of choice.

MI and Other Treatment Methods

In the 1980s and 1990s the clinical style of MI stood in stark contrast to dominant models of addiction treatment (Miller & Rollnick, 1991). There was a widespread belief, never supported by scientific evidence, that people with addictions had a distinctive pathological personality characterized by high levels of immature defense mechanisms such as denial. In fact, in the first two editions of its *Diagnostic and Statistical Manual* the American Psychiatric Association (1968) classified alcohol/drug problems among the personality disorders. This categorization served as a rationale for a highly confrontational treatment style that was thought to be essential for overcoming denial (e.g., Janzen, 2001) but that proved to be largely ineffective or even harmful (White & Miller, 2007). Ultimately even Hazelden, the flagship program of the Minnesota model (Cook, 1988a, 1988b), renounced such confrontational methods (Hazelden Foundation, 1985). The field was ready for a different approach.

Happily, there is now an impressive menu of evidence-based treatment methods available for those seeking help with substance use disorders (Fletcher, 2009; Miller, Forcehimes, & Zweben, 2011). The community reinforcement approach seeks to establish or reestablish natural competing sources of reward that do not depend on substance use (Meyers & Miller, 2001; Meyers & Smith, 1995; Smith, Meyers, & Miller, 2001). Families can learn to support sobriety (Meyers & Smith, 1997; Meyers & Wolfe, 2004), and pharmacotherapies can block some of the incentive properties of alcohol and other drugs (O'Malley & Kosten, 2006). Twelve-step programs provide an immediate social support community for sobriety (Longabaugh, Wirtz, Zweben, & Stout, 1998). MI is thus just one clinical tool within an array of options. It can be combined with other evidence-based treatment methods (e.g., Anton et al., 2006; Obert et al., 2000), and doing so can increase the efficacy of both treatments (Hettema, Steele, & Miller, 2005). MI can also be delivered effectively within brief health care consultations (Rollnick, Miller, & Butler, 2008).

Rationale for MI in Addiction Treatment

Historically many addiction programs have assumed and even required readiness for change as a prerequisite for treatment. The popular (and circular) concept of "hitting bottom" implies a sufficient course of suffering to trigger change, and people who did not appear to be adequately motivated or compliant were sometimes told, "Come back when you're ready."

Dissemination of the transtheoretical model of change (Prochaska & DiClemente, 1984) suggested, in contrast, that people's readiness for change is malleable and that it is an important part of the clinician's task to help increase clients' readiness for change. Initial descriptions of MI proposed that the high levels of "resistance" being experienced in addiction treatment were largely the product of a confrontational counseling style. If people are ambivalent about their substance use, then a counselor strongly voicing prochange arguments would predictably evoke from clients the other side of their ambivalence, namely, counterchange arguments. Within MI the interviewer seeks to arrange the conversation so that it is the client who makes the arguments for change. In essence, clients talk themselves into (rather than out of) change by voicing their own motivations. Subsequent process research supports this relationship of client speech to treatment outcome (Miller & Rose, 2009) and confirms that MI-consistent counseling increases client change talk (Glynn & Moyers, 2010; Moyers, Houck, Glynn, & Manuel, 2011; Moyers & Martin, 2006).

Furthermore, evidence was accumulating that client outcomes vary widely, depending on the therapist who provides treatment (Najavits & Weiss, 1994; Project MATCH Research Group, 1998). In random assignment studies, clients with the most favorable outcomes were those who had been treated by therapists with high levels of empathic and other client-centered counseling skills, as described by Rogers (1965; Truax & Carkhuff, 1967), whereas low therapist empathy was associated with poor outcomes (Miller, Taylor, & West, 1980; Moyers & Miller, 2013; Valle, 1981).

MI is not the only strategy designed to enhance motivation for treatment and change. Coercive interventions were developed to pressure "unmotivated" people into treatment (Johnson, 1986; Trice & Beyer, 1984). Although the traditional Johnson Institute intervention can engage in treatment a minority of those who initially refuse to seek help, many families ultimately refuse to go through with it (Miller, Meyers, & Tonigan, 1999), and the Johnson Institute itself no longer offers this approach. The community reinforcement and family training (CRAFT) approach is effective in engaging about two-thirds of initially unmotivated alcohol/drug users in treatment by working unilaterally through concerned family members (Azrin, Sisson, Meyers, & Godley, 1982; Meyers, Miller, Hill, & Tonigan, 1999; Meyers, Miller, Smith, & Tonigan, 2002; Meyers & Smith, 1997; Meyers & Wolfe, 2004; Miller et al., 1999).

Research on MI and Addictions

Perhaps the most persuasive reason to learn and practice MI is the substantial evidence base for its efficacy as a brief intervention in addiction treatment. Among the more than 200 randomized trials of interventions identified as MI or MI-related, the largest body of trials still focuses on alcohol/drug problems.

One evaluation design has compared MI as a brief intervention with no intervention or simple advice. Meta-analyses reflect significant benefit from MI in addressing alcohol, tobacco, and other substance use problems, with effect sizes varying widely across studies and averaging in the small to medium range (Burke, Arkowitz, & Menchola, 2003; Lundahl et al., 2013; Lundahl, Kunz, Brownell, Tollefson, & Burke, 2010).

A different type of trial contrasts MI with other evidence-based treatment methods, with the MI intervention typically involving fewer sessions. Such studies typically find no difference in client outcomes despite the lesser intensity of MI interventions (Hettema et al., 2005; Project MATCH Research Group, 1997; UKATT Research Team, 2005). That is, briefer MI often (though not always) yields effects similar to those from more intensive treatments and is preferable to placing people on a waiting list for treatment (e.g., Miller, Benefield, & Tonigan, 1993).

Additive designs have tested the value of combining MI with other active treatments. MI can enhance retention and adherence in other evidence-based treatments, and this synergistic effect may account for why MI has been found to exert longer-lasting effects in additive trials (Hettema et al., 2005). Motivational enhancement therapy (MET) combines the clinical style of MI with personalized assessment feedback (Ball et al., 2007; Miller, Zweben, DiClemente, & Rychtarik, 1992; Project MATCH Research Group, 1997; UKATT Research Team, 2005) and may be particularly useful in developing discrepancy (i.e., between where one is and wants to be) with clients who show little or no initial readiness for change (Miller & Rollnick, 2013).

Addiction treatment outcomes often vary widely across therapists working within the same program or therapeutic approach (Anderson, Ogles, Patterson, Lambert, & Vermeersch, 2009; Crits-Christoph et al., 2009; McLellan, Woody, Luborsky, & Goehl, 1988; Valle, 1981), and this is also true with MI (Moyers & Miller, 2013; Project MATCH Research Group, 1998). Differences in therapist fidelity and outcomes may account for why MI has been found in multisite studies to work at some sites and not others (e.g., Ball et al., 2007), because therapists are confounded with the sites in which they work. Variations in therapists' MI skills and fidelity in practice also contribute to variability in findings across MI outcome trials (Miller & Rollnick, 2014).

Special Issues and Challenges

Engaging

Engaging is one of the most overlooked tasks and opportunities in addiction treatment. "Intake" is often conceptualized as a fact-gathering enterprise that precedes treatment. At one time the public treatment agency where I worked required prospective clients to answer 3–4 hours of questions over two or three visits with administrative staff. Not surprisingly, many people dropped out before ever seeing a counselor. I later discovered that the actual amount of information needed in order for us to be paid for a first counseling visit could be gathered in about 20 minutes. Private for-profit programs are less likely to make this mistake as compared to overburdened public programs with long waiting lists. Perhaps running the gauntlet of intake is (consciously or not) a kind of motivational prescreen.

From my perspective, treatment begins with the first contact. Since so many people end up coming for only one session, why not give them something useful in their very first visit? After all, as Carl Rogers observed, clients already know all of the information that we will ask about! Providing MI in the first visit can facilitate change, and ironically it can also increase the likelihood that clients will come back.

Done well, MI begins with a process of engaging, developing a collaborative working alliance. This can begin within a matter of minutes and is fostered primarily by the OARS skills (i.e., open-ended questions, affirmations, reflective lists, and summaries) derived directly from the person-centered approach developed by Rogers and his students. The prime objective in engaging is to understand clients' own experience and perspective on their life situation. Even focusing—let alone, evoking and planning—comes later. Engaging involves establishing trust and a working relationship through good listening.

Focusing

Differing goals is a common issue in specialist addiction treatment. Often the goal(s) espoused by a provider or program may not be shared by the prospective client. This is particularly true when, as has often been the case, the announced goal is always lifelong abstinence from all psychoactive substances (except perhaps tobacco). People can and do make their own choices—so, why not *discuss* the client's own goals rather than presumptuously announcing them? Trying to set people's goals for them is likely to evoke reactance.

The challenges of focusing are somewhat different in service contexts where the client did not come to discuss substance use. In primary health care, for example, people come with more or less specific medical concerns. Asking about tobacco use has become routine in health care, but screening for alcohol and other drug use is now also encouraged and may reveal reason for concern. Substance use may also be related to the presenting medical issues. People with substance use disorders are also overrepresented among those seen for psychotherapy, social services, or in correctional systems. Here the challenge is raising a sensitive topic that the client did not necessarily expect to discuss. Asking permission is useful here when such discussion is indicated: "I wonder if we might talk a bit about your alcohol use. Would it be OK to discuss that for a few minutes?"

Clients' level of motivation for change often varies across the drugs that they use. One person may be eager to stop using stimulants, willing to cut back on drinking, but unwilling to consider tobacco cessation. Another may be ready to quit drinking, contemplating stopping smoking, but reluctant to stop opiate use. Telling such people that we won't help them unless they are willing to quit everything immediately has a rather predictable result. From an MI perspective, one starts with people where they are, working on the changes they are willing to make, an approach sometimes referred to as harm reduction (Marlatt, 1998; Tatarsky & Marlatt, 2010).

For some providers, an ethical concern is whether it is ill advised to work with clients toward any goal other than abstinence. In primary health care it is now common to advise heavy drinkers to reduce their alcohol use, and there are research-based guidelines for estimating the relative likelihood of achieving moderation or abstinence goals, depending on the alcohol problem's severity (Miller & Muñoz, 2013). Pursuing an intermediate goal is much preferable to offering no treatment at all. Focusing, then, involves exploring what changes people are willing to consider and then developing agreed-upon goals.

Suppose, however, that as a mental health professional you are concerned about the person's substance use, whereas he or she does not seem to be. Substance use can contribute to psychological problems and impede their treatment. A client who is depressed may be using alcohol or other depressant drugs. Stimulants complicate treatment for anxiety disorders and schizophrenia. It is appropriate to raise your concern in such situations, but how can this be done in a way that does not elicit pushback and counterchange arguments from the client?

A key here point is to remember that people get to make their own choices and therefore to honor their autonomy. This can best be done by asking permission and prefacing your concern with language that respects client autonomy:

> "There's something that worries me here. It may not concern you, but I wonder if it's OK for me to tell you what's on my mind."
> "I'd like to ask you a little more about your drinking. What you decide to do is up to you, of course, but I wonder if alcohol might be making your depression worse. Can you see how it might?"

In this way you can raise a possible topic for discussion and treatment, but in a very real sense it's not a goal until your client shares it.

Evoking

The process of evoking in MI is about eliciting the client's own reasons for change. Some therapists simply forget to do this, sticking instead with client-centered listening. Others follow their righting reflex and offer their own arguments for the client to change, with the expected result of active or passive resistance. Evoking involves asking and being curious about what clients themselves perceive as possible reasons for change. If you push ahead into planning (how to) before your client is on board and sufficiently motivated to move forward, change is unlikely to occur. Never get ahead of your client's own readiness level.

The most common way of evoking change talk is to ask for it. Ask open-ended questions the natural answer to which is change talk.

> "If you did decide to stop using cocaine, what do you think would be the best way to do it?"
> "What would you say are the three best reasons to cut back on drinking?"
> "How important would you say it is for you to quit smoking? On a scale from 0 to 10, where 0 is not at all and 10 is the most important thing in your life right now, what number would you give yourself? . . . And why do you say _____ and not 0?"
> "You've been using several different drugs—and it's up to you, of course—but I wonder what changes you might be willing to consider in your drug use."

In MI there are also particular ways to respond when you hear change talk that make it more likely to continue:

- *Ask more* about it. Ask for an example or for elaboration ("In what ways . . . ?")
- *Reflect* the change talk. Don't just repeat it, but offer a complex refection that makes a guess about what the person may mean.
- *Affirm* it.
- *Summarize* the change talk you have heard. Think of each self-motivating statement you hear as a flower, and collect the flowers. When you have heard two or three themes that favor change, put them together into a bouquet and ask, "What else?"

Another example of evoking is to ask your client to look ahead. "How would you like for your life to be different, say, 5 years from now?" (For some people, particularly adolescents, a shorter time frame is better.) Explore the person's hopes, goals, and dreams: "And how does your drug use fit into those goals?" Yet another way of looking forward as a trigger for change talk is to ask: "Suppose that you don't make any changes in your drinking/drug use but just keep on the way you have been. What do you think your life would be like down the line?" It is important to ask such questions with open curiosity and no tone of sarcasm or cynicism. Even voice tone can evoke pushback, and your client will tell you if you're doing it right. When you hear change talk, that's your client telling you that you're on the right track. When you begin to hear defensiveness and justification of the status quo, that's your client suggesting that you try a different approach.

For some reason the idea of doing a "decisional balance" became popular in counseling people about substance use. The usual approach is to ask about and explore all the pros and cons, all the reasons to change and the reasons not to change. This has even been confused with MI (Miller & Rollnick, 2009). If you want to maintain neutrality and not influence whether the client moves toward or away from a change, a decisional balance is a reasonable clinical tool. It was originally developed as a nondirective method of helping people make difficult decisions without influencing the choice that they make (Janis & Mann, 1977). If, however, your hope is to help someone who is ambivalent to move toward making a particular change, using MI would be preferable. When done with ambivalent people, a decisional balance intervention tends to *decrease* commitment to change (Miller & Rose, in press). There is no theoretical or empirical justification for systematically evoking and exploring all of the person's counterchange motivations if your goal is to encourage change.

Planning

Once there seems to be sufficient motivation in place, MI moves ahead to the planning process of considering how best to proceed toward change. Some clients do enter treatment with a high level of readiness already in place: "I've decided to quit smoking. How can I do it?" In this case, the client's focus is clear and there may not be much need for the evoking process. With sufficient engagement, you can move on to planning. If planning is premature, it will become clear soon enough.

So often, though, addiction treatment professionals and programs jump right into the how-to planning process with little attention to engaging, focusing (arriving at common goals), and evoking the client's own motivations for change. More than most any other area of behavioral health care, addiction services adopted an expert model: "I know what's best for you, and I'm going to tell you." Unless they are quite ready for change, most people don't respond well to this approach, and the result can be in-session resistance, unaccomplished homework assignments, low compliance with treatment, missed appointments, and treatment dropout. Those behaviors are signals that discussion about planning was premature.

At the other extreme is insufficient planning. "OK, I'll quit" may signal the best of intentions, and for some people the decision to quit is enough. A good planning process, though, thinks through how best to proceed and anticipates possible obstacles along the way. What would be one good next step? When and how will the person do it? Research on implementation intentions indicates that people are more likely to follow through with an action when they have a *specific* plan of action and state their intention to accomplish it (Gollwitzer, Wieber, Myers, & McCrea, 2010).

Addiction treatment has also been rife with black-and-white thinking. Any diversion from a goal is thought of as a "relapse"—a peculiar concept seldom applied to other behaviors. If someone being treated for depression or anxiety comes back with increased symptoms, they are seldom told that they have "relapsed." The process of recovering from an addiction is *normally* progressive, with symptomatic episodes becoming shorter, less severe, and less frequent. Periods of remission get longer, and for any other chronic condition that would be regarded as dramatic success (McLellan, Lewis, O'Brien, & Kleber, 2000; McLellan, McKay,

Forman, Cacciola, & Kemp, 2010). Beware being discouraged (either yourself or your clients) by unfair black-and-white "relapse" thinking that can undermine perfectly good progress (Miller, 1996; Miller, Westerberg, Harris, & Tonigan, 1996).

Planning is not a one-time event but rather a process that occurs over time. In the course of implementing change, people run into obstacles that require new planning. Motivation for change can also fluctuate, indicating a need to return to earlier processes of evoking, focusing, or even engaging (Miller & Rollnick, 2013).

Clinical Illustration

Treatment for addictions should not be just a specialist affair but rather should be part of mainstream psychological and mental health services (Miller & Brown, 1997; Miller et al., 2011). After depression, substance use disorders are the second most common diagnosis encountered in the general population and clinical practice. The following case example occured in a community mental health center, beginning with the initial contact session. A screening questionnaire alerted the interviewing clinician that heavy alcohol use could be an issue, but the presenting problem was depression. After initial greetings and orientation the clinician began with an open-ended question.

Engaging

INTERVIEWER: Well, tell me what brings you here today—what's concerning you.

CLIENT: My doctor said I should see somebody about my depression. I don't actually feel sad or anything, but I'm not sleeping well and I don't seem to have any energy. She said there's nothing wrong with me medically, but she could prescribe an antidepressant or I could go see somebody.

INTERVIEWER: And you chose to come here.

Reflection (continuing the paragraph).

CLIENT: Uh-huh. I don't like to take medication if I don't have to.

INTERVIEWER: You're concerned about how medication might affect you.

Complex reflection making a guess.

CLIENT: I just don't like to rely on drugs. It feels like a crutch.

INTERVIEWER: You like managing on your own. That's important to you.

Complex reflection, making a guess.

CLIENT: Yes, it is.

INTERVIEWER: Well, tell me a bit about what you have been experiencing.

Open question.

CLIENT: I usually sleep right through the night, but I've been having trouble getting to sleep, and also I wake up in the middle of the night. And I'm normally a pretty energetic person, but I don't feel like doing much anymore, so I stay home.

INTERVIEWER: That's a big change for you—not like your normal self. You're not doing things you enjoy much.

Without asking a lot of questions, the interviewer stays with complex reflection as the heart of the engaging process.

CLIENT: It's not like me. I don't even enjoy eating, and I lost some weight—which is what got my doctor's attention.

INTERVIEWER: You're pretty healthy, and yet you don't feel like your usual self. You'd like to get back to normal.

Summary reflection.

CLIENT: Or even better.

INTERVIEWER: Even better than normal! In what ways? How might you be even better?

Simple reflection, followed by an open question to evoke change talk broadly.

CLIENT: I think I've been in a slump, in a rut for quite a while, not really going anywhere. Not accomplishing much.

Focusing

INTERVIEWER: Where would you like to go?	*Open question to begin exploring goals. Focusing overlaps with continued engaging.*
CLIENT: I don't know. I think I'm a creative person, but I'm not doing anything very creative.	
INTERVIEWER: You've got some talents you haven't been using lately. What kinds of talents?	*Complex reflection, affirmation.* *Open question.*
CLIENT: I'm a potter—I even have my own wheel. I can't remember the last time I used it. I like storytelling—I used to do that for children at the library, and I've written some stories.	
INTERVIEWER: Making things from scratch—pots, stories. You really enjoy that. And telling stories to children.	*Complex reflection.*
CLIENT: I used to enjoy it.	
INTERVIEWER: And that's something you'd like to have back.	*Complex reflection.*
CLIENT: Yes.	

This exploration of aspects of the client's depression could go on for some time, and MI could be focused on recovery from depression (see Chapter 6, this volume). The clinician also remembers the screening questionnaire and after a while decides to explore alcohol use.

INTERVIEWER: There's something else I'd like to ask you about—if that's OK. In the waiting room you filled out a questionnaire for us, and I appreciate you taking the time to do that. One of the questions was about how often you have four or	*Asking permission.* *Affirmation.*

more drinks, and I think you said it's more than once a week. Tell me about that.	*Elicit.*
CLIENT: I don't count or anything, and I'm not an alcoholic, but I do drink at home. I like beer and sometimes scotch when I'm watching TV.	
INTERVIEWER: I ask because alcohol is a depressant drug. Do you see where I'm going here?	*Provide.* *Elicit.*
CLIENT: Really? It makes you depressed?	
INTERVIEWER: In larger doses, yes.	*Provide.*
CLIENT: I usually feel better when I drink.	
INTERVIEWER: So, in a way, alcohol seems more like a help than a hindrance.	*Complex reflection (avoiding the righting reflex).*
CLIENT: That's funny since I just said I don't like to rely on drugs.	*Responding with the other side of ambivalence.*
INTERVIEWER: You like to manage without them.	*Reflecting potential change talk about drinking.*
CLIENT: What do you think?	
INTERVIEWER: Well, what you said on the questionnaire caught my eye because alcohol can interfere with sleeping right, and as a drug it is a depressant. Does that make sense to you?	*Provide.* *Elicit.*
CLIENT: Actually I think it helps me get to sleep.	
INTERVIEWER: That's right! It can sedate you enough to get to sleep, but often it's a restless kind of sleep, and you wake up during the night. Just a thought. It looks like that's not an idea you like.	*Provide.* *Reflecting nonverbal cues.*

CLIENT: I just never thought about it.

INTERVIEWER: I wonder if there's any-
    thing else you've wondered about
    how alcohol affects you.

*Open question, seeking
change talk.*

CLIENT: Does it seem to you like I drink
    too much?

Giving permission.

INTERVIEWER: We haven't really talked
    about it much, so I'm not sure.
    The question you answered asks
    about four or more drinks at a time
    because that's an unusual amount
    that can cause health problems.
    Does that surprise you?

Provide.

Elicit.

CLIENT: Yes and no.

INTERVIEWER: No, because . . .

Open question.

CLIENT: Sometimes I can't remember
    things that happened.

*Offering some vulnerable
information—change talk.*

INTERVIEWER: When you've been
    drinking.

Continuing the paragraph.

CLIENT: Right. That bothers me.

Change talk.

INTERVIEWER: It's a little scary when
    you can't remember what happened
    or what you did. What else?

Reflection.

CLIENT: I notice how often I'm buying
    bottles of scotch.

INTERVIEWER: It surprises you.

Reflection.

CLIENT: How much I spend on it.

INTERVIEWER: Oh, I see. The cost of all
    that.

Reflection.

CLIENT: I've heard you shouldn't drink
    by yourself.

INTERVIEWER: Well, my concern is
    whether it's contributing to this
    depression that you're experiencing.
    I don't think eliminating the alcohol
    would solve all these concerns you

Provide.

have, but it might help. It's just one piece of the puzzle.

CLIENT: Oh.

INTERVIEWER: So, let me see if I understand you right on this, and then we can move on. You said on the questionnaire that you're having four or more drinks more than once a week, which medically is a risky level. You've been surprised sometimes how much alcohol you're buying, especially scotch, which you enjoy. You're troubled by depression and sleeping problems, which alcohol can exacerbate. And sometimes you don't remember what happened when you were drinking, and you don't like that. We've puzzled together about whether making a change in your alcohol use could be one piece of the puzzle here. What do you think at this point? It's really up to you.

Recapitulation summary of change talk themes.

Open question. Emphasizing personal choice.

CLIENT: I guess I'm willing to think about it. What do you think I should do?

Client signals openness to some planning.

Planning

INTERVIEWER: Well, I was just wondering what you think you'd be willing to try.

Open question— avoiding giving an immediate solution.

CLIENT: I don't know whether I should cut back or just stop it altogether for a while.

INTERVIEWER: Either cut down or take a vacation from alcohol. Both seem possible to you.

Reflection and reframe.

Reflection of ability.

CLIENT: I'd rather not quit altogether unless I have to.

INTERVIEWER: You'd prefer not to quit completely, but it sounds like you're willing to do whatever is in your best interest.	*Double-sided reflection; the "but" places greater emphasis on the latter (change talk) part.*
CLIENT: I am. Something has to change.	*Change talk.*
INTERVIEWER: It's that important.	*Reflection of change talk.*
CLIENT: I just want to get back to my usual self again.	
INTERVIEWER: Whatever it takes. Good for you!	*Reflection of change talk; affirmation.*

The planning process could proceed to explore whether the client would like some specific support or treatment to make a change in drinking. Planning would also focus, of course, on other possible treatment for the depression itself.

Conclusions

Motivational interviewing is not so much a technique as a specific style for having a conversation about change. It was originally developed to help problem drinkers, and it seems to be particularly useful in the treatment of addictions, where ambivalence is such a central dynamic. It is just one tool, not a comprehensive treatment approach in itself, and it blends well with other therapeutic tools such as cognitive-behavior therapy or 12-step facilitation. I find it is quite compatible with what Bill W., the cofounder of Alcoholics Anonymous, described as "working with others" (AA World Services, 2001). In truth, we do not get to make life choices for our clients, but we can talk with them in a way that evokes their own natural motivations to be healthy and whole.

References

AA World Services. (2001). *Alcoholics Anonymous: The story of how many thousands of men and women have recovered from alcoholism* (4 ed.). New York: Author.

American Psychiatric Association. (1952). *Diagnostic and statistical manual of mental disorders*. Washington, DC: Author.

American Psychiatric Association. (1968). *Diagnostic and statistical manual of mental disorders* (2nd ed.). Washington, DC: Author.

American Psychiatric Association. (2013). *Diagnostic and statistical manual of mental disorders* (5th ed.). Arlington, VA: Author.

Anderson, T., Ogles, B. M., Patterson, C. L., Lambert, M. J., & Vermeersch, D. A. (2009). Therapist effects: Facilitative interpersonal skills as a predictor of therapist success. *Journal of Clinical Psychology, 65*(7), 755–768.

Anton, R. F., O'Malley, S. S., Ciraulo, D. A., Cisler, R. A., Couper, D., Donovan, D. M., et al. (2006). Combined pharmacotherapies and behavioral interventions for alcohol dependence: The COMBINE study: A randomized controlled trial. *JAMA, 295*(17), 2003–2017.

Azrin, N. H., Sisson, R. W., Meyers, R. J., & Godley, M. (1982). Alcoholism treatment by disulfiram and community reinforcement therapy. *Journal of Behavior Therapy and Experimental Psychiatry, 13*, 105–112.

Ball, S. A., Martino, S., Nich, C., Frankforter, T. L., van Horn, D., Crits-Christoph, P., et al. (2007). Site matters: Multisite randomized trial of motivational enhancement therapy in community drug abuse clinics. *Journal of Consulting and Clinical Psychology, 75*, 556–567.

Baumeister, R. F., Heatherton, T. F., & Tice, D. M. (1994). *Losing control: How and why people fail at self-regulation*. New York: Academic Press.

Brown, J. M. (1998). Self-regulation and the addictive behaviors. In W. R. Miller & N. Heather (Eds.), *Treating addictive behaviors* (2nd ed., pp. 61–74). New York: Plenum Press.

Burke, B. L., Arkowitz, H., & Menchola, M. (2003). The efficacy of motivational interviewing: A meta-analysis of controlled clinical trials. *Journal of Consulting and Clinical Psychology, 71*, 843–861.

Cook, C. H. (1988a). The Minnesota model in the management of drug and alcohol dependence: Miracle, method, or myth? Part II. Evidence and conclusions. *British Journal of Addiction, 83*, 735–748.

Cook, C. H. (1988b). The Minnesota model in the management of drug and alcohol dependency: Miracle, method, or myth? Part I. The philosophy and the programme. *British Journal of Addiction, 83*, 625–634.

Crits-Christoph, P., Gallop, R., Temes, C. M., Woody, G., Ball, S. A., Martino, S., et al. (2009). The alliance in motivational enhancement therapy and counseling as usual for substance use problems. *Journal of Consulting and Clinical Psychology, 77*(6), 1125–1135.

Edwards, G., & Gross, M. M. (1976). Alcohol dependence: Provisional description of a clinical syndrome. *British Medical Journal, 1*, 1058–1061.

Fletcher, A. M. (2009). *Sober for good: New solutions for drinking problems—advice from those who have succeeded*. Boston: Houghton-Mifflin.

Glynn, L. H., & Moyers, T. B. (2010). Chasing change talk: The clinician's role in evoking client language about change. *Journal of Substance Abuse Treatment, 39*, 65–70.

Gollwitzer, P. M., Wieber, F., Myers, A. L., & McCrea, S. M. (2010). How to maximize implementation intention effects. In C. R. Agnew, D. E. Carlston, W. G. Graziano, & J. R. Kelly (Eds.), *Then a miracle occurs:*

Focusing on behavior in social psychological theory and research (pp. 137–161). New York: Oxford University Press.

Hazelden Foundation. (1985). You don't have to tear 'em down to build 'em up. *Hazelden Professional Update, 4*(2), 2.

Hettema, J., Steele, J., & Miller, W. R. (2005). Motivational interviewing. *Annual Review of Clinical Psychology, 1,* 91–111.

Institute of Medicine. (1990). *Broadening the base of treatment for alcohol problems.* Washington, DC: National Academy Press.

Janis, I. L., & Mann, L. (1977). *Decision making: A psychological analysis of conflict, choice and commitment.* New York: Free Press.

Janzen, R. (2001). *The rise and fall of Synanon.* Baltimore: Johns Hopkins University Press.

Johnson, V. F. (1986). *Intervention: How to help someone who doesn't want help.* Center City, MN: Hazelden.

Longabaugh, R., Wirtz, P. W., Zweben, A., & Stout, R. L. (1998). Network support for drinking, Alcoholics Anonymous and long-term matching effects. *Addiction, 93,* 1313–1333.

Lundahl, B., Moleni, T., Burke, B. L., Butters, R., Tollefson, D., Butler, C., et al. (2013). Motivational interviewing in medical care settings: A systematic review and meta-analysis of randomized controlled trials. *Patient Education and Counseling, 93*(2), 157–168.

Lundahl, B. W., Kunz, C., Brownell, C., Tollefson, D., & Burke, B. L. (2010). A meta-analysis of motivational interviewing: Twenty-five years of empirical studies. *Research on Social Work Practice, 20*(2), 137–160.

Marlatt, G. A. (Ed.). (1998). *Harm reduction: Pragmatic strategies for managing high-risk behaviors.* New York: Guilford Press.

McLellan, A. T., Lewis, D. C., O'Brien, C. P., & Kleber, H. D. (2000). Drug dependence, a chronic medical illness: Implications for treatment, insurance, and outcomes evaluation. *Journal of the American Medical Association, 284,* 1689–1695.

McLellan, A. T., McKay, J. R., Forman, R., Cacciola, J., & Kemp, J. (2010). Reconsidering the evaluation of addiction treatment: From retrospective follow-up to concurrent recovery monitoring. *Addiction, 100,* 447–458.

McLellan, A. T., Woody, G. E., Luborsky, L., & Gochl, L. (1988). Is the counselor an "active ingredient" in substance abuse rehabilitation? An examination of treatment success among four counselors. *Journal of Nervous and Mental Disease, 176,* 423–430.

Meyers, R. J., & Miller, W. R. (2001). *A community reinforcement approach to addiction treatment.* Cambridge, UK: Cambridge University Press.

Meyers, R. J., Miller, W. R., Hill, D. E., & Tonigan, J. S. (1999). Community reinforcement and family training (CRAFT): Engaging unmotivated drug users in treatment. *Journal of Substance Abuse, 10*(3), 1–18.

Meyers, R. J., Miller, W. R., Smith, J. E., & Tonigan, J. S. (2002). A randomized trial of two methods for engaging treatment-refusing drug users through concerned significant others. *Journal of Consulting and Clinical Psychology, 70,* 1182–1185.

Meyers, R. J., & Smith, J. E. (1995). *Clinical guide to alcohol treatment: The community reinforcement approach.* New York: Guilford Press.

Meyers, R. J., & Smith, J. E. (1997). Getting off the fence: Procedures to engage treatment resistant drinkers. *Journal of Substance Abuse Treatment, 14,* 467–472.

Meyers, R. J., & Wolfe, B. L. (2004). *Get your loved one sober: Alternatives to nagging, pleading and threatening.* Center City, MN: Hazelden.

Miller, W. R. (1983). Motivational interviewing with problem drinkers. *Behavioural Psychotherapy, 11,* 147–172.

Miller, W. R. (1996). What is a relapse? Fifty ways to leave the wagon. *Addiction, 91*(Suppl.), S15–S27.

Miller, W. R. (2006). Motivational factors in addictive behaviors. In W. R. Miller & K. M. Carroll (Eds.), *Rethinking substance abuse; What science shows and what we should do about it* (pp. 134–150). New York: Guilford Press.

Miller, W. R., & Atencio, D. J. (2008). Free will as a proportion of variance. In J. Baer, J. C. Kaufman, & R. F. Baumeister (Eds.), *Are we free?: Psychology and free will* (pp. 275–295). New York: Oxford University Press.

Miller, W. R., Benefield, R. G., & Tonigan, J. S. (1993). Enhancing motivation for change in problem drinking: A controlled comparison of two therapist styles. *Journal of Consulting and Clinical Psychology, 61,* 455–461.

Miller, W. R., & Brown, S. A. (1997). Why psychologists should treat alcohol and drug problems. *American Psychologist, 52*(1269–1272).

Miller, W. R., Forcehimes, A. A., & Zweben, A. (2011). *Treating addiction: Guidelines for professionals.* New York: Guilford Press.

Miller, W. R., Meyers, R. J., & Tonigan, J. S. (1999). Engaging the unmotivated in treatment for alcohol problems: A comparison of three strategies for intervention through family members. *Journal of Consulting and Clinical Psychology, 67,* 688–697.

Miller, W. R., & Muñoz, R. F. (2013). *Controlling your drinking* (2nd ed.). New York: Guilford Press.

Miller, W. R., & Rollnick, S. (1991). *Motivational interviewing: Preparing people to change addictive behavior.* New York: Guilford Press.

Miller, W. R., & Rollnick, S. (2009). Ten things that motivational interviewing is not. *Behavioural and Cognitive Psychotherapy, 37,* 129–140.

Miller, W. R., & Rollnick, S. (2013). *Motivational interviewing: Helping people change* (3rd ed.). New York: Guilford Press.

Miller, W. R., & Rollnick, S. (2014). The effectiveness and ineffectiveness of complex behavioral interventions: Impact of treatment fidelity. *Contemporary Clinical Trials, 37*(2), 234–241.

Miller, W. R., & Rose, G. S. (2009). Toward a theory of motivational interviewing. *American Psychologist, 64,* 527–537.

Miller, W. R., & Rose, G. S. (2015). Motivational interviewing and decisional balance: Contrasting procedures to client ambivalence. *Behavioural and Cognitive Psychotherapy, 43*(2), 129–146.

Miller, W. R., Taylor, C. A., & West, J. C. (1980). Focused versus broad spectrum behavior therapy for problem drinkers. *Journal of Consulting and Clinical Psychology, 48,* 590–601.

Miller, W. R., Westerberg, V. S., Harris, R. J., & Tonigan, J. S. (1996). What predicts relapse? Prospective testing of antecedent models. *Addiction, 91*(Suppl.), S155–S171.

Miller, W. R., Zweben, A., DiClemente, C. C., & Rychtarik, R. (1992). *Motivational Enhancement Therapy manual: A clinical research guide for therapists treating individuals with alcohol abuse and dependence* (Vol. 2). Rockville, MD: National Institute on Alcohol Abuse and Alcoholism.

Moyers, T. B., Houck, J. M., Glynn, L. H., & Manuel, J. K. (2011). Can specialized training teach clinicians to recognize, reinforce, and elicit client language in motivational interviewing? (Abstract). *Alcoholism: Clinical and Experimental Research, 335*(S1), 296.

Moyers, T. B., & Martin, T. (2006). Therapist influence on client language during motivational interviewing sessions. *Journal of Substance Abuse Treatment, 30,* 245–252.

Moyers, T. B., & Miller, W. R. (2013). Is low therapist empathy toxic? *Psychology of Addictive Behaviors, 27*(3), 878–884.

Najavits, L. M., & Weiss, R. D. (1994). Variations in therapist effectiveness in the treatment of patients with substance use disorders: An empirical review. *Addiction, 89,* 679–688.

Nowinski, J. (2003). Facilitating 12–step recovery from substance abuse and addiction. In F. Rotgers, J. Morgenstern & S. Walters (Eds.), *Treating substance abuse* (pp. 31–66). New York: Guilford Press.

Obert, J. L., McCann, M. J., Marinelli-Casey, P., Weiner, A., Minsky, S., Brethen, P., et al. (2000). The matrix model of outpatient stimulant abuse treatment: History and description. *Journal of Psychoactive Drugs, 32*(2), 157–164.

O'Malley, S. S., & Kosten, T. R. (2006). Pharmacotherapy of addictive disorders. In W. R. Miller & K. M. Carroll (Eds.), *Rethinking substance abuse: What the science shows and what we should do about it* (pp. 240–256). New York: Guilford Press.

Peele, S. (1985). *The meaning of addiction.* San Francisco: Jossey-Bass.

Prochaska, J. O., & DiClemente, C. C. (1984). *The transtheoretical approach: Crossing traditional boundaries of therapy.* Homewood, IL: Dow/Jones Irwin.

Project MATCH Research Group. (1997). Matching alcoholism treatments to client heterogeneity: Project MATCH posttreatment drinking outcomes. *Journal of Studies on Alcohol, 58,* 7–29.

Project MATCH Research Group. (1998). Therapist effects in three treatments for alcohol problems. *Psychotherapy Research, 8,* 455–474.

Rogers, C. R. (1965). *Client-centered therapy.* New York: Houghton Mifflin.

Rollnick, S., Miller, W. R., & Butler, C. C. (2008). *Motivational interviewing in health care: Helping patients change behavior.* New York: Guilford Press.

Smith, J. E., Meyers, R. J., & Miller, W. R. (2001). The community reinforcement approach to the treatment of substance use disorders. *The American Journal on Addictions, 10,* 51–59.

Tatarsky, A., & Marlatt, G. A. (2010). State of the art in harm reduction psychotherapy: An emerging treatment for substance misuse. *Journal of Clinical Psychology, 66,* 117–122.

Trice, H. M., & Beyer, J. M. (1984). Work-related outcomes of the constructive-confrontation strategy in a job-based alcoholism program. *Journal of Studies on Alcohol, 45,* 393–404.

Truax, C. B., & Carkhuff, R. R. (1967). *Toward effective counseling and psychotherapy.* Chicago: Aldine.

UKATT Research Team. (2005). Effectiveness of treatment for alcohol problems: Findings of the randomised UK alcohol treatment trial. *British Medical Journal, 331*(7516).

Valle, S. K. (1981). Interpersonal functioning of alcoholism counselors and treatment outcome. *Journal of Studies on Alcohol, 42,* 783–790.

White, W. L., & Miller, W. R. (2007). The use of confrontation in addiction treatment: History, science, and time for change. *Counselor, 8*(4), 12–30.

CHAPTER 11

• • • • • •

Brief Treatments
for Gambling Problems
Using Motivational Approaches

David C. Hodgins
Jennifer L. Swan
Katherine M. Diskin

Gambling is generally understood to incorporate the element of risk in an organized way, in which the individual risks something he or she has in the hope of acquiring more. Forms of gambling have existed across the ages and cultures of humanity. Primitive dice made from the knucklebones of sheep (astralagi) have been found in caves dating from 3500 B.C.E. (Bernstein, 1996), while as of January 2015, over 3,100 online casinos and gambling websites were available to the public (Casino City, 2015). Even when gambling has not been legally sanctioned, illegal gambling opportunities such as floating card and crap games, bookies, numbers, and illegal slot machines have been available. Some forms of gambling are legal in all provinces of Canada and every state in the United States except Utah and Hawaii, with local and regional governments participating in providing gambling opportunities and sharing in gambling revenue.

The majority of gamblers, like the majority of drinkers, do not experience adverse effects from their activities; however, excessive gambling has been a source of serious distress for centuries. Romans who could not pay their gambling debts were sold into slavery (National Research Council, 1999), while gambling-related suicide attempt rates for problem and pathological gamblers currently range from 7 to 26% (Hodgins, Mansley, & Thygesen, 2006).

Although "gambling mania" was identified as a form of "monomania" in the early 1800s, pathological gambling was included in the American Psychiatric Association's *Diagnostic and Statistical Manual of Mental Disorders* (DSM) for the first time in 1980 as a disorder of impulse control (American Psychiatric Association, 1980). The criteria for pathological gambling disorder have continued to be modified in subsequent editions of the manual. At present, DSM-5 (American Psychiatric Association, 2013) defines gambling disorder as "persistent and recurrent problematic gambling behavior leading to clinically significant impairment or distress" (p. 585). The criteria for gambling disorder combine those relating to the effects of gambling (for example, relationship problems, hiding losses) with some encountered in substance abuse (tolerance, withdrawal) and also include the use of gambling as a means of escaping from problems or relieving a dysphoric mood. National estimates of the past-year prevalence of pathological gambling, or gambling disorder, range from 0.2 to 5.3% worldwide, depending on the availability of legal gambling and other cultural factors, but most estimates are between 0.3 to 1%, with another 1 to 2% showing subclinical signs, often labeled problem gambling (American Psychiatric Association, 2013; Hodgins, Stea, & Grant, 2011). Throughout this chapter, the term "disordered gambling" will be used inclusively to describe problem and pathological gambling as well as gambling disorder, as defined by the current DSM.

The effects of disordered gambling are wide-ranging. Gamblers are at high risk for stress-related physical illnesses and comorbid psychiatric disorders. It is clear that disordered gambling affects more than just the gambler. Family, friends, employers, and health and social welfare systems all feel the impact of problem gambling. Gamblers often face serious legal problems as a result of committing illegal acts to finance their gambling. More specifically, disordered gamblers are more likely than recreational gamblers to be divorced, to have received welfare, to have experienced bankruptcy, to have been arrested, and to have physical and psychological health problems (The National Gambling Impact Study Commission Final Report, cited in Volberg, 2001). The relative speed at which increased gambling opportunities have become available has made it difficult to accurately estimate the extent of the financial and social costs of gambling problems.

Usual Treatments

Based on various understandings of the factors that cause and maintain problem gambling, modalities used in its treatment have included psychoanalysis, client-centered supportive therapy, various forms of group therapy, marital therapy, behavioral and cognitive therapies including self-help manuals, Gamblers Anonymous (GA) groups, and pharmacological treatments (Hodgins et al., 2011; Stea & Hodgins, 2011). A recent systematic review of face-to-face individual psychological therapies for gambling identified 14 randomized controlled trials examining brief, moderate, or intensive therapies (Cowlishaw et al., 2012). Of the 14 studies, 11 examined cognitive-behavioral interventions, four examined therapies using motivational interviewing (MI), two studies evaluated an integrative therapy, and one study evaluated group therapy modeled after the 12 steps of Gamblers Anonymous. The authors concluded that cognitive-behavioral approaches currently have the strongest empirical support of the treatments reviewed. However, the authors note that several of the treatments reviewed, including MI, showed promise for the treatment of gambling problems, although additional research to further examine their potential benefits is needed.

Recently, a systematic review and meta-analysis of randomized controlled trials included both face-to-face, Internet, and telephone-based MI for disordered gambling (Yakovenko, Quigley, Hemmelgarn, Hodgins, & Ronksley, 2015). The meta-analysis included five controlled trials comparing MI to non-MI interventions such as cognitive-behavioral therapy, and found a significant positive effect for MI interventions posttreatment for both days and dollars gambled. Over the course of follow-up, the effect of MI interventions was still significantly greater for days gambled but not for dollars gambled. The results of this meta-analysis suggest there are positive short-term benefits of MI for disordered gambling; however, the long-term maintenance of the effect is less clear.

Rationale for Using MI with Gambling Problems

MI is a natural fit to the area of disordered gambling for a number of reasons. First, it is clear that impairment of control and motivation are important features of the disorder. The conceptualization of disordered gambling is a matter of some debate, with some theorists focusing on its similarity to addictive disorders such as substance abuse. Some view disordered gambling as an impulse control disorder, while others consider it to fall within the obsessive–compulsive spectrum (Mudry et al., 2011). The diagnostic criteria of previous and current versions of the DSM reflect the lack of a clear consensus: the criteria are modeled after those of substance dependence, but until recently the disorder was placed within the impulse disorders section of the manual (American Psychiatric Association, 2000, 2013). Currently, DSM-5 places gambling disorder in a new section for substance-related and other addictive disorders. Regardless, the various conceptualizations share the recognition that impairment of control over gambling is a central feature of the disorder, and, as a result, a struggle with motivational factors is pivotal in outcome. It is common to use treatment approaches for pathological gambling that are adapted from substance abuse treatment models such as cognitive-behavioral treatments.

Heather (2005) has suggested that addiction may be a "disorder of motivation," based on the idea that the "addict" is choosing to behave in a way that is against his or her long-term interests. This definition includes more than the idea that the person is doing something that society finds unacceptable—this is something that the individual him- or herself (at least sometimes) wants to change, resulting in "a motivational conflict composed of the contrasting incentives and disincentives. . . . The resolution of such a conflict is, of course, at the heart of MI" (Heather, 2005, pp. 4–5).

A second reason that MI fits well with disordered gambling is the observation that recovery from gambling problems without treatment (i.e., natural recovery) is common (Hodgins, Wynne, & Makarchuk, 1999). The existence of self-directed recovery is consistent with the notion that motivation is central in the change process. Interviews with recovered disordered gamblers confirm that cognitive-motivational factors are perceived to be primary in maintaining abstinence from gambling (Hodgins & el-Guebaly, 2000).

Clinical Applications

As with many mental health disorders, rates of treatment seeking are low relative to the prevalence estimates of the number of people suffering from the disorder. Less than 10% of disordered gamblers seek out the available treatments (Cunningham, 2005; Suurvali, Hodgins, Cordingley, & Cunningham, 2009). To the extent that low treatment seeking is related to motivation and lack of access to treatment, two potential complementary solutions are to increase the motivation of individuals to seek formal treatment and to broaden the treatment options by offering more accessible types of treatment. We present examples of both of these approaches that use MI. First, we present the use of a brief motivational intervention to increase the efficacy of a self-help workbook for disordered gambling. Second, we provide a description of a one-session motivational intervention to encourage reduction of gambling behavior.

A third application of MI to gambling treatment relates to treatment compliance. Dropout rates in both psychosocial and pharmacological clinical trials are unacceptably high (Grant, Kim, & Potenza, 2003; Hodgins & Petry, 2004; Toneatto & Ladouceur, 2003). An Australian study illustrated the value of a variety of compliance-improving interventions in increasing attendance in outpatient cognitive-behavioral therapy for problem gambling (Milton, Crino, Hunt, & Prosser, 2002). The compliance-improving interventions included providing written and verbal reinforcement for attendance, encouraging a sense of optimism and self-efficacy about the outcome, providing feedback on assessment results, the regular use of decisional balance exercises between sessions, and the discussion of barriers to treatment involvement. A number of these strategies were adapted from the MI literature. Together these compliance-improving interventions increased treatment completion rates to 65% from a baseline of 35% completion before the changes.

Promoting Self-Recovery in Disordered Gamblers by Using Motivational Enhancement

To capitalize on the desire of some disordered gamblers to recover without formal help (Cunningham, Cordingley, Hodgins, & Toneatto, 2011; Cunningham, Hodgins, & Toneatto, 2009), a self-help workbook was developed that incorporated techniques that recovered gamblers identified in interviews as significant in the recovery process (Hodgins & Makarchuk, 2002). The content of the workbook includes sections on self-assessment, goal setting, cognitive-behavioral strategies, relapse prevention strategies, and information about more formal treatment resources.[1]

We assessed the efficacy of providing self-help materials to pathological gamblers who did not wish to enter formal treatment in a clinical trial. Media recruitment was used to identify individuals concerned

---

[1]The workbooks are available through *www.addiction.ucalgary.ca.*

about their gambling but not wanting treatment, and two alternative self-help protocols were compared to a 1-month waiting-list control (see Hodgins, Currie, & el-Guebaly, 2001, for details). The first approach involved simply providing a self-help workbook via the mail (workbook-only group) after a brief telephone assessment; the second involved a telephone motivational interview prior to receiving the workbook (motivational group). The workbook was distributed as a bound booklet, with the instruction that the participant work through the exercises at his or her own pace. Participants were followed for 24 months to track their progress with the self-help protocols.

The motivational interview took between 20 to 45 minutes and was conducted using MI (Miller & Rollnick, 2002, 2013). In addition to collecting basic assessment information, the interview had four goals that aligned with the central processes of MI: engaging, focusing, evoking, and planning (Miller & Rollnick, 2013). The general aim of the interview was to be supportive and empathic and to demonstrate interest in the client's problem to enhance engagement. The interviewer attempted to elicit the gamblers' concerns, including the difficulties they were experiencing (focusing). For example:

> "What worries have you had about your gambling? What makes you think you need to change your gambling?"

The interviewer's queries focused on the effects on financial and legal status, relationships, and emotional functioning and elicited gamblers' thoughts about the advantages of quitting. The second and third goals of the interview followed the central process of evoking and were intended to explore the gambler's ambivalence about change and to promote self-efficacy:

> "What might make it difficult to accomplish a change in your gambling? How successful do you think you will be? Looking back, what makes you think you can accomplish it?"

Finally, the interviewer suggested specific strategies for the individual based on past successful change attempts (planning). These strategies were tied to a section of the workbook. For example:

> "It sounds like starting exercising was helpful when you quit drinking. There is a section in the workbook that recommends taking on new activities—that might be helpful."

After the interview, the clinicians prepared a brief personalized note to the gambler that was sent in the mail along with the workbook. The note focused on affirming the individual's goal regarding gambling.

Many U.S. states and Canadian provinces offer problem gambling helplines to provide treatment information and personal support to individuals. This motivational intervention protocol is ideally suited to be integrated into such a service, as has been done in the statewide gambling treatment system in Oregon and the national helpline in New Zealand. Our research experience is that it does successfully attract individuals not interested in formal treatment.

Description of a Typical Participant

Belinda is married and in her late 40s. Her husband is in charge of their finances and has recently told her that if she doesn't get her slot machine gambling under control he will leave her. She has tried Gamblers Anonymous, but found that she didn't like the religious aspect of it and that listening to other people talk about gambling made her gambling urges even stronger. She also found it difficult to identify herself as the type of person who goes to GA. The idea of a treatment approach in which she can work at her own pace and speak with someone over the phone really appealed to her.

During the motivational interview, Belinda spoke a lot about her self-image and how she did not see herself as the type of person who would get addicted. She identified a sense of challenge and the pleasure of escaping the boredom of life for a while as significant positive aspects of playing the slots for her, although she recognized the negative impact on her marriage, finances, and self-esteem. Belinda described herself as being highly self-directed and having a reasonable amount of self-control. She was interested to hear that many people successfully recover from gambling. When asked about previous behavior changes, she described how she had lost a great deal of weight when she was a teen. The therapist linked the strategies that she had used to lose weight—setting short-term goals, exercising regularly with friends, and reminding herself of her long-term goals—to the contents of the workbook.

The telephone interview lasted about 40 minutes and ended with the therapist giving a summary statement, as recommended in MI. At the end of the interview, the therapist told Belinda:

> "I am impressed with how open you are to talking about your struggles. It sounds like you like the challenge of playing the slots and like

the fact that it gives you time alone. On the other hand, it has caused you a number of problems—both you and your husband are upset with the financial cost, and you are starting to spend your savings, which will have implications for your long-term goal of retiring to the coast. As well, you are a strong person, so the gambling takes its toll on your self-esteem. You find it hard to believe that you would continue to gamble. You have tackled hard personal issues before—your weight—and it sounds like you might be ready to tackle this one."

Belinda did, in fact, set some short-term gambling goals, following the suggestions in the workbook. These goals included not gambling for 2 weeks as an evaluation period. She changed her behavior by arranging to go for daily walks with a friend right after work, which was when she typically would visit the casino. She decided to track her finances more closely to monitor her "savings" from not gambling. She also prepared herself for how she would handle the urges to gamble through distraction and reminding herself about her long-term goals.

Belinda gambled once after the 2-week period but immediately felt that she wanted to make it her last time. She recommitted herself to her goals and strategies and did not gamble again.

Research Outcomes

The study described earlier constitutes a randomized clinical trial comparing motivational enhancement plus workbook to a workbook-only condition and a waiting-list control. The results showed a significant advantage for the group receiving the motivational intervention. For example, at 3 months 42% of the motivational group was abstinent and an additional 39% were categorized as improved, compared with 19% and 56% of the workbook-only group (Hodgins et al., 2001). At 24 months, although 37% of the people were abstinent across groups, 54% of the motivational group had improved compared with 25% of the workbook only group (Hodgins, Currie, el-Guebaly, & Peden, 2004). These results suggest that the brief telephone motivational intervention is a wise investment of resources in enhancing the likelihood of individual success.

To replicate and extend these findings, a study comparing a waiting-list group to a workbook-only group, a motivational telephone intervention plus workbook group (brief group), and a group that, in addition to the initial motivational telephone call, received a monthly booster call for 5 months (brief booster group) has been conducted (Hodgins, Currie, Currie, & Fick, 2009). The rationale for this last condition was to determine whether a motivational booster would maintain and improve outcomes over time. The results indicated a short-term advantage for the brief and brief booster groups. For example, at 6 weeks posttreatment, 25% of participants in the brief group and 23% of participants in the brief booster group were abstinent, compared to 14% in both the workbook-only and waiting-list control groups. During the first 6 months of study follow-up, participants in both the brief and brief booster groups gambled significantly fewer days than participants in the workbook-only control group; however, there were no significant differences in dollars spent gambling between the groups. By the 12-month follow-up, all three groups showed improvement, with no significant differences among them. While inclusion of booster calls over the follow-up period did not yield greater improvements for participants, the results of this study provide additional support for brief MI interventions for problem gambling.

One-Session MI for Disordered Gambling

The promoting self recovery approach that was described earlier was focused on providing a telephone contact and written materials to individuals seeking to change their behavior. The next study involved comparing a face-to-face motivational intervention with a clinical interview that did not contain motivational components in order to determine whether the MI elements of the contact specifically accounted for the response (see Diskin & Hodgins, 2009, for details). We advertised for participants who were experiencing some concerns about their gambling. Participants were not required to be wanting to reduce their gambling but simply to be experiencing some level of concern. The inclusion criteria for the study were intentionally as broad as possible. The only exclusion criteria for participation were that potential participants must have gambled within the preceding 2 months and that they had obtained a score of 3 or higher on the Problem Gambling Severity Index of the Canadian Problem Gambling Index (Ferris, Wynne, & Single, 1998), which is indicative of an "at-risk" level of problem. Participants were randomly assigned to one of two groups. Half the participants were given the motivational interview (described in detail below). The other half spent a similar amount of time with an interviewer talking about their gambling and completing various semistructured personality measures. Two clinicians conducted both the motivational and nonmotivational interviews. All participants were given a copy of the self-help workbook and were followed for a 12-month period with follow-up calls at 1, 3, 6, and 12 months.

    In developing a brief interview that could be used with a wide range of individuals with varying levels of gambling problems and varying levels of concern about their gambling, we sought, as our primary goal, to incorporate the spirit and four central processes of MI into the intervention. The interview was intended as an opportunity for a collaborative encounter—a dialogue about gambling. We hoped to provide an opportunity for gamblers to explore their concerns and ambivalence about gambling in a nonjudgmental setting. To this end, it was necessary for the interviewers to commit sincerely to the idea that the impetus and responsibility for change had to come from the gambler. We found that gamblers who received a motivational intervention reduced their gambling significantly more over a 12-month period following the interview than gamblers receiving the nonmotivational interview.

The Interview

The intervention closely adhered to the four central processes that make up MI. These basic components included a brief discussion about gambling habits (engaging); a discussion of the things people liked and disliked about gambling (focusing); a normative and personalized feedback section; a decisional balance exercise, an exploration of self-efficacy, a future-oriented imagination exercise, and ratings of motivation to change and of confidence (evoking); and, if appropriate, a discussion of the participant's thoughts about changing his or her gambling behavior (planning). The discussion about potential changes was left to the discretion of the interviewer in order to tailor the interview to the client. Some participants were not ready to consider change or didn't feel they had a problem. Insisting on a discussion of possible change strategies might have alienated the participant and would have served to detract from the purpose of the interview, which was to allow the participant time to access and reflect on his or her thoughts and feelings about what he or she was doing. Although all of the components were expected to be included in the interview if possible, the order and relative emphasis of each were at the discretion of the interviewer, to promote flexibility. If, for example, a question about the "good things" about gambling evoked a litany of worries, we did not require that individuals stop expressing their concerns. Instead, we followed their lead and asked for more information. We would ask about the "good things" at a later point in the interview, perhaps framing the question historically, for example:

> "You've told me a lot about the problems you've been having with gambling, but I'm wondering what was it about gambling that attracted you when you started—what did you like about it?"

The intention was for the interviewer to retain control of the direction of the encounter while allowing the participant to discuss what was important to him or her. We often employed brief summaries of the discussion to shift to the next section of the interview.

HOW DID THE INTERVIEW PROCEED?

All the interviews began with a very general question about each participant's gambling. After describing their gambling preferences and the frequency of their gambling, gamblers often started to describe their current difficulties, which led smoothly to an initial discussion of current problems. For people who had some difficulty warming up to the interview, we asked what had prompted them to participate in the study. For people who seemed unconcerned or unsure about why they had volunteered, we asked if other people had "said anything" about their gambling. If others had voiced concerns, we would then ask if the gambler had any concerns or if he or she did not feel that the issues identified were a problem. For less talkative gamblers we sometimes asked for a description of a typical gambling day, which often generated a discussion about employment (or lack of it), situational factors that made gambling attractive on certain days, and their feelings before and after gambling.

The interviews typically started as follows:

> "We advertised for people who have been wondering about their gambling. Can you tell me a bit about your gambling?"

- "Well, I started off going to Vegas for fun, but now it's not fun anymore."
- "I go to the bar and play the machines and spend money that I need for other things."
- "My wife and I separated about 2 years ago, and I'm lonely, so I want to go out; but I know I should be spending more time with the kids and not wasting my money."

Good and Not-So-Good Things about Gambling

We next took time to explore what the gambler enjoyed about gambling. Often this line of questioning would generate mixed responses—gamblers would start out talking about some positive aspects of gambling but would begin to introduce negative elements. We tried to make sure that gamblers got the opportunity to explore their attraction to gambling—what drew them to it initially and what they still enjoyed. For example:

> "Tell me what you like [or liked] about gambling—what's the best part . . . what else . . . ?"

- "It gives me somewhere to go and meet people—I often see the same people there."
- "I like the rush—the feeling that I might win this time."
- "It's a really good feeling when I win. I get excited and imagine that I can get out of debt."
- "I get to forget what's going on at home."

We would then move into a discussion of the not-so-good things about gambling. For example:

> "You already told me about some concerns you have had about your gambling [summarize]. What else is a concern? What else is not so good about your gambling?"

- "I get depressed when I lose, I feel stupid, I feel like a loser."
- "I think of the things I could have bought for the kids."
- "I'm going further into debt, don't know how I'm going to pay the bills."
- "I never have any extra money."
- "I'm afraid people will find out and think I'm stupid."

During this discussion of good and not-so-good things about gambling, the interviewers were encouraged to remain sensitive and attentive, using reflective listening to encourage exploration of emotional responses and multiple issues. During the discussion of the "not-so-good things," emotions were often quite close to the surface, and the interviewer could often use an initial statement to explore the effects of gambling. For example, in response to "I think of the things I could have bought for the kids," the interviewer could simply reflect perceived emotion—"It makes you sad to think that your kids are missing out because of gambling"—and allow the participant time to sit with this feeling. Alternatively, the interviewer could choose to delve further into the impact of gambling on the family. For example:

> "It sounds like gambling has impacted your ability to buy things for your kids. Has gambling affected your relationship with them in other ways?"

FEEDBACK

After giving the gamblers an opportunity to talk about gambling and explore ambivalence, they were asked if they were interested in receiving information about how their scores on a measure of gambling problems compared with others who had taken the survey. We used data from a recent local survey to provide comparisons with participants' scores on a measure of gambling severity. Such information is available in the majority of states and provinces and in many locations worldwide. The feedback section was the only component of the intervention that is not part of the "classic" motivational interview as described by Miller and Rollnick (2002, 2013), although it is described as a critical element of related brief intervention approaches known as "motivational enhancement therapy" (Miller & Rollnick, 2013). The approach to feedback delivery was consistent with the general MI approach. Participants were first asked if they were interested in finding out how their scores compared with other adult Albertans. After they were told how their scores compared to others and the risk category associated with their score, participants were asked for their reaction to the feedback.

None of the study participants declined the offer of comparing their scores to the general population. Some responded without surprise, and some were quite distressed. Some had difficulty believing that their level of gambling was as unusual as it appeared from the comparison. We did not argue with participants who felt this way or who suggested that other respondents must have minimized their own gambling habits. Instead, we reflected their responses—for example: "It seems to you that lots of people gamble about as much as you do," or "It's hard to believe some people don't gamble at all." Reflections rather than arguments allowed for further exploration of their perceptions of whether or not their level of gambling involvement was unusual as compared to others and allowed for a consideration of how and with whom they spent time. If participants indicated that the feedback confirmed their concerns, the interviewer would reinforce their concern and ask for more—for example, "This is something you have been thinking about for a while—have you thought about what you might want to do about it?" At the end of the 12-month follow-up we asked if gamblers remembered receiving the normative feedback. About two-thirds of the gamblers who had received normative feedback remembered it, and all but one felt it had been helpful.

NORMATIVE FEEDBACK

"When you called in response to the ad, the research assistant asked you some questions about your gambling—that was a questionnaire that has been given to thousands of people. Would you like to see how your score compares to others? You are in the group that is considered to be [either at moderate risk for developing gambling problems or having a substantial level of gambling-related problems]. Does that surprise you at all?"

- "It depresses me a little. . . . "
- "No, that's why I came in."
- "Wow! That's scary."
- "That confirms I have a problem."
- "People were lying when they answered this—I told the truth."
- "I know lots of people who gamble as much as I do."

PERSONALIZED FEEDBACK

"We have another way to look at what's going on with you and your gambling if you're interested. We can look at how much you're spending as compared to how much you take home in a month. You told the research assistant that you take home about $____ per month. You also talked about how much you spent gambling in the last 2 months, which would average about $____. Does that sound about right? If we divide what you spend by the amount you make, we can see what percentage of your income goes to gambling each month. It looks like you are spending about ____% of what you take home on gambling. What do you make of that?"

- "It makes me feel even worse, but committed to change."
- "It depresses me a little—I might cut out scratch cards, but I really like the casino."
- "I'm not sure why I do this, I'm an intelligent person."

DECISIONAL BALANCE

The decisional balance exercise was introduced. This was done in a paper-and-pencil format, and a copy was given to the gambler to take home. The decisional balance was done as a hypothetical cost–benefit exercise. Participants were asked to think about the costs to them if they chose to stay the same and continue gambling at the same level (a further exploration of the not-so-good things about gambling). They were then asked to think about the benefits if their gambling stayed the same (another chance to explore what was important to them about their gambling). We next asked them about the costs of changing—providing an exploration of what they would be giving up if they did make changes (this gave them an opportunity to express some of their fears and concerns about changing their gambling). And finally they were asked to consider the benefits of changing their gambling (giving them an opportunity to imagine a future without gambling). This discussion was framed in terms of the thought that that they might be entertaining the possibility of making some kind of change in their gambling—quitting or cutting down was not introduced unless the gambler brought it up. By maintaining the hypothetical nature of the discussion, participants were free to talk about what might be different without having to commit to any changes at all.

> "We have talked a bit about the good and not-so-good things about gambling for you—this is an exercise that is a little bit the same but gives us a different way to look at things. We can look at these questions even if you aren't sure you want to quit or cut down."

Costs of Staying the Same. We started with thinking about what life would be like if no changes were made in gambling—what the costs would be to the gambler if he or she made no changes at all in behavior, including some of the previously discussed problems.

- "I'm leading a double life—lying to family and friends."
- "Stealing."
- "Feeling guilty."
- "Growing debts."
- "I will go broke."
- "I worry about money all the time."
- "I could go bankrupt."

Benefits of Staying the Same. Next we talked about the benefits of not changing—what are the important things about maintaining their gambling? This is an opportunity to understand what people like about gambling, what purpose it serves in their lives.

- "I might win."
- "It's entertainment."
- "It's a chance to dream."
- "I like the excitement, rush."
- "Getting away from home, socializing."
- "It's an escape."

Many people could not think of anything that would be good about staying the same—often this question would generate a quick response— "There's nothing good about it." After reflecting the feeling we would proceed to the next quadrant. We often found that when people moved to thinking about the costs of changing their gambling (what they would be giving up) they were more able to identify their reasons for persisting with gambling, and these were discussed as perceived benefits when the thoughts were generated.

Costs of Making Changes. This was a very useful area to explore— it provoked a great deal of thought in terms of what the gambler would be giving up and what might be difficult about changing. It also was a springboard for the gamblers to generate alternatives to their current activities.

- "I would lose the chance to go out, boredom."
- "I would lose the chance to escape from stuff at home."
- "It's hard to change."
- "It's hard to be responsible."
- "I'd have to give up the chance of winning."

Benefits of Making Changes. What would he or she imagine would be different if a change were made? This was an opportunity to imagine a hypothetical future—an opportunity to think about the things besides gambling that are important. Again, some of the items raised from the previous discussion could be discussed and expanded.

- "I could trust myself more, not feel guilty."
- "I could do things with the money: eat healthier food, travel, give kids more, pay debts, buy a house."
- "I could have less stress, be healthier, spend time with kids, friends."
- "My spouse wouldn't divorce me."

ENCOURAGEMENT OF SELF-EFFICACY

This was an opportunity to talk about change more generally, to ask about how this individual makes changes in his or her life. People could usually think of something that they had had some success with, even if they hadn't been totally successful. Even if they had not succeeded in changing a behavior, they could often generate some thoughts about what had and hadn't worked. This was an opportunity to restate that the client is the best authority on him- or herself and is the person most likely to know what he or she is willing to undertake. Often people would start to generate ideas about how they could change their gambling if they wanted to by using previously successful strategies. If they had no personal experience or ideas around change, we might ask if they knew of any strategies other people had used. We also asked about situations where they had the opportunity to gamble but chose not to, exploring what they had done differently in those situations.

> "We've been talking about the idea of making changes—have you ever made changes in other areas of your life? What works best for you?"

- "I need to do it cold turkey."
- "Telling people, being open with them, getting help."
- "Getting counseling."
- "Just deciding—made a decision I didn't want it."
- "I have to cut ties with people who were involved in the same things [e.g., drinking, drugs]."

FUTURE-ORIENTED IMAGINATION EXERCISE

We asked people to think about their lives in 5 or 10 years. What did they imagine their lives would be like based on two scenarios—if they did make changes in their gambling and if they didn't?

> "If you decided you don't want to change anything about your gambling, what do you imagine your life would be like in 5 or 10 years?"

- "The same, maybe worse."
- "I'd be homeless."
- "I would disappear, be lonely."
- "I would get more depressed."
- "I would lose my family."

> "If you decide you want to make some changes in your gambling, what do you imagine your life would be like in 5 or 10 years?"

- "I could have a different house."
- "I would be healthy, less anxious."
- "Better marriage."

- "I could help my kids, take care of grandkids."
- "Get married, have a family, have a nice house."
- "I would be debt-free."

RATINGS OF MOTIVATION AND CONFIDENCE

This exercise was introduced as another way to get an idea of how the gambler was feeling about his or her gambling and the possibility of change. We asked people to imagine a ruler with markings from 0 to 10 and asked them two questions:

> "If we had a ruler in front of us, and 0 on the ruler was 'not at all motivated to change anything about my gambling,' and 10 on the ruler was 'absolutely motivated to make changes in my gambling'— where would you put yourself right now?"

> "If you decided you did want to make changes in your gambling, how confident are you that you could—with 0 being not at all confident and 10 being absolutely confident you could do it if you set your mind to it?"

After each exercise we explored why a particular number had been chosen. If the person rated his or her motivation as a 5, we might ask more questions. If they seemed quite negative and yet chose a 5, we might comment, "Wow, it sounds like, even though you're worried about what changing would be like, you still rate your motivation as a 5." This could be followed with questions such as "Why are you a 5 and not a 0?" or "What would it take for your motivation to move to a 7 or 8? What would have to happen?" Responses ranged from enthusiastic—some even said 12 on the 10-point scale, for example—to extremely doubtful. This was another opportunity for the gamblers to think about whether or not changing gambling was something they were really interested in doing at this time.

DECISION DISCUSSION

At the end of the interview we summarized the discussion and acknowledged that talking about their gambling with a stranger could be very difficult. This was not only intended to continue the practice of affirming the clients, a central MI concept, but also to let them know that we were aware that they had allowed us to share in painful and difficult areas of their lives. We also expressed our appreciation for their willingness to take part in the interview, acknowledging that by doing so they were not only helping with our research but also doing something to care for themselves. Next we asked participants to tell us their thoughts after having gone through the interview. We encountered a wide range of responses to this question. At this point gamblers often expressed ambivalence about change. Some people were quite clear that they wanted to quit or cut down substantially and made statements about fairly specific changes they wanted to make. We reinforced these plans and encouraged further thought and planning about how change could take place. Others were not ready to consider any changes. People who were not ready to change were encouraged to continue to think about the discussion and refer to the workbook if they were interested at a later date. We acknowledged that we had covered a lot of territory in the interview and that the participant was the person who was the best authority on what he or she should be doing (or not doing).

"We've talked about a lot of things today—what do you think about all this?"

- "I feel overwhelmed, it makes me sick."
- "I'd quit if I really thought it was a problem or it started to affect my health."
- "I really have to do something."
- "I would have to stay away from the casino/bar, those friends."
- "I would have to make some different arrangements about money."
- "I would have to start exercising."
- "I have to do it cold turkey."
- "I could make a list of things I want to spend my money on instead of wasting it."
- "It made me think about everything I could lose."
- "I'm not wanting to change right now."

Research Outcomes

This study involved a randomized clinical trial comparing a face-to-face motivational intervention with a control interview that consisted of traditional close-ended assessment questions (Diskin & Hodgins, 2009). We intended this to be a fairly stringent test of the effectiveness of MI with problem gamblers. Everyone received a workbook, and everyone spent about 45 minutes to an hour speaking with a clinically trained interviewer. We used a 12-month follow-up period in order to take into account the high rate of natural recovery in this population.

Immediately after the interviews participants were asked to evaluate their experiences of the interview and of their interviewer. The two groups did not differ in their ratings of their interviewer, with both groups rating their interviewers quite highly in terms of empathy, trustworthiness, respect, and understanding. However, the groups did differ in their ratings of the interview they received. Gamblers rated the motivational intervention higher in terms of several variables, including helpfulness, overall satisfaction, and whether problems were worked on effectively.

Since participation in the study did not require that participants intend to quit gambling (or even intend to make any change in their gambling), we decided to use the number of days gambled per month and monthly gambling expenditures as the dependent variables of interest. Both groups were gambling a mean amount of approximately $1,300 Cdn per month in the 2 months preceding the interview and both groups were gambling about 7 days per month.

For the participants who completed the study, we found that over the 12-month period the gamblers who had received a motivational intervention gambled less often and spent less money gambling than the control group. In the 3 months preceding the final interview the motivational group gambled approximately 2.2 days per month, whereas the control group gambled about 5 days per month. In the final 3-month period preceding the 12-month interview, the motivational group also gambled less money on a monthly basis as compared to the attention control group. The motivational intervention participants spent an average of about $340 gambling per month, but the control group participants spent an average of $912 monthly.

A very interesting and unexpected result was related to the level of problem gambling severity. Almost all the gamblers in the study were experiencing significant levels of gambling problems. We had expected that gamblers with comparatively less severe problems would likely find the motivational intervention more helpful than those that were experiencing more severe problems. Instead, we found that for the people who completed the 12-month follow-up, those with less severe problems improved in a similar fashion whether they received a motivational interview or were in the control condition. Those with more severe problems reduced their gambling significantly if they received a motivational intervention but did not do so if they were in the attention control group.

Over the course of the study gamblers in the comparatively lower severity group who received a motivational interview spent about $325 per month on gambling, while those in the control group spent about $265 per month (this difference was not statistically significant). It seems that for those whose gambling problems were comparatively less severe, the motivational intervention did not have a significant effect over and above receiving the self-help manual and participating in the study. Lower severity participants in both groups reduced the amount of money they spent over 12 months considerably.

However, gamblers in the higher severity group who received a motivational interview spent about $300 dollars gambling per month. Those in the control group spent about $1,100 dollars per month. For those in the comparatively more severe group, the motivational intervention was helpful in reducing both dollars and days spent gambling. All of the participants in the study were willing to make some effort to explore their concerns about gambling (enough to make and keep an appointment for an interview). For those with less severe problems, this effort and the availability of the manual may have been enough. For those with more severe problems, participating in the MI made a significant difference. It is unclear at this point which elements of the interview were effective in helping people with severe problems maintain changes in their gambling behavior over the course of 12 months. To the extent that we were able to adhere to the spirit of MI, it may be that the opportunity to explore their ambivalent feelings about gambling in a nonjudgmental atmosphere was helpful in empowering them to decide to make significant changes.

Problems and Suggested Solutions

Generally the MI approach appears to work well with disordered gambling with many individuals. One potential complication, however, is the extremely high prevalence of comorbid mental health disorders (substance abuse, mood and anxiety, personality) with gambling disorders, which can impact the course and outcome of the gambling problem (Hodgins & el-Guebaly, 2010; Lorains, Cowlishaw, & Thomas, 2011). To date, little is known about the implications of comorbidity for gambling treatment. It is not clear whether one or the other disorder should be tackled first or whether treatment should be concurrent (separate interventions) or integrated, or whether client preference should dictate the sequencing. In the absence of evidence-based guidelines, the solution is flexibility on the part of the therapist to move where the client needs to move, which requires a broad base of training and experience. Being able to summon expertise in each of the comorbid disorders is the ideal situation. As the chapters in this book illustrate, the general MI approach can be tailored to the unique characteristics of a diverse range of mental health disorders.

Another complication with gambling disorders is the need to focus on financial issues as part of therapy. Individuals cannot typically pay down huge debt loads quickly and therefore must learn to manage them effectively over time. Financial pressures, if not dealt with, can erode motivation and be a risk for relapse (Hodgins & el-Guebaly, 2004). Therapists working with gambling problems must either develop financial counseling expertise or provide concurrent help in this area, even when just offering a brief MI intervention.

Access and convenience of treatment presents another potential complication. Online gambling opportunities are increasing, providing convenient and accessible means of gambling without ever leaving one's own home. Web-based treatments represent a convenient, accessible, and potentially cost-effective method for reaching problem gamblers and can be incorporated into shared and stepped-care models of treatment (Gainsbury & Blaszczynski, 2011). We are currently conducting a study examining the effect of a web-based, self-directed motivational enhancement intervention for problem gamblers (Hodgins, Fick, Murray, & Cunningham, 2013). The program is a text-based interactive tool developed using transcribed motivational interviews from previous research (Hodgins et al., 2009). While the delivery of self-help tools to gamblers in a web-based format has shown promise (e.g., Carlbring & Smit, 2008), the provision of motivational enhancement interventions for problem gamblers in a web-based format has not been previously explored. This ongoing study compares the motivational program to a web-based tool providing brief assessment and feedback to gamblers. Recruitment is under way, and participants will be followed over a 12-month period to track their gambling involvement.

Conclusions

The research we have presented here and our clinical experience support the value of MI for disordered gambling. In three studies a motivationally based intervention plus a self-help workbook was clearly associated with better outcomes than a comparison workbook-only condition. In two studies the intervention was via telephone, and in the other it was face to face. Two studies recruited individuals who were seeking to address their gambling problem, albeit without using formal treatment, and the other recruited individuals who were concerned but not necessarily ready to change. Further, a meta-analysis of five controlled trials examining MI interventions for disordered gambling (including the three we discussed) found promising short-term effects for MI and disordered gambling, although long-term effects of the interventions were unclear. Brief motivational interventions appear to be a way of extending the options provided by traditional treatment and encouraging reluctant gamblers to initiate the change process.

Further refinement and research are required in a number of areas. Comorbidity rates are high, and the implications of comorbidity for recovery and treatment are unclear. It is possible that for more complicated clinical presentations imbedding MI in a more intensive treatment intervention is more beneficial than offering brief interventions. Further development of treatment compliance methods using motivational principles is also important, given the high dropout rates reported. Dropping out may be more likely among those with comorbid disorders as well.

MI has the potential to play an important role in the gambling disorder treatment system as it continues to evolve. Treatment for pathological and problem gambling, as compared to other mental health disorders, is still in its infancy. As a result, the system may be more readily influenced by empirical effectiveness and efficacy research than in other areas of mental health.

References

American Psychiatric Association. (1980). *Diagnostic and statistical manual of mental disorders* (3rd ed.). Washington, DC: Author.

American Psychiatric Association. (2000). *Diagnostic and statistical manual of mental disorders* (4th ed., text rev.). Washington, DC: Author.

American Psychiatric Association. (2013). *Diagnostic and statistical manual of mental disorders* (5th ed.). Arlington, VA: Author.

Bernstein, P. L. (1996). *Against the gods: The remarkable story of risk*. New York: Wiley.

Carlbring, P., & Smit, F. (2008). Randomized trial of Internet-delivered self-help with telephone support for pathological gamblers. *Journal of Consulting and Clinical Psychology, 76*, 1090–1094.

Casino City. (2015). Retrieved January 15, 2013, from *http://onlinecasinocity.com*.

Cowlishaw, S., Merkouris, S., Dowling, N., Anderson, C., Jackson, A., &

Thomas, S. (2012). Psychological therapies for pathological and problem gambling. *Cochrane Database of Systematic Reviews, 11.*

Cunningham, J. A. (2005). Little use of treatment among problem gamblers. *Psychiatric Services, 56,* 1024–1025.

Cunningham, J. A., Cordingley, J. C., Hodgins, D. C., & Toneatto, T. (2011). Beliefs about gambling problems and recovery: Results from a general population survey. *Journal of Studies on Gambling, 27*(4), 625–631.

Cunningham, J. A., Hodgins, D. C., & Toneatto, T. (2009). Natural recovery from gambling problems: Results from a general population survey. *Sucht, Journal of Addiction Research and Practice, 55,* 99–103.

Diskin, K. M., & Hodgins, D. C. (2009). A randomized controlled trial of a single session motivational intervention for concerned gamblers. *Behaviour Research and Therapy, 47*(5), 382–388.

Ferris, J., Wynne, H., & Single, E. (1998). *Measuring problem gambling in Canada: Interim report to the inter-provincial task force on problem gambling.* Toronto: Canadian Interprovincial Task Force on Problem Gambling.

Gainsbury, S. M., & Blaszczynski, A. (2011). Online self-guided interventions for the treatment of problem gambling. *International Gambling Studies, 11,* 289–308.

Grant, J. E., Kim, S. W., & Potenza, M. N. (2003). Advances in the pharmacological treatment of pathological gambling disorder. *Journal of Gambling Studies, 19,* 85–109.

Heather, N. (2005). Motivational interviewing: Is it all our clients need? *Addiction Research and Theory, 13,* 1–18.

Hodgins, D. C., Currie, S. R., Currie, G., & Fick, G. H. (2009). Randomized trial of brief motivational treatments for pathological gamblers: More is not necessarily better. *Journal of Consulting and Clinical Psychology, 77*(5), 950–960.

Hodgins, D. C., Currie, S. R., & el-Guebaly, N. (2001). Motivational enhancement and self-help treatments for problem gambling. *Journal of Consulting and Clinical Psychology, 69,* 50–57.

Hodgins, D. C., Currie, S. R., el-Guebaly, N., & Peden, N. (2004). Brief motivational treatment for problem gambling: A 24-month follow-up. *Psychology of Addictive Behaviors, 18,* 293–296.

Hodgins, D. C., & el-Guebaly, N. (2000). Natural and treatment-assisted recovery from gambling problems: A comparison of resolved and active gamblers. *Addiction, 95,* 777–789.

Hodgins, D. C., & el-Guebaly, N. (2004). Retrospective and prospective reports of precipitants to relapse in pathological gambling. *Journal of Consulting and Clinical Psychology, 72,* 72–80.

Hodgins, D. C., & el-Guebaly, N. (2010). The influence of substance dependence and mood disorders on outcome from pathological gambling: Five year follow. *Journal of Studies on Gambling, 26*(1), 117–127.

Hodgins, D. C., Fick, G., Murray, R., & Cunningham, J. A. (2013). Internet-based interventions for disordered gamblers: Study protocol for a randomized controlled trial of online self-directed cognitive-behavioral motivation therapy. *BMC Public Health, 13,* 10.

Hodgins, D. C., & Makarchuk, K. (2002). *Becoming a winner: Defeating problem gambling.* Edmonton: AADAC.

Hodgins, D. C., Mansley, C., & Thygesen, K. (2006). Risk factors for suicide ideation and attempts among pathological gamblers. *American Journal on Addictions, 15*(4), 303–310.

Hodgins, D. C., & Petry, N. M. (2004). Cognitive and behavioral treatments. In J. E. Grant & M. N. Potenza (Eds.), *Pathological gambling: A clinical guide to treatment.* New York: American Psychiatric Association Press.

Hodgins, D. C., Stea, J. N., & Grant, J. E. (2011). Gambling disorders. *The Lancet, 378,* 1874–1884.

Hodgins, D. C., Wynne, H., & Makarchuk, K. (1999). Pathways to recovery from gambling problems: Follow-up from a general population survey. *Journal of Gambling Studies, 15,* 93–104.

Lorains, F. K., Cowlishaw, S., & Thomas, S. A. (2011). Prevalence of comorbid disorders in problem and pathological gambling: Systematic review and meta-analysis of population surveys. *Addiction, 106,* 490–498. doi:10.1111/j.1360–0443.2010.03300.x

Miller, W. R., & Rollnick, S. (2002). *Motivational Interviewing: Preparing people for change* (2nd ed.). New York: Guilford Press.

Miller, W. R., & Rollnick, S. (2013). *Motivational Interviewing: Helping people change* (3rd ed.). New York: Guilford Press.

Milton, S., Crino, R., Hunt, C., & Prosser, E. (2002). The effect of compliance-improving interventions on the cognitive-behavioral treatment of pathological gambling. *Journal of Gambling Studies, 18,* 207–230.

Mudry, T. E., Hodgins, D. C., el-Guebaly, N., Wild, T. C., Colman, I., Patten, S. B., et al. (2011). Conceptualizing excessive behaviour syndromes: A systematic review. *Current Psychiatry Reviews, 7,* 138–151.

National Research Council. (1999). *Pathological gambling. A critical review.* Washington, DC: National Academy Press.

Stea, J. N., & Hodgins, D. C. (2011). A critical review of treatment approaches for gambling disorders. *Current Drug Abuse Reviews, 4,* 67–80.

Suurvali, H., Hodgins, D. C., Cordingley, J., & Cunningham, J. A. (2009). Barriers to seeking help for gambling problems: A review of the empirical literature. *Journal of Gambling Studies, 25,* 407–424.

Toneatto, T., & Ladouceur, R. (2003). Treatment of pathological gambling: A critical review of the literature. *Psychology of Addictive Behaviors, 17,* 284–292.

Volberg, R. A. (2001). *When the chips are down: Problem gambling in America.* New York: Century Foundation Press.

Yakovenko, I., Quigley, L., Hemmelgarn, B. R., Hodgins, D. C., & Ronksley, P. (2015). The efficacy of motivational interviewing for disordered gambling: Systematic review and meta-analysis. *Addictive Behaviors, 43,* 72–82.

CHAPTER 12

• • • • • •

Motivational Interviewing for Smoking Cessation with Adolescents

Suzanne M. Colby

Cigarette smoking continues to be the leading cause of morbidity and premature mortality in the United States, accounting for the death of roughly 440,000 people per year (U.S. Department of Health and Human Services, 2010). A recent analysis of 50-year trends in smoking-related mortality among men and women in the United States documents the strong associations between smoking and deaths from lung cancer, chronic obstructive pulmonary disease, ischemic heart disease, and stroke. However, the odds of smoking-related death are reduced dramatically by smoking cessation at any age (Thun et al., 2013). In particular, quitting by age 40 has recently been shown to reduce the odds of smoking-related death nearly to never-smoker levels, whereas those continuing to smoke can expect to lose a decade of life on average as a result of their smoking (Jha et al., 2013).

The vast majority of adult smokers initiated their smoking during adolescence, a phenomenon in 1995 that led David Kessler, then commissioner of the Food and Drug Administration, to describe nicotine addiction as a "pediatric disease" (Hilts, 1995). According to the most recent findings from the national Monitoring the Future study, nearly half of all high school students have tried cigarette smoking, and about 1 in 10 adolescents (in grades 8, 10, and 12) report smoking in the past month; in 2013, about 1 in 11 high school seniors reported regular daily smoking (Johnston, O'Malley, Bachman, & Schulenberg, 2014). Prevalence varies widely, however, with higher rates of smoking seen in white adolescents (as compared to black/African American and Latino youth) and in rural areas. Overall, current rates of smoking reflect substantial progress since the late 1990s, when past-month smoking prevalence among adolescents was more than double (at 28%) and regular daily smoking among high school seniors was 25%. Most of that progress can be attributed to lower rates of smoking initiation and progression among adolescents owing to tobacco control efforts such as taxation of tobacco products, smoke-free indoor air laws, advertising restrictions, antitobacco media campaigns, and youth-access enforcement. Research has demonstrated that such strategies tend to work synergistically and are less effective when implemented in isolation, underscoring the need for comprehensive and multifaceted tobacco control policy (Lantz et al., 2000; Levy, Chaloupka, & Gitchell, 2004). To maximize public health benefit, a strong case has been advanced for widely promoting effective cessation treatments as one component of tobacco control; that is, effective treatments are needed to increase quitting and maximally reduce smoking prevalence (Aveyard & Raw, 2012).

While experimentation with substance use may be considered normal adolescent behavior, the high dependence liability associated with nicotine results in high levels of smoking maintenance into adulthood. So, for example, while the use of alcohol and other drugs tends to begin in adolescence, peak in early adulthood, and then decline, smoking follows a different trajectory, steadily increasing over the life course. When adolescents begin experimenting with smoking, they expect their smoking to be short-lived. In one study of high school smokers, only 5% expected to be smoking after high school graduation whereas, in reality, 75% were still smoking 5 years later (Charlton, Media, & Moyer, 1990).

Compared to smoking among adults, adolescent smoking tends to be characterized by fewer cigarettes per day, more intermittent day-to-day patterns, less intense inhalation, and shorter smoking histories. Studies of smoke exposure biomarkers (e.g., exhaled carbon monoxide [CO] levels and levels of cotinine, a nicotine metabolite) also indicate lower levels of exposure among adolescent smokers as compared with adult smokers. One might reasonably assume that lighter smoking patterns with less exposure to nicotine would lead to better treatment outcomes in adolescents as compared with adults, but in fact the opposite is true. There are many treatments that are effective for treating adult smokers, including pharmacological treatments like nicotine replacement therapies and other medications including Varenicline and Bupropion, and yet none of these treatments has received strong support in studies with adolescents. The reasons for these discrepancies are not known, but several factors have been implicated, including lower levels of treatment motivation, participation, and retention among adolescents as compared to adults.

The state of the adolescent smoking cessation research literature is poor. Compared to treatment research involving adult smokers, the adolescent smoking cessation literature is composed of dramatically fewer clinical trials overall and fewer trials testing each specific intervention. Even those trials that have been completed tend to be smaller, have lower rates of retention, and much lower cessation rates achieved as compared to adult trials. Most reviews of the adolescent smoking treatment literature conclude that delivering treatment leads to better smoking outcomes than not delivering treatment, but there is no *one* treatment that can be definitively recommended at this time. Effective treatment of adolescent smokers remains an urgent priority because, for every three adolescents who take up smoking, two will continue to smoke into adulthood, and one will die prematurely as a direct result of smoking.

Usual Treatments

Adolescent smoking cessation interventions have been systematically reviewed by the Cochrane Collaboration (Grimshaw & Stanton, 2010). which conducts comprehensive reviews of treatments for various health conditions and is internationally recognized as the gold standard in evidence-based treatment evaluation. A total of 24 randomized trials were identified, involving over 5,000 adolescent smokers as participants. The authors found that most of the interventions tested were multifaceted, combining different approaches from various theoretical backgrounds. The strongest evidence for treatment success was from 11 trials that incorporated a specific therapeutic focus on enhancing adolescents' motivation to change. The content of these trials varied, but the majority used motivational interviewing (MI) or motivational enhancement therapy (MET) with or without additional treatment components like cognitive-behavioral therapy (CBT). These motivation-focused interventions were significantly more likely to lead to smoking abstinence at follow-up compared with interventions that did not specifically focus on increasing adolescents' motivation. Trials using the transtheoretical model (TTM; Prochaska & Velicer, 1997), in which intervention messages and strategies were tailored to the adolescent's readiness to change showed a comparable effect on quitting, but there were only two such trials. Four trials tested the American Lung Association's Not-on-Tobacco (N-O-T) (see Horn, Dino, Kalsekar, & Mody, 2005), a multisession cognitive-behavioral intervention, which received qualified support. The increased likelihood of quitting associated with N-O-T interventions was marginally significant. Finally, there was insufficient evidence to recommend any type of pharmacological interventions for adolescent cessation, owing both to having too few trials but also because the trials that were undertaken failed to demonstrate support for medications' effectiveness in adolescents.

The Cochrane Review highlighted some important methodological points to keep in mind when evaluating adolescent cessation approaches. First, it is important to consider the specific *outcome measure* used to evaluate each program. The most rigorous trials use a measure of extended abstinence (for example, 30 days of continuous abstinence) at follow-up. But many trials use less stringent evaluation criteria, as short as past 24-hour abstinence. Also, trials involving adolescents have convincingly shown that self-reported outcomes are not always reliable. Adolescents tend to claim more quitting success than biomarker analysis demonstrates (for example, an adolescent's report of having quit smoking may be disconfirmed by high levels of cotinine in his or her saliva), and the discrepancies between self-report and biomarker data can be quite dramatic. Thus, trials that rely exclusively on self-reported outcomes in adolescent smokers may lead to incorrect conclusions about treatment success. This point will be revisited later.

What do we know about the types of treatment that are actually available to young smokers in their communities? A unique study by Dr. Susan Curry and her colleagues (Curry et al., 2007) documented the characteristics and availability of community-based cessation programs for youth (ages 12–24) in the United States. Drawing on a stratified random sample of 408 U.S. counties, the researchers individually interviewed program administrators of 591 programs that had treated over 36,000 young smokers in the prior year. Over a third of counties had no cessation programs for young smokers. These counties were disproportionately economically disadvantaged and/or outside metropolitan areas. Among the counties that had adolescent smoking cessation programs, most had just one or two programs with limited reach. Most programs treated fewer than 50 smokers per year; roughly half treated just 20 or fewer youth. Program administrators said that enrolling sufficient numbers of young smokers, and keeping them in the program once they start, are among the most challenging aspects of running these programs. As the authors concluded, the number of participants served by the identified treatment programs "represents a miniscule proportion of young smokers" in the counties sampled.

For those young smokers in the United States who do have access to treatment, though, what is usually provided and how is it provided? According to the Curry study, the large majority (about 90%) of cessation programs offered to young people are school-based. The remaining programs are not concentrated in one particular type of setting, but rather, are scattered across a variety of settings that include community centers, health clinics, hospitals, and (least frequently) churches or other religious centers. Treatment for young smokers is primarily delivered in multisession in-person groups, and many programs have additional components, including one-on-one counseling, self-help materials, telephone counseling, and/or web-based support. Encouragingly, most program administrators reported selecting their programs based on research evidence. Administrators typically purchased prepackaged programs such as N-O-T through the American Lung Association (Horn, Dino, Kalsekar, & Fernandez, 2004; Horn et al., 2005) or "Project EX" (Sussman, Dent, & Lichtman, 2001), both designated as model programs by the U.S. Substance Abuse and Mental Health Services Administration's National Registry of Evidence-based Programs and Practices. Treatment is usually delivered by teachers, nurses, school counselors, or social workers, in addition to their other job responsibilities. Most of these treatment providers receive specific training in implementing the program, follow a written manual, and assess smoking outcomes at follow-up (typically relying on self-reported outcomes).

The content of youth smoking treatment was very similar across most programs. Nearly all programs discuss the short- and long-term consequences of smoking as well as tobacco industry tactics designed to get young people to smoke. Most teach a variety of cognitive-behavioral strategies recommended in the literature for both adult and adolescent cessation. Also, programs for youth smokers incorporate topics that are relevant to their developmental stage, such as discussing their life goals, and the relationship of smoking to other problem behaviors like drug use. Few programs for youth offer medications for smoking cessation.

The report by Curry and colleagues (2007) highlights important points about accessing treatment by adolescents. First, most young smokers do not seek treatment to support their cessation efforts. This is problematic since nearly all unassisted quit attempts among adolescent smokers end in failure (Gwaltney, Bartolomei, Colby, & Kahler, 2008). Second, there is a great need to increase the availability of these programs. Consider this illustration. My state, Rhode Island, has five counties. I live in Kent County. Based on the Curry study, my county is most likely to have one to two cessation programs, probably based in high schools. Who does not have access to these programs? Kent County has a total of 33 public and private middle and high schools; if 2 have cessation programs, then the students attending any of the remaining 31 schools would not have any access to cessation treatment. Young smokers who have graduated from or dropped out of high school similarly would not have access. Even among the students who attend the one or two schools that run a cessation program, those who attempt to quit smoking during the summer or even during the school year but at times other than when the program is being offered will not have access to treatment to support their efforts to quit. In sum, the quality of treatment programs being offered to young smokers is encouraging, but most young smokers either do not have access to treatment or do not seek it out to support their efforts to quit. Adolescent smoking cessation would be more effectively promoted if adolescents were screened proactively regarding their smoking status and then linked to treatments that enhance motivation to quit and support efforts to quit.

Rationale for Using MI for Youth Smoking Cessation

Considering the landscape of adolescent smoking cessation services, MI provides a strong fit for a number of reasons. First, MI's *flexibility* is an important feature. MI could serve as a useful adjunct to the typical multicomponent, multisession interventions offered. MI can be readily incorporated into existing programs since many already offer adjunctive one-on-one counseling. For example, MI might serve as a prelude to group treatment, enhancing subsequent treatment engagement and completion rates. Additionally, MI could be implemented as a stand-alone intervention where treatment programs are not otherwise offered, such as in rural settings where it is challenging to enroll large enough numbers of adolescent smokers to deliver group-based interventions. In our research, we have shown that MI is feasible to administer and acceptable to adolescent patients in hospital settings, health clinics, and pediatricians' offices (Colby et al., 2012). In contrast to a multisession group treatment offered once or twice per year, MI could be more readily delivered as a "drop-in" treatment as needed.

Another advantage of MI for youth smoking is its *orientation toward resolving ambivalence and increasing motivation to make changes* related to smoking. Adolescent smoking and quitting behaviors are characterized by a high degree of ambivalence. Studies consistently show that most adolescent smokers want to quit smoking and most have attempted to do so in the past year (Breland, Colby, Dino, Smith, & Taylor, 2009). But major factors that motivate quitting in adults, such as health consequences, may not motivate adolescents in the same way (Apodaca, Abrantes, Strong, Ramsey, & Brown, 2007), perhaps because the most serious illnesses caused by smoking take decades to emerge. Also, despite their lighter and more intermittent smoking patterns, adolescents experience adult-like adverse effects when they stop smoking, including substantial increases in craving, negative affect, and withdrawal symptoms (Bidwell et al., 2012; Colby et al., 2010). We have shown that smoking a single cigarette provides immediate relief from these symptoms in adolescents (Colby et al., 2010), which can undermine adolescents' motivation to quit during the initial days of a quit attempt. Because MI recognizes the ambivalence typically associated with making difficult behavior changes, it is well suited to addressing these motivational challenges.

Other characteristics of existing adolescent smoking cessation treatment programs lend themselves well to MI's *collaborative approach* and *emphasis on treatment engagement.* The MI process of *engaging,* that is, developing a healthy connection and working relationship between the adolescent and the counselor (Miller & Rollnick, 2013), can facilitate their working together in challenging treatment contexts. For example, at times adolescent participation in smoking treatment is mandated as a punishment for a legal infraction like possession of tobacco or underage smoking (Curry et al., 2007). Being mandated or coerced to attend treatment can result in hostility and defensiveness on the part of treatment participants. Although MI has not been tested specifically for mandated adolescent smokers, there is good evidence from the college student drinking literature that MI is efficacious in reducing alcohol-related harm among students similarly mandated to treatment (Borsari & Carey, 2005; Borsari et al., 2012). MI also has been recommended as a way of reducing defensiveness and hostility in domestic violent offenders mandated to treatment (Carbajosa, Boira, & Tomás-Aragonés, 2013) and has shown initial promise in that regard (Kistenmacher & Weiss, 2008). Apart from mandated treatment, there are good data to suggest that more directive approaches, which are often used in smoking cessation treatment, are more likely to elicit resistance while treatments like MI are less likely to do so (Miller, Benefield, & Tonigan, 1993).

Even adolescents who voluntarily participate in smoking cessation treatment tend to be nontreatment seekers who were proactively recruited into treatment programs with the assurance that motivation to quit was not a prerequisite. That most research trials with adolescent smokers proactively enroll adolescents who are not necessarily motivated to quit smoking may partially account for lower rates of treatment engagement and poorer smoking outcomes reported in adolescent versus adult trials. The MI processes of client-centered *engaging* and *evoking* adolescents' own motivations can be particularly important in these types of interventions.

Clinical Applications and Relevant Research

The evidence supporting the use of MI for adolescent smoking cessation treatment is evolving; though the earliest studies provided initial support for the promise of MI (Colby et al., 1998), individual trials have tended to be small, underpowered, and unable to detect significant differences between MI and comparison treatments. However, more recently a meta-analysis by Hettema and Hendricks (2010) and a pooled analysis by Heckman and her colleagues (Heckman, Egleston, & Hofmann, 2010) have clarified our understanding of the effects of MI and have provided more compelling support for the use of MI for smoking cessation generally and with adolescent smokers specifically. Two additional trials of MI for adolescent smoking cessation (Audrain-McGovern et al., 2011; Colby et al., 2012) have been published since 2010. Below I review the evidence from 10 trials and two reviews.

Table 12.1 summarizes the characteristics of the 10 randomized clinical trials of MI for adolescent smoking cessation published between 1998 and 2012. All 10 of these trials randomly allocated participants to treatment conditions (nearly all of them on an individual basis, with the exception of Woodruff, Conway, Edwards, Elliott, & Crittenden, 2007, which randomized by site), and all reported sufficient data to calculate intent-to-treat abstinence rates. The first seven trials were included in the Hettema and Hendricks (2010) meta-analysis; the first eight were included in the Heckman and colleagues (2010) pooled analysis. Findings from both analyses indicated that MI led to significantly higher rates of smoking cessation in adolescents than in comparison conditions

TABLE 12.1. Description of Randomized Clinical Trials of MI for Adolescent Smoking Cessation (1998–2012)

#	Study	Sample	MI condition	Comparison condition(s)
1	Colby et al. (1998)	40 ED and outpatient clinic patients	1 30-min MI	5-min Brief Advice (BA)
2	Brown et al. (2003)	191 patients with psychiatric disorders	2 45-min. MI + NRT	BA + NRT
3	Lipkus et al. (2004)	402 adolescents recruited from malls/amusement park	3 MI calls	Self-help materials
4	Colby et al. (2005)	85 ED and outpatient clinic patients	1 35-min MI	BA
5	Hollis et al. (2005)	589 primary care patients (past 30-day smokers)	1 5-min MI + 10-min computer program + 1–2 10-min boosters	Dietary BA
6	Horn et al. (2007)	75 ED patients	1 15–30 min MI + 3 calls	BA
7	Woodruff et al. (2007)	136 smokers recruited from high schools	7 45-min virtual reality Internet chat sessions	Assessment only
8	Helstrom et al. (2007)	81 juvenile offenders	1 session MI	Tobacco education session
9	Audrain-McGovern et al. (2011)	355 adolescent medicine patients	3 45-min MI + 2 30-min MI	BA
10	Colby et al. (2012)	162 adolescents recruited from ED, clinics, and high school students	1 45-min MI + 10-min call + 10-min parent MI call	BA

Note. ED, emergency department; NRT = nicotine replacement therapy; calls, telephone calls. Full citations appear in the References.

such as brief advice to quit smoking, tobacco education, or self-help materials. Heckman and colleagues (2010) found that at moderately long-term follow-ups (5.5–6 months), rates of smoking abstinence were significantly greater among adolescents who received MI as compared to those in the comparison conditions (11.5 vs. 6.0%, respectively). Furthermore, after analyzing data from adolescent and adult MI trials together, these authors found that MI effects did not differ by participant characteristics, including race and gender, baseline smoking rate, or— importantly—whether participants had been seeking smoking treatment or not. MI effects were also comparable regardless of who delivered the treatment (counselors/therapists, staff/interventionists, nurses/mid-wives, psychologists, physicians, health educators, or trainees)—also important, considering the range of community-based providers who currently provide cessation treatments to adolescents.

Hettema and colleagues (2010) took a different analytic approach but came to similar conclusions. First, their analyses of the adolescent MI trials showed that MI significantly increased smoking abstinence as compared to alternative conditions at both short- and longer-term follow-ups. Analyzing data from adolescent and adult trials together, these authors also found that MI effects did not differ based on the total duration of treatment or whether MI was combined with other treatments such as pharmacotherapy or behavioral skills training.

Looking at the data from all 10 trials, the value of biochemically verifying self-reported smoking abstinence by analyzing breath samples for CO level (or saliva samples for cotinine) becomes clear. Figures 12.1 and 12.2 contrast the rates of smoking abstinence by treatment group at various follow-up junctures when based on self-report alone (Figure 12.1) or self-report with biochemical confirmation (Figure 12.2). The data do not align perfectly, because not all of the studies reported both indices. However, the available data show that abstinence rates based on self-report alone tend to be much higher than rates that are bio-chemically confirmed (i.e., adolescents overreport quitting smoking). Further, evaluating *confirmed* rates of abstinence more consistently supports MI over comparison conditions. In other words, using more accurate abstinence data helps demonstrate MI's efficacy for smoking intervention.

Although MI effects on smoking cessation are admittedly small, they are consistent across settings, providers, and participant characteristics. Because the duration of the intervention tends to be quite brief (1.5 hours, on average), widespread application of MI is feasible and has the potential to create a cost-effective positive impact on public health.

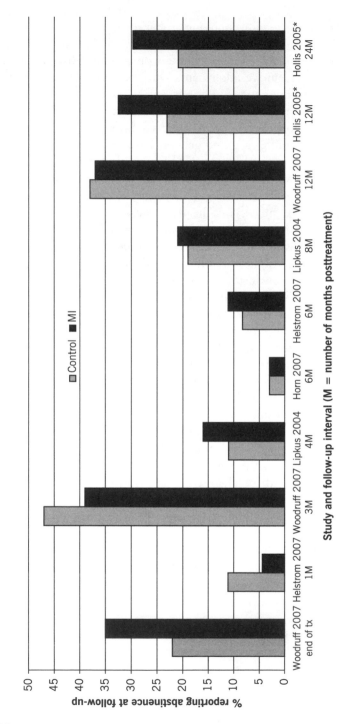

FIGURE 12.1. Rates of self-reported smoking abstinence by study, follow-up interval, and treatment. *Rates exclude baseline non-smokers and experimenters.

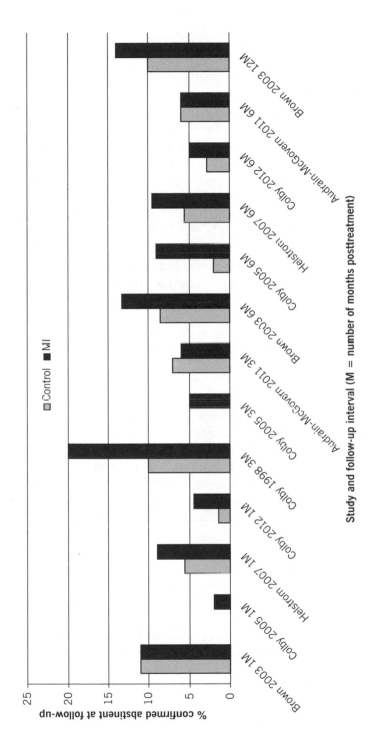

FIGURE 12.2. Rates of biochemically verified smoking abstinence by study, follow-up interval, and treatment.

Clinical Applications

The genesis of our research group's focus on applying MI to adolescent smoking traces back to our early days testing MI for reducing alcohol-related harm among adolescents who presented to the emergency department (ED) for treatment resulting from an alcohol-related event such as a car crash, assault, or severe intoxication (Monti, Barnett, O'Leary, & Colby, 2001). During the screening and enrollment phase of that trial, we noted the higher-than-average prevalence of smoking among adolescent ED patients and considered whether the MI for alcohol use might be adapted for smokers in the ED setting. In the ED, the MI process of *focusing* was approached differently for smoking than it had been for alcohol. The focus for the conversation about alcohol was set up well by the context for the ED visit—an alcohol-related event. In contrast, the smoking intervention was more opportunistic; adolescents came to the ED for treatment for any type of urgent care—usually unrelated to smoking. In this context, the adolescent may not share a concern about his or her smoking with the counselor; the process of focusing is used to identify mutually acceptable goals for the session.

The Protocol

Below, each section of the intervention protocol is described as delivered in our three published randomized trials. Because we incorporated providing personalized feedback as part of the session, the intervention is considered to be MET. Sessions lasted approximately 30–45 minutes, following a standardized assessment which took about 20–25 minutes to complete. Interventions were delivered by research interventionists at various levels of education and clinical training, from bachelors-level counselors with 1–2 years' clinical research experience to postdoctoral fellows and licensed clinical psychologists. Because of the great diversity in interventionists' clinical experience, and because this MET was delivered as a standardized research intervention, the treatment protocol was manualized and semiscripted, but interventionists could use their own discretion in the extent to which they diverted from scripted material, skipped sections that were inappropriate for the participant, or covered topics in a different order. This flexibility is consistent with MI's emphasis on conducting sessions in the overall spirit of MI; rigidly following manuals can undermine effective use of MI (for example, trying to create a change plan with an adolescent who is not yet open to making changes can be countertherapeutic, running the risk of moving an adolescent from ambivalence to arguing against change).

The MET sessions include the following processes:

1. *Engaging.* This involves building rapport with the adolescent and developing a therapeutic alliance that will facilitate collaboration. Client-centered skills are used, which honor the adolescent's values and ideas and support his or her personal authority and responsibility to make decisions about the youth's own health behavior.
2. *Focusing.* The goals of the conversation and the counseling are clarified.
3. *Evoking.* This is the process used to elicit each adolescent's feelings about smoking and his or her own motivations for change. The counselor strategically evokes and reinforces change talk from the adolescent, reflecting and summarizing it.
4. *Providing personalized feedback.* In MET, adolescents are given feedback based on their results from standardized assessments. Feedback is delivered only with the adolescent's permission and expressly in an MI style.
5. *Planning.* When an adolescent expresses sufficient readiness for making changes, the counselor and adolescent collaboratively generate a change plan, including goals and strategies consistent with the adolescent's level of interest in making changes.

Orientation

The session begins with an orientation, which involves *engaging* and *focusing.* The orientation sets the tone for the session, letting the adolescent know what to expect and to ask any questions or voice any concerns early on. The goal is to begin to build rapport and establish the counselor as empathic, concerned, nonauthoritarian, and nonjudgmental. The focusing process is used to identify the goals of the conversation and to ensure that these are mutually acceptable. The session begins by introducing the interview as a chance for the adolescent to talk about his or her thoughts and feelings about smoking. The counselor emphasizes that the intention is not to tell him or her what to do; rather, it is up to him or her to make decisions and choices about smoking.

"What I'd like to do now is talk about your smoking. I want you to know, before we begin, that I'm not here to tell you what to do.

Only you can make those decisions. But I would like to hear what you think and how you feel about smoking, and how you make decisions to smoke or not to smoke. Then, if you like, we can talk about whether you are interested in cutting down or stopping, but that will be up to you. Is that OK? Can we try this out?"

During the process of engaging, the counselor uses client-centered counseling skills and a nonjudgmental style from the start to minimize defensiveness on the part of the adolescent, increasing openness to considering new information and working collaboratively with the counselor. The emphasis is on understanding smoking from the adolescent's point of view and supporting the adolescent's autonomy in making decisions about smoking.

Assessing Motivation

Early in the session, the pros and cons of smoking, from the adolescent's perspective, are explored. Because none of the participants in our trials had been seeking smoking treatment, with most being in the precontemplation (i.e., not considering quitting) or very early in the Contemplation stage of change, we found this exercise to be a helpful way to understand the role of smoking in the adolescent's life, to appreciate his or her personal concerns about smoking, and to develop discrepancy. The adolescent is encouraged to generate as many responses as possible and to talk about the effects that matter most to him or her. Open-ended questions are used, such as:

"What do you like about your smoking? What else?"
"What don't you like as much about your smoking? What else?"
"Of the things you like about smoking, [such as . . .], which effect matters most to you?"
"Of the things you don't like so much about smoking, [such as . . .], which effect matters most you to?"

During this conversation, the counselor uses reflective listening techniques, experiencing and communicating accurate empathy. The goal is for the counselor to understand how the adolescent is experiencing his or her smoking and to reflect that understanding back to him or her in a way that encourages therapeutic momentum. In summing up this part of the discussion, the counselor summarizes information about salient pros and cons, using double-sided reflections to highlight the adolescent's ambivalence about smoking. The counselor strategically links together information and emphasizes certain points, particularly highlighting change talk that has been elicited during the conversation. [Let us note here that in the third edition of *Motivational Interviewing* (Miller & Rollnick, 2013) such a decisional balance exercise is no longer used, in order to minimize sustain talk; our protocol in this study, however, preceded its publication.]

Providing Personalized Feedback

Next, the counselor offers to review personalized feedback from the standardized assessments the adolescent completed related to his or her smoking. This information is presented only after soliciting permission from the adolescent.

"May I share with you some information about the questionnaires you answered?"

Personalized feedback was provided in a number of domains, including information about normative influence, social consequences, effects on health, addiction, and the financial costs of smoking. The goal is to provide personally relevant information based on questionnaire responses rather than generic educational information about the effects of smoking. So, information is provided in each of the various domains only when responses indicate that the information is relevant to the individual.

The *normative influence* section is designed to correct normative misperceptions about how many adolescents smoke. Most adolescents overestimate the percentage of their (same-age same-gender) peers that smoke; in this section, the adolescent is shown figures illustrating the percentage of adolescents they thought were smokers alongside the actual rate of smoking. As relevant, the false consensus effect is explained (people who smoke tend to have more contact with other smokers and therefore may believe that smoking is more common than it actually is).

Feedback on *social consequences* is prompted by adolescents' responses to questions about: (1) their parents' and friends' concerns about smoking; (2) feeling pressure to smoke or feeling more confident socially when smoking; (3) concerns about effects of their second-hand smoke on others; and (4) concerns about how modeling smoking behavior might affect younger children.

Feedback on *health consequences* reflects the extent to which the adolescent reported health effects related to smoking, the exacerbation of other health conditions (like asthma) affected by smoking, or concerns about future effects on health. Although life-threatening conditions such as lung cancer and chronic obstructive pulmonary disease (COPD) take decades to develop in smokers, adolescents often report immediate health effects, such as more difficulty breathing while exercising. Our emphasis in this section is to discuss the health effects of personal concern to the adolescent rather than provide general educational information on the negative health effects of smoking. Adolescents were also given information about their own exhaled alveolar carbon monoxide (CO) level, the physiological effects of CO at various levels, and how their level compares to the average CO for nonsmokers.

Feedback on the *addiction* topic covered any items endorsed by the adolescent reflecting signs of nicotine dependence, such as the development of tolerance, withdrawal, smoking more cigarettes early in the day, and difficulty during past quit attempts. Open-ended questions are used to encourage the adolescent to talk about personal experiences related to these indices of nicotine dependence.

Finally, feedback on the *financial costs* of smoking calculates how much the adolescent spends on cigarettes in a year, contrasting that amount with how much it costs tobacco manufacturers to produce them. The annual and monthly costs of tobacco at various levels of use (e.g., the adolescent's current use vs. the current level of use reduced by half) are provided.

For each topic, the counselor discusses the feedback with the adolescent, asks for the adolescent's reaction, and provides clarification as appropriate. The adolescent's autonomy is supported throughout (e.g., "This may or may not be a concern for you. What do you think about it?"). Information is offered in small amounts, checking in with the adolescent and eliciting his or her own perceptions and reactions, following the "elicit–provide–elicit" sequence (Rollnick, Miller, & Butler, 2008). The counselor finishes the feedback section with a summary of the main points discussed and elicits the adolescent's reactions with open-ended questions such as "What information that we discussed surprised you the most? Which of the areas we've talked about concerns you the most?" Throughout, the counselor is alert to expressions of concern about smoking and its consequences, indications of intention to change, and statements related to self-efficacy related to quitting. Change talk is explored in more detail, reflected, and summarized by the counselor.

Envisioning the Future

Following the feedback discussion, the counselor elicits the adolescent's thoughts about what might happen in the future if his or her smoking were to stay the same and what might happen if it were to decrease or even stop completely. This is an evoking strategy in which the adolescent may consider and articulate the advantages of making changes in his or her smoking behavior or concerns about what might happen if he or she continues to smoke at the same level. Prompts in this section might include:

Imagine Life without Cigarettes

"Tell me what you imagine your life would be like one year from now if you gave up smoking."
"What might be difficult about not smoking one year from now?"
"What would be the best thing you could imagine happening?"
(If adolescent has difficulty):
"How were things different before you started smoking?"
"What was life like then?"

Imagine Life with Cigarettes

"Tell me what you imagine your life would be like one year from now if you continued smoking."
"What would be the good aspects and the not-so-good aspects?"
"May I tell you some of my own concerns?"

In this section, the counselor may refer back to earlier topic areas in which concerns about smoking had been raised. Areas of difficulty presented by not smoking can be noted by the counselor as potential barriers to successful behavior change and addressed in the goals section (below). While considering good things that might result from quitting smoking, if the adolescent leaves out important factors elicited earlier, the counselor can raise them again. As change talk is elicited, the counselor reflects, reinforces, and further explores it, affirming and encouraging the adolescent. The counselor summarizes this part of the session, accurately reflecting the adolescent's statements while strategically connecting points in support of change.

Planning

The final section of the intervention involves helping the adolescent determine what he or she would like to do differently with regard to smoking. This portion includes identifying goals for behavior change, exploring barriers to those changes, and providing advice and a menu of strategies (when appropriate) from which the client can choose. This conversation starts with open-ended questions about the adolescent's interest in change:

> "Where does this leave you now?"
> "Where do you go from here?"
> "How would you like things to be different?"
> "What might be a good first step for you?"
> "What are your options? . . . How do you think that [first option] would work?"
> "Would you be interested in learning more about how to cut down or resist cigarettes?"

Based on responses, the counselor works collaboratively with the adolescent to develop a plan for behavior change that is appropriate to his or her readiness to make changes. If an adolescent is ready to consider reducing or quitting smoking, the counselor will help to elicit steps that are acceptable to the adolescent and then explore how these can be accomplished. The key is that the plan should come from the adolescent rather than the counselor. An adolescent may be interested in making changes but unsure how to proceed. The adolescent and counselor may complete a worksheet titled "Which Goals Do You Want to Try?" There is a list of short- and longer-term goals appropriate to various stages of readiness to change, from which the adolescent can choose. For each goal, there is a space to write in when he or she will try to achieve it and a check box to record when it was accomplished. There is also space to write in additional or alternative change goals that the adolescent creates. Potential barriers to accomplishing goals are elicited, and the counselor and client work together to find ways to overcome them.

> "What might get in the way of you making these changes?"
> "What has it been like before when you've tried to quit (or cut down)?"
> "When do you think it will be hardest not to smoke?"
> "What do you think you can do to resist the urges or pressure to smoke?"

In this section, the counselor aims to help the adolescent to learn from past experiences, to anticipate challenges (such as withdrawal), and to discuss new ways to cope. If appropriate, handouts are provided for common challenges like managing withdrawal symptoms and for strategies for quitting successfully. The counselor seeks to support the adolescent's self-efficacy for making changes. The adolescent's personal responsibility for deciding what to do about smoking is reiterated. Past successes, either in abstaining from smoking or in overcoming other obstacles, are elicited by the counselor ("What helps you to believe in yourself that you can make these changes?"). Responses provide opportunities to affirm the adolescent's strengths and support his or her self-efficacy.

Finally, the counselor summarizes the session, tying together salient points and reinforcing the adolescent's commitment to the change plan, reflecting the adolescent's decisions, and affirming his or her desire and ability to implement the selected goals.

Problems and Suggested Solutions

A challenge we encountered while adapting our alcohol MET session to smoking was how to approach the behavior change target. In contrast to alcohol, which can be consumed safely in moderation, cigarette smoking at any level is unsafe (U.S. Department of Health and Human Services, 2010). Accordingly, smoking interventions tend to be strongly abstinence-oriented (Lawson, 2012); outcomes other than complete smoking abstinence (such as smoking reduction, for example, or switching to smokeless tobacco) are considered unacceptable. In developing our MI treatment for smoking, we sought to provide (with participant permission) objective and accurate information on the harmful consequences of smoking and the benefits of complete cessation. At the same time, consistent with MI, we emphasized that it was the adolescent's responsibility to make personal decisions about his or her own smoking, and counselors supported behavior change goals that fell short of cessation (for example, cutting down the number of cigarettes per day), reasoning that progress toward quitting was still progress. In most of our trials of MET for smoking, we have contrasted MET with traditional brief advice that consists of strong directive advice to quit smoking completely as soon as possible, along with self-help materials and treatment referrals designed to support quitting. In this way, we have been able to empirically test the relative merits of each approach in samples of proactively recruited adolescent smokers mostly unmotivated to quit smoking.

Conclusions

Though significant progress has been made in reducing smoking prevalence among adults and adolescents, rates of smoking remain unacceptably high and increasingly concentrated in vulnerable individuals commonly characterized by economic disadvantage, low access to treatment, and mental health problems. Treatment for smoking and other tobacco use is an essential component of comprehensive tobacco control, but access is low for adolescents, and the evidence in support of treatment efficacy tends to be limited.

In the past several years, evidence has emerged in support of MI and MET for treating smoking in both adults and adolescents. Most evidence indicates that MI has small but consistent effects on smoking, and the consistency of effects does not appear to depend on the setting in which it is administered, the type of professional delivering it, whether it is combined with other treatments or not, or whether clients are motivated to quit smoking or not. The orientation toward resolving ambivalence is a good fit for smokers generally and adolescent smokers specifically, and MI's flexibility with respect to implementation contexts makes it a good fit for the existing treatment delivery system for adolescents. Although most existing smoking interventions for youth are delivered in schools, there is a pressing need to increase the number of schools that deliver treatment. In addition, a number of studies have shown that MI or MET could be readily integrated into health care delivery systems, and health care reform changes are making it easier for providers to get reimbursed for treating their patients who smoke. Integrating MI for smoking into health care delivery in a comprehensive way could dramatically expand access to treatment for adolescent smokers.

References

Apodaca, T. R., Abrantes, A. M., Strong, D. R., Ramsey, S. E., & Brown, R. A. (2007). Readiness to change smoking behavior in adolescents with psychiatric disorders. *Addictive Behaviors, 32,* 1119–1130.

Audrain-McGovern, J., Stevens, S., Murray, P. J., Kinsman, S., Zuckoff, A., Pletcher, J., et al. (2011). The efficacy of motivational interviewing versus brief advice for adolescent smoking behavior change. *Pediatrics, 128,* e101–e111.

Aveyard, P., & Raw, M. (2012). Improving smoking cessation approaches at the individual level. *Tobacco Control, 21,* 252–257.

Bidwell, L. C., Leventhal, A. M., Tidey, J. W., Brazil, L., Niaura, R. S., & Colby, S. M. (2013). Effects of abstinence in adolescent tobacco smokers:

Withdrawal symptoms, reactive irritability and cue reactivity. *Nicotine and Tobacco Research, 15*, 457–464.

Borsari, B., & Carey, K. B. (2005). Two brief alcohol interventions for mandated college students. *Psychology of Addictive Behaviors, 19*, 296–302.

Borsari, B., Hustad, J., Mastroleo, N. R., O'Leary Tevyaw, T., Barnett, N. P., Kahler, C. W., Short, E. E., & Monti, P. M. (2012). Addressing alcohol use and problems in mandated college students: A randomized clinical trial using stepped care. *Journal of Consulting and Clinical Psychology, 80*, 1062–1074.

Breland, A. B., Colby, S. M., Dino, G., Smith, G., & Taylor, M. (2009). *Youth smoking cessation interventions: Treatments, barriers, and recommendations for Virginia.* Richmond, Viginia: Virgina Commonwealth University, Institute for Drug and Alcohol Studies. Unpublished manuscript.

Brown, R. A., Ramsey, S. E., Strong, D. R., Myers, M. G., Kahler, C. W., Lejuez, R., et al. (2003). Effects of motivational interviewing on smoking cessation in adolescents with psychiatric disorders. *Tobacco Control, 12*(Suppl 4), iv3–iv10.

Carbajosa, P., Boira, S., & Tomás-Aragonés, L. (2013). Difficulties, skills and therapy strategies in interventions with court-ordered batterers in Spain. *Aggression and Violent Behavior, 18*, 118–124.

Charlton, A., Melia, P., & Moyer, C. (1990). *A manual on tobacco and young people for the Industrialized World International Union Against Cancer (UICC).* Geneva, Switzerland.

Colby, S. M., Leventhal, A. M., Brazil, L., Lewis-Esquerre, J., Stein, L. A. R., Rohsenow, D. J., et al. (2010). Smoking abstinence and reinstatement effects in adolescent cigarette smokers. *Nicotine and Tobacco Research, 12*, 19–28.

Colby, S. M., Monti, P. M., Barnett, N. P., Rohsenow, D. J., Weissman, K., Spirito, A., et al. (1998). Brief motivational interviewing in a hospital setting for adolescent smoking: A preliminary study. *Journal of Consulting and Clinical Psychology, 66*, 574–578.

Colby, S. M., Monti, P. M., O'Leary-Tevyaw, T. A., Barnett, N. P., Spirito, A., et al. (2005). Brief motivational intervention for adolescent smokers in a hospital setting. *Addictive Behaviors, 30*, 865–874.

Colby, S. M., Nargiso, J., Tevyaw, T., Barnett, N. P., Metrik, J., Woolard, R. H., et al. (2012). Enhanced motivational interviewing versus brief advice for adolescent smoking cessation: A randomized clinical trial. *Addictive Behaviors, 37*, 817–823.

Curry, S. J., Emery, S., Sporer, A. K., Mermelstein, R., Flay, B. R., Berbaum, M., et al. (2007) A national survey of tobacco cessation programs for youths. *American Journal of Public Health, 97*, 171–177.

Grimshaw, G., & Stanton, A. (2010). Tobacco cessation interventions for young people. *Cochrane Database of Systematic Reviews, 4*, Art. No. CD003289.

Gwaltney, C. J., Bartolomei, R., Colby, S. M., & Kahler, C. W. (2008). Ecological momentary assessment of adolescent smoking cessation: A feasibility study. *Nicotine and Tobacco Research, 10*, 1185–1190.

Heckman, C. J., Egleston, B. L., & Hofmann, M. T. (2010). Efficacy of motivational interviewing for smoking cessation: A systematic review and meta-analysis. *Tobacco Control, 19,* 410–416.

Helstrom, A., Hutchison, K., & Bryan, A. (2007). Motivational enhancement therapy for high-risk adolescent smokers. *Addictive Behaviors, 32,* 2404–2410.

Hettema, J. E., & Hendricks, P. S. (2010). Motivational interviewing for smoking cessation: a meta-analytic review. *Journal of Consulting and Clinical Psychology, 78,* 868–884.

Hilts, P. J. (1995, March 9). F.D.A. head calls smoking a pediatric disease. *New York Times,* pp. A22.

Hollis, J. F., Polen, M. R., Whitlock, E. P., Lichtenstein, E., Mullooly, J. P., Velicer, W. F., et al. (2005). Teen reach: Outcomes from a randomized, controlled trial of a tobacco reduction program for teens seen in primary medical care. *Pediatrics, 115,* 981–989.

Horn, K., Dino, G., Hamilton, C., & Noerachmanto, N. (2007). Efficacy of an emergency department-based motivational teenage smoking intervention. *Preventing Chronic Disease, 4*(1), 1–12.

Horn, K. A., Dino, G. A., Kalsekar, I. D., & Fernandes, A. W. (2004). Appalachian teen smokers: Not On Tobacco 15 months later. *American Journal of Public Health, 94,* 181–184.

Horn, K., Dino, G., Kalsekar, I., & Mody, R. (2005). The impact of Not on Tobacco on teen smoking cessation: End-of-program evaluation results, 1998–2003. *Journal of Adolescent Research, 20,* 640–661.

Jha, P., Ramasundarahettige, C., Landsman, V., Rostron, B., Thun, M., Anderson, R. N., et al. (2013). 21st-century hazards of smoking and benefits of cessation in the United States. *New England Journal of Medicine, 368,* 341–350.

Johnston, L. D., O'Malley, P. M., Bachman, J. G., & Schulenberg, J. E. (2014). *Monitoring the Future national survey results on adolescent drug use: Overview of key findings, 2013.* Ann Arbor: Institute for Social Research, The University of Michigan.

Kistenmacher, B. R., & Weiss, R. L. (2008). Motivational interviewing as a mechanism for change in men who batter: A randomized control trial. *Violence and Victims, 23,* 558–570.

Lantz, P. M., Jacobson, P. D., Warner, K. E., Wasserman, J., Pollack, H. A. Berson, J., et al. (2000). Investing in youth tobacco control: A review of smoking prevention and control strategies. *Tobacco Control, 9,* 47–63.

Lawson, G. P. (2012). Tobacco harm reduction: Thinking the unthinkable. *British Journal of General Practice, 62,* 314.

Levy, D. T., Chaloupka, F., & Gitchell, J. (2004). The effects of tobacco control policies on smoking rates: A tobacco control scorecard. *Journal of Public Health Management Practice, 10,* 338–353.

Lipkus, I. M., McBride, C. M., Pollak, K. I., Schwartz-Bloom, R. D., Tilson, E., & Bloom, P. N. (2004). A randomized trial comparing the effects of self-help materials and proactive telephone counseling on teen smoking cessation. *Health Psychology, 23,* 397–406.

Miller, W. R., Benefield, R. G., & Tonigan, J. S. (1993). Enhancing motivation for change in problem drinking: A controlled comparison of two therapist styles. *Journal of Consulting and Clinical Psychology, 61,* 455.

Miller, W. R., & Rollnick, S. (2013). *Motivational interviewing: Helping people change* (3rd ed.). New York: Guilford Press.

Monti, P. M., Barnett, N. P., O'Leary, T. A., Colby, S. M. (2001). Brief motivational enhancement for alcohol-involved adolescents. In P. M. Monti, S. Colby, & T. A. O'Leary (Eds.). *Adolescents, alcohol and substance abuse: Reaching teens through brief interventions* (pp. 145–182). New York: Guilford Press.

Monti, P. M., Colby, S. M., Barnett, N. P., Spirito, A., Rohsenow, D. J., Myers, M. G., et al. (1999). Brief interventions for harm reduction with alcohol-positive older adolescents in a hospital emergency department. *Journal of Consulting and Clinical Psychology, 67,* 989–994.

Prochaska, J. O., & Velicer, W. F. (1997). The transtheoretical model of health behavior change. *American Journal of Health Promotion, 12,* 38–48.

Rollnick, S., Miller, W. R., Butler, C. C. (2008). *Motivational interviewing in health care.* New York: Guilford Press.

Sussman, S., Dent, C. W., & Lichtman, K. L. (2001). Project EX: Outcomes of a teen smoking cessation program. *Addictive Behaviors, 26,* 425–438.

Thun, M. J., Carter, B. D., Feskanich, D., Freedman, N. D., Prentice, R., Lopez, A. D., et al. (2013). 50–year trends in smoking related mortality in the United States. *New England Journal of Medicine, 368,* 351–364.

U.S. Department of Health and Human Services. (2010). *How tobacco smoke causes disease: The biology and behavioral basis for smoking-attributable disease: A report of the surgeon general.* Atlanta, GA: U.S. Department of Health and Human Services, Centers for Disease Control and Prevention, National Center for Chronic Disease Prevention and Health Promotion, Office on Smoking and Health.

Woodruff, S. I., Conway, T. L., Edwards, C. C., Elliott, S. P., & Crittenden, J. (2007). Evaluation of an Internet virtual world chat room for adolescent smoking cessation. *Addictive Behaviors, 32,* 1769–1786.

CHAPTER 13

• • • • • •

Motivational Interviewing
for Intimate Partner Violence

Erica M. Woodin

Intimate partner violence (IPV) has evolved from being considered a private family matter to being recognized as a major public health concern. IPV can take many forms, including physical types of aggression as well as verbally and psychologically abusive behaviors that are perpetrated against a current or previous intimate partner. As our understanding of the importance of IPV has changed over time, so too have the attempts to ameliorate the impact of IPV on society. Unfortunately, many early interventions have met with only limited success, and thus researchers, clinicians, and public policy experts are actively searching for empirically informed approaches that might be better suited to improving behavior regulation in the context of close relationships. Motivational interviewing (MI) is one approach that shows considerable promise in preventing and treating IPV across a range of populations.

The Clinical Problem

IPV is a commonly occurring interpersonal behavior that has significant negative consequences for victims. In a review of 111 articles reporting on IPV perpetration, the pooled prevalence rates for engaging in physical IPV, including such behaviors as pushing, shoving, and grabbing, were approximately 22% for men and 28% for women (Desmarais, Reeves, Nicholls, Telford, & Fiebert, 2012). Nonphysical forms of IPV are even more common, with at least 40% of women and 32% of men reporting verbal or emotional IPV, such as shouting, swearing, and insulting, and 41% of women and 43% of men reporting the use of coercive control, including emotional abuse, sexual coercion, and stalking (Carney & Barner, 2012). Exposure to psychological and physical IPV is associated with substantial impact on the victim, including poor physical health, mental health, cognitive functioning, and economic and social well-being (Lawrence, Orengo-Aguayo, Langer, & Brock, 2012). Further, psychological IPV has a significant impact above and beyond exposure to physical IPV (Coker et al., 2002).

IPV can take many forms. One of the most well-established distinctions is that between *intimate terrorism*, which consists of primarily male unilateral physical IPV combined with a pattern of controlling and abusive behaviors, versus *situational couple violence*, which consists of noncontrolling and primarily bidirectional forms of violence that often emerge as an outgrowth of conflict between partners (Johnson, 1995). Intimate terrorism is associated with a greater risk of severe IPV and greater physical and psychosocial impacts as compared to situational couple violence (Johnson & Leone, 2005). Intimate terrorism is most likely to be identified through the legal system, whereas situational couple violence is more likely to be identified in clinical and community samples (Graham-Kevan & Archer, 2003). Hence, approaches to treatment vary considerably, based on the form and impact of IPV.

Usual Treatments

A common component of IPV perpetration is that individuals are often unaware that the behavior is a problem. Even in the context of marital therapy, men and women often believe that IPV is a transient or unimportant issue (Ehrensaft & Vivian, 1996). Given this lack of concern, treatment for IPV is often compelled by court order or by other external forces such as pressure from a partner (Saunders, 2000). The oldest and most commonly utilized treatment approach for IPV is court-mandated group treatment programs; however, these programs have met with only limited success. Alternative treatments that attempt to address some of the shortcomings of traditional approaches include couple therapy and universal prevention programs; however, these approaches have their limitations as well.

Group Treatment

Criminal sanctions alone do not appear to be an effective deterrent to repeated IPV offenses (Maxwell & Garner, 2012). Thus, many states and provinces have enacted mandatory treatments for individuals, primarily men, who have been criminally convicted of an IPV offense. The earliest group treatments for IPV drew from the feminist perspective that IPV is a reflection of a larger patriarchal social system that supports the male domination of women (Dobash & Dobash, 1979). Thus, most common treatments based on this approach, such as the Duluth model (Pence & Paymar, 1993), explicitly targeted patriarchal beliefs and value systems through directive and confrontational interventions designed specifically to break down resistance. Many state regulations now explicitly require that court-mandated IPV treatments employ a feminist perspective (Maiuro & Eberle, 2008).

More recently, some group treatment programs have also incorporated interventions based on cognitive-behavioral therapy (CBT), with a focus on interventions such as cognitive restructuring, skills building, and the development of greater emotion regulation (e.g., Wexler, 2006). Although typically less confrontational than the Duluth model, the CBT approach is also primarily directive and assumes a readiness to change on the part of participants. Currently, many group treatment programs incorporate elements of both feminist theory and CBT approaches, making the distinctions between the two approaches difficult to disentangle.

High-quality randomized controlled trials are rare in the IPV group treatment field, and thus we know very little about the effectiveness of traditional treatments. In the most recent review (Eckhardt et al., 2013), only 20 experimental or quasi-experimental studies were located that included measures of recidivism (criminal or partner report of IPV perpetration). The Duluth model was evaluated in 14 of the studies, and the remainder were models with CBT or other skills-based elements included. Only about half of all studies demonstrated a significant effect of group treatment on IPV, compared to a no-treatment control condition, and several of these studies contained significant methodological flaws. Further, in a meta-analysis of IPV group treatment programs (Babcock, Green, & Robie, 2004), an examination of 22 experimental or quasi-experimental studies found that group treatment demonstrated a small but significant effect on IPV recidivism, with no significant differences across treatment modalities (e.g., Duluth, CBT).

In addition to negligible outcomes for group treatments of IPV, dropout rates are extremely high, with many individuals attending only one session or less (Daly & Pelowski, 2000). Further, early dropout is related to greater risk of future IPV (Bennett, Stoops, Call, & Flett, 2007). For instance, in a sample of 199 men court-mandated to batterers' interventions, the dropout rate was 40%, and the risk of reoffense was more than twice as great for participants who dropped out of treatment (Eckhardt, Holtzworth-Munroe, Norlander, Sibley, & Cahill, 2008). Thus, group treatment for IPV produces only small change for individuals who complete treatment and also suffers from extremely high treatment refusal rates.

Possible reasons for the limited efficacy of group treatments for IPV include a lack of intrinsic motivation to change, co-occurring conditions such as mental illness or substance use disorders that hamper change, the multiplicity of important targets for treatment, and the risk of contagion effects from exposure to antisocial peers (Murphy & Meis, 2008). Not surprisingly, court-referred individuals report particularly low intrinsic motivation to change. Of 199 men court-mandated to batterers' treatment, for instance, 76% reported being primarily in either the precontemplative or contemplative stage of change (Eckhardt et al., 2008), based on the transtheoretical model of change (Prochaska & DiClemente, 1984). Similarly, in a group of 292 men attending batterers' treatment, only 13% reported being in the action stage of change (Levesque, Gelles, & Velicer, 2000). Thus, individuals may often attend group treatment for IPV with very low intrinsic motivation to change, suggesting that directive and confrontational intervention approaches might be a particularly poor fit for most attendees.

Couple Therapy

Given that IPV is often bidirectional between partners (Langhinrichsen-Rohling, Misra, Selwyn, & Rohling, 2012) and that relationship distress is strongly linked to IPV perpetration (Stith, Smith, Penn, Ward, & Tritt, 2004), couple therapy approaches have also been developed to treat IPV. Of the limited randomized-controlled trials that exist, couple therapy group treatment is generally equal or superior to gender-specific group treatment (O'Leary, Heyman, & Neidig, 1999) and couple therapy individual treatment (Stith, Rosen, McCollum, & Thomsen, 2004) in reducing IPV perpetration and increasing relationship adjustment. Owing to concerns regarding the risk of violence escalation during treatment, couple therapy is generally recommended only for couples in intact relationships who are engaging in low to moderate levels of IPV, with no history of serious injury and no significant fear of the partner, and as such is not suitable for many individuals with a history of IPV perpetration. Couple therapy programs are also often grounded in feminist and CBT principles, with correspondingly confrontative or directive interventions, and hence issues of low motivation to change may still hamper success within traditional couple therapy approaches.

Universal Prevention

Given the limited effectiveness of interventions designed to treat IPV, increased attention has turned in recent years to the prevention of IPV in young adult populations. IPV prevention programs are primarily universal (e.g., delivered to all members of a group regardless of their risk of IPV perpetration) and psychoeducational in nature, and are targeted toward adolescents and young adults who are just beginning to navigate close relationships. Many programs are delivered in school settings, and some are also delivered in other community contexts or directly to couples or parents (O'Leary, Woodin, & Fritz, 2006). In general, universal psychoeducational programs, particularly those administered in school settings, show very little effectiveness in reducing IPV perpetration (Whitaker, Murphy, Eckardt, Hodges, & Cowart, 2013). Universal prevention programs tend to be standardized and didactic in nature and thus may fail to address the heterogeneity of IPV perpetrators. Further, because these interventions are targeted to large groups of primarily nonaggressive young adults, the dose tends to be quite limited and the effect size is negligible. Targeted IPV prevention programs delivered to at-risk individuals tend to yield larger effect sizes than universal prevention programs, possibly because they employ a greater degree of tailoring and individualization, including the use of more interactive and high-intensity interventions (O'Leary et al., 2006).

Rationale for Using MI to Treat IPV

Given the limited effectiveness of many treatment approaches for IPV, there is a pressing need for the development of empirically informed and flexible treatment models to address the challenges and heterogeneity of IPV perpetration. As stated above, low motivation to change is seen as a primary problem in traditional IPV treatments, and indeed motivation is an important consideration. For example, in a sample of 107 men court-mandated to treatment, motivational readiness to change was the strongest predictor of the working alliance (Taft, Murphy, Musser, & Remington, 2004). Further, Alexander and Morris (2008) demonstrated that men entering group treatment who scored lower in readiness to change also reported less self-reported distress, violence, and problems with anger, despite their partners reporting equal levels of violence perpetration relative to other attendees. Thus, individuals lower in readiness to change may underreport their own level of impairment and have more difficulty in establishing a strong working alliance and therefore be less likely to engage successfully with the treatment process.

Behaviors indicative of resistance (e.g., anger, irritability, opposition, and suspicion) are related to poor outcomes across a range of disorders (e.g., Beutler, Moleiro, & Talebi, 2002); however, there is no empirical evidence that confrontation is the best solution to resistance. Rather, coercive and hostile therapist behaviors often lead to mistrust on the part of clients (Ackerman & Hilsenroth, 2001), and resistant individuals are least likely to benefit from directive forms of therapy (Beutler et al., 2002). Further, brief interventions for alcohol use that employ a directive-confrontational style produce high levels of client resistance that then actually predict increased drinking rates following treatment (Miller, Benefield, & Tonigan, 1993). Thus, confrontational strategies may be a key limitation to the effectiveness of traditional group treatment approaches and may even re-create the very hierarchical and controlling dynamics they are seeking to overcome (Murphy & Baxter, 1997). More recently, interventionists have argued that the structure of the treatment program should be used to facilitate greater intrinsic motivation as treatment progresses, even for participants who begin treatment with very low motivation to change (McMurran, 2002).

The alcohol treatment field experienced a very similar history of largely unsuccessful attempts to use confrontational interventions to break down denial and compel change (e.g., Polich, Armor, & Braiker, 1981). The development of the transtheoretical model of change (Prochaska & DiClemente, 1984) and the therapeutic technique of motivational interviewing (Miller, 1983) were in large part responses to the limitations of existing treatments. The similarities between the alcohol and IPV treatment fields in terms of frequent treatment resistance and the limited efficacy of confrontational approaches have led to a call for the use of motivational methods to treat IPV as well (e.g., Daniels & Murphy, 1997; Murphy & Baxter, 1997). Further, the prevalence of IPV and risky alcohol use both peak in early adulthood during a time of considerable impulsive risk taking and identity formation (Arnett, 2000; O'Leary & Woodin, 2005), suggesting that both behaviors may share some common underlying risk factors and therefore might be amenable to similar forms of treatment.

Clinical Applications

Given the aforementioned limitations with existing treatments, Stuart, Temple, and Moore (2007) argued that systematic empirically informed modifications need to be made to existing treatments. They suggested incorporating motivational strategies into existing treatments to facilitate a stronger working alliance with participants, who are often not yet ready to engage in concrete behavioral change strategies. To date, MI has been incorporated into existing treatment programs in a variety of ways, including as an adjunct treatment for substance use or compliance issues in IPV group treatment programs, as an additional component interwoven into existing IPV group treatment programs, and as a stand-alone targeted prevention approach for at-risk individuals.

MI for Substance Use as an Adjunct to Traditional Treatments

Given that harmful substance use is significantly related to IPV perpetration (Foran & O'Leary, 2008), one natural outgrowth of MI for substance use is as an adjunct to treatments for IPV. In an early trial, 22 men court-mandated to anger management training received one group MI session on substance use (Easton, Swan, & Sinha, 2000). The MI session consisted of a focus on substance-related problems and possible solutions, using an MI-consistent framework. Results demonstrated that motivation to change substance use increased significantly from before to after the MI intervention; however, the researchers did not assess changes in substance use behavior in any subsequent follow-ups.

An MI-inspired brief intervention for substance use has also been developed as an adjunct to couples treatment for IPV (McCollum, Stith, Miller, & Ratcliffe, 2011). Participants with at-risk alcohol or drug use participated in one MI intervention during the sixth couple therapy session. The MI intervention, which was delivered in either a group or individual format and separately for men and women, consisted primarily of psychoeducation related to ways of talking about substance use and recommended drinking guidelines, exploration of the pros and cons of substance use, the administration of a questionnaire to encourage participants to consider possible consequences of substance use, and a worksheet designed to enable participants to decide what changes, if any, they wished to make in their substance use. Throughout the intervention, the therapists responded to clients in an MI-informed fashion. To date, there are no published evaluations of this approach.

MI combined with individualized feedback, referred to as motivational enhancement therapy (MET), has also been examined as a method to reduce alcohol use. The most ambitious study to date randomly assigned 252 hazardous drinking men in batterer intervention programs to receive either 90 minutes of MET for hazardous alcohol use or a no-intervention control condition before attending a standard IPV group treatment (Stuart et al., 2013). At the 3-month follow-up, men in the MET condition reported significantly less alcohol consumption, greater abstinence, less severe physical IPV, less severe psychological IPV, and fewer injuries to partners; however, the effects had largely faded by the 6- and 12-month follow-ups. Thus, MET for substance use is a promising adjunct to increase the efficacy of standard IPV treatment protocols, but its efficacy may diminish over time.

MI as an Adjunct to Improve Compliance with IPV Group Treatment

In the first examination of MI directly targeting IPV as an adjunct to IPV group treatment, Kistenmacher and Weiss (2008) randomly assigned 33 court-mandated men to receive either a two-session IPV-focused MET intervention or a no-intervention control condition before IPV group treatment. The MET sessions consisted of individualized feedback on participants' self-reports of IPV perpetration and stages of change, followed by a second session in which the therapist further discussed their IPV and entry into treatment, using an MI-consistent stance. Men in the MET condition demonstrated greater growth in stages of change and a greater decrease in external attributions for their IPV following the MET intervention; however, the researchers did not report behavioral outcomes, such as compliance with group treatment or rate of IPV recidivism.

A larger study similarly evaluated a two-session MET-focused intake process as compared to a structured intake control completed prior to a court-mandated group CBT treatment (Musser, Semiatin, Taft, & Murphy, 2008). The MET sessions consisted of the completion of the Safe-at-Home Instrument for Assessing Readiness to Change Intimate Partner Violence (SIRC; Begun et al., 2003), followed by a 45-minute MI session and the completion of a self-report questionnaire packet. The second session consisted of MET utilizing personalized written and verbal feedback regarding participants' self-reports of IPV, anger, relationship functioning, and risky substance use, followed by a second motivational interview. In addition to the in-session procedures, therapists also sent a personalized motivational note to the participants between the first and second sessions and also contacted participants by phone and mail following missed appointments. Compared to the control condition, the MET condition was associated with more constructive in-session behaviors, greater homework compliance, better therapist-rated working alliance, and greater outside help-seeking behaviors. No significant effects were found for session attendance, self-reported readiness to change, or client-rated working alliance. Finally, there was a marginally significant effect favoring the MET condition for partner reports of IPV 6 months after the CBT intervention. The authors noted that, because the target behavior was session attendance and not IPV per se, MET might not have been as effective at reducing IPV as it otherwise could have been.

In a follow-up examination of moderators of change, Murphy, Linehan, Reyner, Musser, and Taft (2012) found that men with high initial reluctance to change were more likely to report forward movement in their stage of change following the MET intervention than men who were already motivated to change. In addition, for men who initially claimed to have already solved their problems, MET was actually related to greater backward movement in stages of change and greater homework compliance, suggesting that MET facilitated these men's reconsidering the effort they might still need to expend. MET was also related to greater working alliance for men high in contemplation to change and better attendance for men with high trait anger.

Scott, King, McGinn, and Hosseini (2011) developed a six-session group pretreatment for highly resistant court-mandated men that incorporated themes from motivational interviewing, including a focus on empathy, creating discrepancies, and building self-efficacy. The men then attended a Duluth model group treatment program. The authors found that dropout rates were lower for highly resistant men receiving the motivational pretreatment group as compared to highly resistant men completing the standard group treatment only; however, there were no significant differences in group leaders' ratings of in-session treatment engagement. Further, there was no follow-up to examine rates of IPV recidivism after the intervention.

Crane and Eckhardt (2013) evaluated a single session of MI as an adjunct to court-mandated group treatment. The MI session consisted of 45–55 minutes spent discussing the most recent IPV event, exploring participants' responses to the Safe at Home Scale (Begun et al., 2003), and in some cases completing a standardized change plan. Therapists responded to participants in a manner consistent with the tenets of MI.

Results indicated that MI was related to better session attendance and treatment compliance relative to a control condition. Further, readiness to change moderated these findings, with participants low in readiness to change demonstrating significant effects in session attendance and treatment compliance, whereas participants high in readiness to change participated well regardless of the intervention condition. The authors found no significant differences in recidivism 6 months following the intervention; however, IPV-specific recidivism was very low in both conditions. The authors also noted that the effects of MI seemed to dissipate by midtreatment as rates of compliance became more similar between conditions, and they suggested that a second booster session of MI midtreatment might be an effective addition.

MI Themes Incorporated into Group Treatment

Alexander, Morris, Tracy, and Frye (2010) responded to the limitations of existing approaches to group treatment by randomly assigning 528 male batterers to a 26-week stages-of-change motivational interviewing (SOCMI) group intervention or a standard CBT gender reeducation group intervention. The first 14 sessions of the SOCMI intervention utilized experiential change processes consistent with precontemplation and contemplation stages of change, whereas the final 12 sessions consisted of behavioral change process. Group leaders delivered all SOCMI sessions in an MI-consistent manner. Findings indicated that members of the SOCMI group perpetrated less posttreatment physical IPV as compared to members of the CBT condition. Consistent with theoretical predictions, men lower in readiness to change engaged in significantly less physical IPV after the SOCMI condition than the CBT condition, whereas men higher in readiness to change engaged in significantly less physical IPV in the CBT condition as compared to the SOCMI condition.

Summary

To summarize, MI and MET have most often been used as an adjunct to IPV group treatments, with a focus on either substance use or IPV behaviors. Most studies demonstrate an increase in readiness to change as a result of MI and MET interventions, and many studies have also documented improved session attendance and compliance. Few studies reported on changes in IPV after the MI/MET intervention; however, there is some evidence that these approaches lead to at least temporary reductions in IPV perpetration. Finally, MI/MET approaches appear to produce larger changes in behavior for individuals with lower motivation to change, whereas more structured interventions such as CBT produce equal or even larger changes for individuals with high motivation to change.

Clinical Illustration

We developed the Dating Checkup Program as a stand-alone MET intervention for at-risk college dating couples (Woodin & O'Leary, 2010). We were interested in creating a program that would be helpful for intact couples experiencing low to moderate levels of physical IPV in their relationship, with the goal of providing a brief tailored intervention that could serve as a targeted prevention approach for couples who might not generally be aware of or interested in more intensive interventions. We were specifically interested in intervening with couples in the "emerging adulthood" period of development, which tends to be characterized by a high degree of risk taking and identity development (Arnett, 2000) as well as a high-risk time for IPV (O'Leary & Woodin, 2005). Further, we were particularly interested in intervening with male IPV, as past research has shown male IPV is particularly detrimental to the victim (Lawrence et al., 2012). At the same time, we were cognizant that the majority of our couples would likely report bidirectional IPV (Magdol et al., 1997), and as such we specifically designed our assessment and intervention procedures to be flexible and equally applicable to men and women.

Based on these goals, we designed a study comparing a MET session with a control condition consisting of brief nonmotivational feedback and psychoeducation (Woodin & O'Leary, 2010). We recruited couples from the campus of Stony Brook University. Our inclusion criteria were that both partners were between 18 and 25 years old, they had shared a nonmarried and noncohabiting dating relationship for at least 3 months, and they had experienced at least one episode of mild physical IPV (threw something that could hurt, twisted an arm or hair, pushed or shoved, grabbed, or slapped) perpetrated by the male partner during the past 3 months.

The Assessment Session

Couples who met the inclusion criteria were invited to a 2-hour assessment session. In the first hour, partners were separated and completed a series of computerized questionnaires in nonadjoining rooms. We assessed levels of physical IPV during the preceding months (reported separately for perpetration and victimization) with the Revised Conflict Tactics Scales (CTS2; Straus, Hamby, Boney-McCoy, & Sugarman, 1996). We also assessed for common risk factors for IPV, including psychological IPV with the CTS2, patterns of verbal conflict with the Communication Patterns Questionnaire (CPQ; Christensen & Sullaway, 1984), perceptions of stress with the Life Experiences Survey (LES; Sarason, Johnson, & Siegel, 1978), and hazardous alcohol use with the Alcohol Use Disorders Identification Test (AUDIT; Saunders, Aasland, Babor, de la Puente, & Grant, 1993). Finally, we also assessed for common consequences of IPV, including relationship satisfaction with the Dyadic Adjustment Scale (DAS; Spanier, 1976), depression symptoms with the Beck Depression Inventory—Revised (BDI-II; Beck, Steer, & Brown, 1996), and anxiety symptoms with the Beck Anxiety Inventory (BAI; Beck, Epstein, Brown, & Steer, 1988).

After the computerized assessments were completed, we first examined the assessment results for any history of serious IPV-related injury, as measured by the CTS2, or any significant fear of the partner, using the Fear of Partner Scale (FPS; O'Leary, Foran, & Cohen, 2013). For safety reasons, couples reporting injury or significant fear were excluded from participation in the feedback session. Our exclusion protocol entailed an individual and confidential debriefing with each partner regarding the person's immediate and long-term safety, with a referral to the undergraduate counseling center, a local emergency shelter, and a violence hotline.

In the last step of the assessment session, a master's-level therapist interviewed both partners together about the history and course of their relationship, using the Oral History Interview (OHI; Buehlman, Gottman, & Katz, 1992). The OHI is a semistructured interview that includes questions regarding how the partners first met, what attracted them to each other, and how their relationship has progressed. To maintain confidential reporting, we did not ask any questions specifically about IPV, and hardly any couples voluntarily discussed IPV during the interview. We chose to have couples complete the OHI, which is generally considered a pleasant and enjoyable interview, to build rapport with the study therapist and to provide the therapist context for the feedback session.

The MET Feedback Session

Participants assigned to the MET feedback session, which lasted up to 45 minutes for each partner, first received written individualized feedback regarding the IPV perpetration (based only on each partner's own self-report for confidentiality reasons) as well as written feedback on risk factors for physical IPV (psychological IPV, verbal conflict, stress, alcohol use) and possible consequences of IPV (relationship satisfaction, depression, anxiety). The feedback was tailored to provide the partners with information on how their self-reports compared to the "average college student" of their gender, based on normative data collected from other college student populations for each questionnaire. The feedback was generally provided as "low," "medium," or "high" on each measure, and a brief description of the meaning of each partner's score was provided. In addition, the IPV feedback was presented as percentile scores relative to other students at Stony Brook University, based on past research with our laboratory group. Our provision of this tailored normative feedback is consistent with evidence that changes in normative perceptions of alcohol use are important mechanisms of change in brief interventions for harmful alcohol use (Borsai & Carey, 2000), as well as with evidence from the IPV field that young adults who report a discrepancy between their current IPV and their attitudes toward IPV (i.e., cognitive dissonance) are most likely to reduce IPV over time, even after controlling for attitude change (Schumacher & Slep, 2004).

During the feedback session, the therapist provided the individualized feedback in an empathic and nonconfrontational manner, discussed the current impact and possible future risks to the individual and to the relationship as a result of the IPV, and facilitated a discussion of possible means of behavior change. Common precipitating events for IPV were discussed as appropriate (e.g., heavy alcohol use, psychological IPV, relationship conflict, stress). Further, the potential impact of the IPV on the well-being of the individual and the relationship were highlighted. Participants were asked to respond to this feedback, and any statements indicating motivation to change these behaviors were attended to and reinforced.

The last interview of the motivational feedback session was 15 minutes long and included both partners, and therefore no specific mention of individual feedback was made. Instead, the therapist asked the couple to discuss their overall impressions of the strengths and concerns in their relationship. As in the individual interviews, the therapist attended to and reinforced statements indicating motivation to change any risk factors for physical IPV (e.g., frequent conflict, alcohol use).

Outcome Results

Woodin and O'Leary (2010) reported the treatment outcome findings from the Dating Checkup Program as a stand-alone MET intervention for at-risk college dating couples. Compared to a nonmotivational control condition, the MET condition was associated with less physical IPV, less harmful alcohol use, and less acceptance of psychological IPV in the 9 months following the intervention. In a follow-up analysis, Woodin, Sotskova, and O'Leary (2012) found that therapist behaviors consistent with competency in MI predicted significantly greater reductions in physical IPV following the MET feedback session, suggesting that MET procedures exerted their effects through the hypothesized mechanism.

Description of a Typical MET Feedback Session

Carly and Adam have been dating for 8 months. Carly is a first-generation college student who is originally from Cambodia, and Adam is a second-generation Ukrainian American. They met through mutual friends, and both live in on-campus student housing. They are both graduating at the end of the semester but are experiencing some stress because they are not sure where their paths will take them after graduation. They are also under pressure from their families, who do not approve of their dating outside of their cultural group and who would like to see them break up before their relationship gets more serious. Carly reported that she was initially drawn to Adam because of his good looks and friendly demeanor, and Adam reported that he was drawn to Carly because she was outgoing and personable. They describe their relationship as generally strong and loving but that they also struggle with issues of jealousy, particularly at social gatherings, and often experience conflict that "gets out of hand."

During Carly's motivational feedback session, she was not surprised by much of the individualized feedback, particularly that she and Adam have a great deal of verbal conflict and psychological IPV in their relationship. In contrast, she was quite surprised and alarmed by the feedback that both she and Adam scored above the 90th percentile for their frequency of physical IPV as compared to the average Stony Brook student. Her initial response was "Is this domestic violence?" She went on to say that she had never thought of their pushing and shoving as anything very serious, as she assumed that most couples engaged in such behavior from time to time. The therapist reflected back her surprise and worked to help her further develop and explore the discrepancy she had unearthed. The therapist then worked to elicit self-motivational statements from Carly, which particularly revolved around her goal to solve conflict effectively so that their relationship would not be so stressful. Carly was able to generate several ideas about ways she could handle conflict more effectively, particularly when she felt jealous of Adam talk-ing to other women. With the therapist's assistance, she was able to iden-tify areas of self-efficacy, and she felt that her strong interpersonal skills would help her communicate more effectively.

During Adam's motivational feedback session, he was less surprised than Carly regarding the feedback on his physical IPV perpetration but reported feeling saddened that it was the case. He described having regu-larly witnessed his father and mother fighting physically when he was a child, and he had sworn to never repeat the same pattern in his own rela-tionships. He said that he often felt overwhelmed during fights with Carly and that their fights would become physical when he abruptly attempted to leave the room to "cool off." Adam quickly recommitted to his goal of remaining violence-free in his relationship, saying, "That's not the man I want to be." The therapist then asked Adam to come up with some ideas for what he could do instead when feeling overwhelmed, and Adam was able to generate several strategies, including telling Carly that he needed a break from the conversation before things got too heated.

In the final conjoint feedback session, the therapist guided the cou-ple to think about some of the overall strengths and challenges in their relationship and to explore how they might deal with their challenges. Carly and Adam both identified their strong bond and determination to make their relationship work as their greatest strengths, and they jointly focused on their problems with conflict and jealousy as important chal-lenges. The partners expressed a desire to find a better way to resolve conflict, and each described some of the key strategies he or she would use when feeling upset. The therapist reflected these self-motivational statements and reiterated the couple's areas of strengths as evidence of self-efficacy to make these changes happen.

The MI Process

The motivational feedback session is designed to be flexible and indi-vidualized so that the therapist is able to move through the stages of MI at an appropriate pace for each participant. Throughout the session, therapists focus explicitly on maintaining an empathic and noncon-frontational stance while maintaining the standards of high-quality MI administration. Therapists concentrate on asking primarily open-ended questions, on using more reflections than questions, and using complex reflections whenever possible. Therapists also avoid providing advice without permission.

Providing Normative Feedback

The first stage in the feedback process is generally to ask permission to provide written normative feedback to the participant and to then ask for his or her reaction to this feedback. "Based on how you filled out the survey, you scored in the high range in your level of alcohol use. Typically we say that a score above 7 places people at risk for drinking problems, and your score of 18 is quite a bit above that." The therapist provides this feedback in a flexible manner and might skip to various sections as needed if the participant is resonating with a particular theme. Conversely, if the participant scores low on certain sections (e.g., their alcohol use is within healthy limits), the therapist will reinforce this source of strength and then move on to issues that might be more salient to the individual.

Exploring the Participant's Reactions

After providing feedback on each measure, the therapists then ask for a reaction from the participant. "What do you make of this?" "How does this fit with how you see yourself?" Many participants are particularly surprised by their scores on the physical IPV measure, and quite a few mention that they believe the behavior is much more common in their social circles. The therapists respond empathically and nonconfrontationally to these assertions with statements such as "It seems to you like a lot of your friends fight physically from time to time."

Eliciting Change Talk

Throughout the session, the therapists work to elicit and selectively attend to client change talk, including times when participants are open to talking about their IPV perpetration, considering problems related to the IPV, and directly commenting on their wish to stop engaging in IPV. The therapists elicited these statements through open-ended questions such as:

> "Tell me a bit more about what it's like when you push and shove your partner. What's positive about it? And what's the other side? What are your worries about the conflict and fighting for yourself and your relationship?"
> "Tell me what you've noticed about times when you fight with your partner. What concerns you, what could be problems or might become a problem?"

"What makes you think that you might need to make a change in your relationship?"

The therapist attempts to elicit as much change talk as possible while acknowledging that the sources of motivation might vary considerably from one person to another. Common motivations for college dating couples typically revolve around the impact of IPV on their relationship, on their own mental and physical health and well-being, or on their academic performance and ability to cope with the demands of school. The therapist then reflects back those change talk statements to the client, typically immediately after each statement is made, and then as a summary reflection at the end of this process.

"Derek, for you the biggest issue is that when you fight physically it doesn't actually solve the problem but tends to make it much worse in the long run. You're worried about how the stress is affecting your relationship, and it makes it hard for you to concentrate when you're trying to study. It also makes you feel bad about yourself because it goes against your belief that 'men don't hit.'"

Eliciting Ideas about Changing

After the therapist has solicited and reflected change talk, the next step is generally to ask the participant about his or her ideas about changing the IPV behavior. Conversely, many participants will start to spontaneously generate their own ideas for changing, which the therapist can then reinforce through the use of reflections. Common therapist questions might include:

"Now that you've thought about the problems with your aggression, what do you think you'll do the next time you're feeling jealous?"
"Where does this leave you now in terms of how you want to act in your relationship?"
"What do you make of all this? What's next for you? What might help?"
"What do you hope for in the future? How would things look if they were a lot better than they are now? How would you get there?"

During this process, the therapist refrains from making suggestions or recommendations but, rather, solicits the participant's own ideas for change and then reflects upon those ideas. The therapist also emphasizes that it is the participant's decision about how and if to make any changes in his or her behavior. The therapist also does not make a recommendation regarding whether the participant should remain in the relationship or terminate the relationship, but rather responds in a neutral manner to any thoughts the participant has in this regard.

If the participant directly solicits advice or asks a direct question of the therapist, the therapist will then respond with objective advice if possible but will often reiterate the theme of personal responsibility and autonomy.

> "It's your choice to decide what works for you, but I can say that for many people taking a brief time out can make a big difference when you're feeling really upset."
> "Since you mentioned that most of your worst fights happen when you're both drinking a lot, one thing that might help is to cut down on your drinking when you're out together at night."

Providing a Menu of Options

The final stage of the motivational feedback session involves providing participants with a pamphlet on building healthy relationships along with a referral list with on-campus and off-campus resources. Participants are again reminded that these are options that may or may not be helpful in their particular case, but that they are resources that are sometimes useful for individuals who are dealing with violence in their relationships.

Problems and Suggested Solutions

Owing to the empathic and nonconfrontational nature of MI, this approach is generally more effective than standard treatment approaches in engaging individuals who are hesitant to label themselves as having a problem with IPV (Alexander et al., 2010; Crane & Eckhardt, 2013; Kistenmacher & Weiss, 2008; Murphy et al., 2012; Scott et al., 2011). That being said, there are certain issues that can arise with MI for IPV that require additional problem solving.

A key issue that can arise in any MI session—but that might be more likely in MI sessions with court-mandated or coerced individuals—is the high degree of "resistance" that an individual might express to the process of receiving MI or MET. In this circumstance, the traditional MI tools are key. Therapists can simply acknowledge the hesitation directly ("You really don't want to be here") or even amplify the participant's concern ("This is the last thing on earth you want to be doing right now!"). Double-sided reflections on the ambivalence can also be helpful ("There's a part of you that thinks this process is a waste of time, but on the other hand some of this really surprises you"). Sometimes changing the topic is effective ("Let's switch gears and talk a bit about the stress you've been under lately"). Throughout this process, the therapist reminds the participant about his or her own personal autonomy and responsibility, always maintaining an empathic and nonjudgmental stance toward the participant's experience. Above all else, the therapist avoids direct confrontation, arguing, or advice giving, as these behaviors will likely increase the participant's mistrust and hesitancy.

Another issue that can often emerge with MI for IPV is that the participant might be experiencing comorbid conditions that may make behavior change more difficult. Indeed, substance use and mental health concerns significantly predict poorer response for men in batterers' treatment (Tollefson & Gross, 2006). In this case, MI techniques can also be useful for increasing motivation to access other services such as substance use and/or mental health treatment. This is related to the menu-of-options approach and can be considered part of a participant's individualized plan to stop IPV.

Finally, MI as a stand-alone treatment for IPV is likely contraindicated if there is acute risk of injury to the partner. As described previously, I recommend using MI as a stand-alone treatment only for individuals with no history of severe injury or extreme coercion of the partner and only for couples in which neither partner is fearful of engaging in the process. If there is elevated risk, participants should be encouraged to attend a longer-term treatment program with the goal of learning greater behavioral regulation in a context in which ongoing safety issues can be addressed routinely. Further, partners should receive treatment separately to mitigate the risk of violence escalation and injury, at least until such time as behavior regulation is improved considerably.

Conclusions

MI is a flexible and accessible approach to IPV that overcomes many of the limitations of existing treatments. Although there is still a need for additional randomized controlled trials to examine the efficacy and utility of various uses of MI and MET for IPV, initial results appear promising. One caveat is that very few studies have examined change in actual IPV behavior following an intervention (see Alexander et al., 2010; Crane & Eckhardt, 2013; Musser et al., 2008; Stuart et al., 2013; and Woodin & O'Leary, 2010, for exceptions), and even fewer have been able to obtain partner reports of IPV, which tend to be the most reliable indicator of recidivism but which are not always available (particularly in the case of men court-mandated to treatment). Another possible limitation of MI for IPV is that results seem to fade within the first year. As recommended by several authors, booster sessions given 6 months after the initial MI session might prove beneficial in prolonging the gains achieved. Alternatively, the reduction in effectiveness seen in some studies might be the result of combining one or two sessions of MI with a confrontational and directive group treatment program. In this case, an essential point of intervention refinement may be to maintain an MI-consistent stance *throughout* the treatment process. Finally, as with other conditions, MI for IPV is likely most useful for individuals with low awareness of IPV as a problem and/or low motivation to change IPV behaviors. Thus, individuals high in readiness to change are likely to benefit more from change-oriented directive approaches. Despite these caveats and limitations, MI is clearly an exciting intervention approach that moves the field of IPV intervention forward to the next stage of empirically informed treatment programs that have the potential to significantly improve outcomes for a wider range of individuals currently struggling to remain violence-free.

References

Ackerman, S. J., & Hilsenroth, M. J. (2001). A review of therapist characteristics and techniques negatively impacting the therapeutic alliance. *Psychotherapy: Theory, Research, Practice, Training, 38*, 171–185.

Alexander, P. C., & Morris, E. (2008). Stages of change in batterers and their response to treatment. *Violence and Victims, 23*, 476–492.

Alexander, P. C., Morris, E., Tracy, A., & Frye, A. (2010). Stages of change and the group treatment of batterers: A randomized clinical trial. *Violence and Victims, 25*, 571–587.

Arnett, J. J. (2000). Emerging adulthood: A theory of development from the late teens through the twenties. *American Psychologist, 55*, 469–480.

Babcock, J. C., Green, C. E., & Robie, C. (2004). Does batterers' treatment work? A meta-analytic review of domestic violence treatment. *Clinical Psychology Review, 23*, 1023–1053.

Beck, A. T., Epstein, N., Brown, G., & Steer, R. A. (1988). An inventory for measuring clinical anxiety: Psychometric properties. *Journal of Consulting and Clinical Psychology, 56,* 893–897.

Beck, A. T., Steer, R. A., & Brown, G. K. (1996). *Beck Depression Inventory—Second Edition (BDI-II), Manual.* San Antonio, TX: Psychological Corp.

Begun, A. L., Murphy, C., Bolt, D., Weinstein, B., Strodthoff, T., Short, L., et al. (2003). Characteristics of the Safe at Home instrument for assessing readiness to change intimate partner violence. *Research on Social Work Practice, 13,* 80–107.

Bennett, L. W., Stoops, C., Call, C., & Flett, H. (2007). Program completion and re-arrest in a batterer intervention system. *Research on Social Work Practice, 17,* 42–54.

Beutler, L. E., Moleiro, C., & Talebi, H. (2002). Resistance in psychotherapy: What conclusions are supported by research? *Journal of Clinical Psychology, 58,* 207–217.

Borsai, B., & Carey, K. B. (2000). Effects of a brief motivational intervention with college student drinkers. *Journal of Consulting and Clinical Psychology, 68,* 728–733.

Buehlman, K. T., Gottman, J. M., & Katz, L. F. (1992). How a couple views their past predicts their future: Predicting divorce from an oral history interview. *Journal of Family Psychology, 5,* 295–318.

Carney, M., & Barner, J. R. (2012). Prevalence of partner abuse: Rates of emotional abuse and control. *Partner Abuse, 3,* 286–335.

Christensen, A., & Sullaway, M. (1984). *Communication Patterns Questionnaire.* Unpublished manuscript, University of California, Department of Psychology, Los Angeles.

Coker, A. L., Davis, K. E., Arias, I., Desai, S., Sanderson, M., Brandt, H. M., et al. (2002). Physical and mental health effects of intimate partner violence for men and women. *American Journal of Preventive Medicine, 23,* 260–268.

Crane, C. A., & Eckhardt, C. I. (2013). Evaluation of a single-session brief motivational enhancement intervention for partner abusive men. *Journal of Counseling Psychology, 60,* 180–187.

Daly, J. E., & Pelowski, S. (2000). Predictors of dropout among men who batter: A review of studies with implications for research and practice. *Violence and Victims, 15,* 137–160.

Daniels, J. W., & Murphy, C. M. (1997). Stages and processes of change in batterers' treatment. *Cognitive and Behavioral Practice, 4,* 123–145.

Desmarais, S. L., Reeves, K. A., Nicholls, T. L., Telford, R. P., & Fiebert, M. S. (2012). Prevalence of physical violence in intimate relationships, Part 2: Rates of male and female perpetration. *Partner Abuse, 3,* 1–54.

Dobash, R. E., & Dobash, R. (1979). *Violence against wives: A case against the patriarchy.* New York: Free Press.

Easton, C., Swan, S., & Sinha, R. (2000). Motivation to change substance use among offenders of domestic violence. *Journal of Substance Abuse Treatment, 19,* 1–5.

Eckhardt, C., Holtzworth-Munroe, A., Norlander, B., Sibley, A., & Cahill, M.

(2008). Readiness to change, partner violence subtypes, and treatment outcomes among men in treatment for partner assault. *Violence and Victims, 23,* 446–475.

Eckhardt, C. I., Murphy, C. M., Whitaker, D. J., Sprunger, J., Dykstra, R., & Woodard, K. (2013). The effectiveness of intervention programs for perpetrators and victims of intimate partner violence. *Partner Abuse, 4,* 196–231.

Ehrensaft, M. K., & Vivian, D. (1996). Spouses' reasons for not reporting existing marital aggression as a marital problem. *Journal of Family Psychology, 10,* 443–453.

Foran, H. M., & O'Leary, K. (2008). Alcohol and intimate partner violence: A meta-analytic review. *Clinical Psychology Review, 28,* 1222–1234.

Graham-Kevan, N., & Archer, J. (2003). Intimate terrorism and common couple violence: A test of Johnson's predictions in four British samples. *Journal of Interpersonal Violence, 18,* 1247–1270.

Johnson, M. P. (1995). Patriarchal terrorism and common couple violence: Two forms of violence against women. *Journal of Marriage and the Family, 57,* 283–294.

Johnson, M. P., & Leone, J. M. (2005). The differential effects of intimate terrorism and situational couple violence: Findings from the National Violence against Women Survey. *Journal of Family Issues, 26,* 322–349.

Kistenmacher, B. R., & Weiss, R. L. (2008). Motivational interviewing as a mechanism for change in men who batter: A randomized controlled trial. *Violence and Victims, 23,* 558–570.

Langhinrichsen-Rohling, J., Misra, T. A., Selwyn, C., & Rohling, M. L. (2012). Rates of bidirectional versus unidirectional intimate partner violence across samples, sexual orientations, and race/ethnicities: A comprehensive review. *Partner Abuse, 3,* 199–230.

Lawrence, E., Orengo-Aguayo, R., Langer, A., & Brock, R. L. (2012). The impact and consequences of partner abuse on partners. *Partner Abuse, 3,* 406–428.

Levesque, D. A., Gelles, R. J., & Velicer, W. F. (2000). Development and validation of a stages of change measure for men in batterer treatment. *Cognitive Therapy and Research, 24,* 175–199.

Magdol, L., Moffitt, T. E., Caspi, A., Newman, D. L., Fagan, J., & Silva, P. A. (1997). Gender differences in partner violence in a birth cohort of 21-year-olds: Bridging the gap between clinical and epidemiological approaches. *Journal of Consulting and Clinical Psychology, 65,* 68–78.

Maiuro, R. D., & Eberle, J. A. (2008). State standards for domestic violence perpetrator treatment: Current status, trends, and recommendations. *Violence and Victims, 23,* 133–155.

Maxwell, C. D., & Garner, J. H. (2012). The crime control effects of criminal sanctions for intimate partner violence. *Partner Abuse, 3,* 469–500.

McCollum, E. E., Stith, S. M., Miller, M., & Ratcliffe, G. (2011). Including a brief substance-abuse motivational intervention in a couples treatment program for intimate partner violence. *Journal of Family Psychotherapy, 22,* 216–231.

McMurran, M. (2002). *Motivating offenders to change: A guide to enhancing engagement in therapy.* New York: Wiley.

Miller, W. R. (1983). Motivational interviewing with problem drinkers. *Behavioural Psychotherapy, 11,* 147–172.

Miller, W. R., Benefield, R. G., & Tonigan, J. S. (1993). Enhancing motivation for change in problem drinking: A controlled comparison of two therapist styles. *Journal of Consulting and Clinical Psychology, 61,* 455–461.

Murphy, C. M., & Baxter, V. A. (1997). Motivating batterers to change in the treatment context. *Journal of Interpersonal Violence, 12,* 607–619.

Murphy, C. M., Linehan, E. L., Reyner, J. C., Musser, P. H., & Taft, C. T. (2012). Moderators of response to motivational interviewing for partner-violent men. *Journal of Family Violence, 27,* 671–680.

Murphy, C. M., & Meis, L. A. (2008). Individual treatment of intimate partner violence perpetrators. *Violence and Victims, 23,* 173–186.

Musser, P. H., Semiatin, J. N., Taft, C. T., & Murphy, C. M. (2008). Motivational interviewing as a pregroup intervention for partner-violent men. *Violence and Victims, 23,* 539–557.

O'Leary, K. D., Foran, H., & Cohen, S. (2013). Validation of Fear of Partner Scale. *Journal of Marital and Family Therapy, 39,* 502–514.

O'Leary, K., Heyman, R. E., & Neidig, P. H. (1999). Treatment of wife abuse: A comparison of gender-specific and conjoint approaches. *Behavior Therapy, 30,* 475–505.

O'Leary, K., & Woodin, E. M. (2005). Partner aggression and problem drinking across the lifespan: How much do they decline? *Clinical Psychology Review, 25,* 877–894.

O'Leary, K., Woodin, E. M., & Fritz, P. T. (2006). Can we prevent the hitting?: Recommendations for preventing intimate partner violence between young adults. *Journal of Aggression, Maltreatment and Trauma, 13,* 121–178.

Pence, E., & Paymar, M. (1993). *Education groups for men who batter: The Duluth model.* New York: Springer.

Polich, J. M., Armor, D. J., & Braiker, H. B. (1981). *The course of alcoholism four years after treatment.* New York: Wiley.

Prochaska, J. O., & DiClemente, C. C. (1984). *The transtheoretical approach: Crossing traditional boundaries of change.* Homewood, IL: Dorsey.

Sarason, I. G., Johnson, J. H., & Siegel, J. M. (1978). Assessing the impact of life changes: Development of the Life Experiences Survey. *Journal of Consulting and Clinical Psychology, 46,* 932–946.

Saunders, G. B. (2000). Feminist, cognitive, and behavioral group interventions for men who batter: An overview of rationale and methods. In D. B. Wexler (Ed.), *Domestic violence 2000: An integrated skills program for men: Group leader's manual* (pp. 21–31). New York: Norton.

Saunders, J. B., Aasland, O. G., Babor, T. F., de la Puente, J. R., & Grant, M. (1993). Development of the Alcohol Use Disorders Screening Test (AUDIT). WHO collaborative project on early detection of persons with harmful alcohol consumption—II. *Addiction, 88,* 791–804.

Schumacher, J. A., & Slep, A. M. S. (2004). Attitudes and dating aggression: A cognitive dissonance approach. *Prevention Science, 5,* 231–243.

Scott, K., King, C., McGinn, H., & Hosseini, N. (2011). Effects of motivational enhancement on immediate outcomes of batterer intervention. *Journal of Family Violence, 26*, 139–149.

Spanier, G. B. (1976). Measuring dyadic adjustment: New scales for assessing the quality of marriage and similar dyads. *Journal of Marriage and the Family, 38*, 15–28.

Stith, S. M., Rosen, K. H., McCollum, E. E., & Thomsen, C. J. (2004). Treating intimate partner violence within intact couple relationships: Outcomes of multi-couple versus individual couple therapy. *Journal of Marital and Family Therapy, 30*, 305–318.

Stith, S. M., Smith, D. B., Penn, C. E., Ward, D. B., & Tritt, D. (2004). Intimate partner physical abuse perpetration and victimization risk factors: A meta-analytic review. *Aggression and Violent Behavior, 10*, 65–98.

Straus, M. A., Hamby, S. L., Boney-McCoy, S., & Sugarman, D. B. (1996). The revised Conflict Tactics Scales (CTS2): Development and preliminary psychometric data. *Journal of Family Issues, 17*, 283–316.

Stuart, G. L., Shorey, R. C., Moore, T. M., Ramsey, S. E., Kahler, C. W., O'Farrell, T. J., et al. (2013). Randomized clinical trial examining the incremental efficacy of a 90-minute motivational alcohol intervention as an adjunct to standard batterer intervention for men. *Addiction, 108*, 1376–1384.

Stuart, G. L., Temple, J. R., & Moore, T. M. (2007). Improving batterer intervention programs through theory-based research. *JAMA, 298*, 560–562.

Taft, C. T., Murphy, C. M., Musser, P. H., & Remington, N. A. (2004). Personality, interpersonal, and motivational predictors of the working alliance in group cognitive-behavioral therapy for partner violent men. *Journal of Consulting and Clinical Psychology, 72*, 349–354.

Tollefson, D. R., & Gross, E. R. (2006). Predicting recidivism following participation in a treatment program for batterers. *Journal of Social Service Research, 32*, 39–62.

Wexler, D. B. (2006). *Stop domestic violence: Innovative skills, techniques, options, and plans for better relationships.* New York: Norton.

Whitaker, D. J., Murphy, C. M., Eckhardt, C. I., Hodges, A. E., & Cowart, M. (2013). Effectiveness of primary prevention efforts for intimate partner violence. *Partner Abuse, 4*, 175–195.

Woodin, E. M., & O'Leary, K. (2010). A brief motivational intervention for physically aggressive dating couples. *Prevention Science, 11*, 371–383.

Woodin, E. M., Sotskova, A., & O'Leary, K. (2012). Do motivational interviewing behaviors predict reductions in partner aggression for men and women? *Behaviour Research and Therapy, 50*, 79–84.

CHAPTER 14

· · · · · ·

Motivational Interviewing
in the Treatment
of Disordered Eating

Stephanie E. Cassin
Josie Geller

Eating disorders refer to a wide range of clinical features associated with the overvaluation of weight or shape, including dietary restriction, binge eating, and compensatory behaviors. Bulimia nervosa and binge-eating disorder are both characterized by repeated episodes of binge eating, defined as consuming a large amount of food within a 2-hour period and experiencing a loss of control over eating (American Psychiatric Association, 2013). They are primarily distinguished according to the presence or absence of compensatory behaviors intended to prevent weight gain. Individuals whose self-evaluation is heavily influenced by their weight and shape and who regularly engage in compensatory behaviors including self-induced vomiting, fasting, excessive exercise, or the misuse of laxatives, diuretics, or enemas are diagnosed with *bulimia nervosa*, whereas individuals who experience significant distress regarding their binge eating but do not regularly engage in compensatory behaviors are diagnosed with *binge-eating disorder.*

Anorexia nervosa is characterized by persistent restriction of energy intake, leading to a significantly low body weight for sex, age, and height. Weight loss is accomplished through dieting, fasting, and excessive exercise. Despite having a low body weight, individuals with anorexia nervosa experience an intense fear of gaining weight or engage in persistent behaviors that interfere with weight gain, and they display a disturbance in the way they experience their bodies. For example, body size may be overestimated or may become one of the primary determinants of self-evaluation. Individuals with anorexia nervosa who do not engage in regular binge eating and/or compensatory behaviors are diagnosed with *anorexia nervosa, restricting type*, whereas those who do engage in such behaviors are diagnosed with *anorexia nervosa, binge eating/purging type*.

In contrast to DSM-5-diagnosed eating disorders, which range in prevalence from 0.5% for anorexia nervosa to 3% for binge eating disorder (American Psychiatric Association, 2013), the prevalence of "disordered eating" is much higher. The term "disordered eating" encompasses a much broader conceptualization of eating behaviors that cause significant distress or impairment. For example, an individual might meet all of the criteria for bulimia nervosa or binge-eating disorder with the exception that purging or compensatory behaviors occur at a lower frequency (less than once per week) or for a shorter duration (less than 3 months), or might meet all of the criteria for anorexia nervosa with the exception that body weight is within a normal range, or might engage in regular compensatory behaviors despite the absence of binge eating. In addition to these other specified feeding or eating disorders (American Psychiatric Association, 2013), some additional forms of disordered eating include attempting to follow strict dietary rules regarding when, what, or how much to eat, regardless of whether these attempts are actually successful (i.e., high levels of dietary restraint). For example, an individual might attempt to abstain from eating after dinner, avoid all "forbidden foods," and eat fewer than 1000 calories every day.

Motivational interviewing (MI) holds great appeal in the treatment of eating disorders for several reasons. First, there are many parallels between disordered eating and the addictions for which MI was originally developed. Second, disordered eating often fulfills important and valued functions. Third, it can be difficult to engage individuals with disordered eating in treatment, and therefore dropout from treatment and relapse following treatment are very common. The usual treatments for disordered eating and the rationale for using MI are discussed below, followed by an overview of the clinical application of MI to disordered eating.

Usual Treatments

The National Institute for Health and Care Excellence (NICE, 2004) recommends outpatient cognitive-behavioral therapy (CBT) or interpersonal therapy (IPT) lasting at least 6 months for the treatment of anorexia nervosa, or family-based interventions in the case of children and adolescents with anorexia nervosa. If an individual experiences significant deterioration during outpatient treatment (e.g., significant weight loss or physical complications) or significant improvements are not noted during a course of treatment, more intensive forms of treatment are recommended. For example, intensive inpatient or day treatment focused on refeeding, weight restoration, and psychological rehabilitation may be required. Following weight restoration, individuals with anorexia nervosa should continue to receive outpatient psychological treatment and physical monitoring for a period of at least 12 months.

In the treatment of bulimia nervosa and binge-eating disorder, individuals should be encouraged to follow an evidence-based self-help program as a first step, such as consulting one of several cognitive-behavioral self-help workbooks available. Guided self-help using a book such as *Overcoming Binge Eating* (Fairburn, 1995) has been found to be effective for a subset of individuals with bulimia nervosa (Wilson, 2005). If symptoms persist following self-help or guided self-help interventions, 16–20 sessions of CBT should be offered over a period of 5–6 months. CBT has been shown to eliminate bingeing and purging in 30–50% of clients and to improve bingeing, purging, dysfunctional dieting, and body image in a substantial number of the remaining clients (NICE, 2004). In addition, symptom improvement is typically well maintained across follow-up periods spanning 1 year and beyond. However, not all clients respond well to CBT, and IPT can be considered as an alternative to CBT despite it typically requiring a longer period of 8–12 months to achieve the same effects (NICE, 2004). More intensive forms of treatment may be required for bulimia nervosa, such as inpatient hospitalization or day treatment, if symptoms persist following outpatient treatment and the individual requires closer monitoring for symptom disruption.

In the treatment of "disordered eating" more broadly, including other specified feeding or eating disorders, it is recommended that treatment be offered for the clinical problem that most closely resembles the individual's eating problem (NICE, 2004). For example, CBT would be recommended for an individual with lower-frequency eating binges and compensatory behaviors.

Rationale for Using MI

Individuals with disordered eating often describe their eating behavior as similar to an addiction (Cassin & von Ranson, 2007). A number of parallels have been noted between binge eating and the addictions for which MI was originally developed, including preoccupation with, cravings for, and repeated urges to consume the substance (i.e., psychoactive substances or food), as well as a mounting sense of tension until the substance is consumed, and subsequent loss of control over the behavior— often resulting in excessive consumption of the substance (Cassin & von Ranson, 2007; Gold, Frost-Pineda, & Jacobs, 2003; Wilson, 1991). In addition, individuals typically have great difficulty in either reducing or stopping the behavior, whatever their knowledge of the adverse physical or psychological effects might be.

Dietary restriction, binge eating, and compensatory behaviors often fulfill important and valued functions; therefore, individuals experiencing disordered eating often feel ambivalent about engaging in treatment and addressing their symptoms. On the one hand, individuals with anorexia nervosa report that dietary restrictions and the associated weight loss allow them to feel in greater control, provide a sense of safety and protection, and make them feel thinner and more attractive (Serpell, Treasure, Teasdale, & Sullivan, 1999), while those with bulimia nervosa report that bingeing and then purging allow them to eat "forbidden foods" without gaining weight, as well as to avoid or regulate their emotions (Serpell & Treasure, 2002). On the other hand, they also acknowledge many costs associated with disordered eating, such as damaging their physical health, limiting their social and academic/occupational opportunities, and paradoxically making them feel more emotionally dysregulated and out of control (Serpell et al., 1999; Serpell & Treasure, 2002). MI is ideally suited to help individuals with disordered eating explore and resolve their ambivalence as well as enhance their intrinsic motivation for making changes in their eating behaviors before engaging in action-oriented treatments.

The action-oriented treatments typically used to treat disordered eating, such as CBT, are efficacious for many individuals who engage in and complete treatment (NICE, 2004; Wilson, 2005). However, these action-oriented treatments assume, perhaps incorrectly, that individuals who present for treatment are ready to make changes. Readiness for change fluctuates not only over time but also across symptoms (Geller, Cockell, & Drab, 2001). For example, individuals might seek treatment to reduce eating binges but feel highly ambivalent about reducing their dietary restrictions, laxative use, and exercise. Similarly, individuals might feel ready to change their disordered eating behaviors but not their cognitions (such as overvaluation of weight and shape). As a result, engagement in treatment may be low, and treatment dropout and relapse may be high. Of patients who enroll in CBT for bulimia nervosa, fewer than half make significant improvements in their bingeing and purging behavior and maintain the changes over time (Wilson & Fairburn, 2007). Similarly, a 33% dropout rate was reported in a large trial of CBT for anorexia nervosa, and only 38% of those who enrolled in treatment reached a BMI of 18.5 kg/m^2 posttreatment (Fairburn et al., 2013). Readiness for change is an important target for treatment because it has been shown to prospectively predict enrollment in intensive day treatment, completion of recovery-related activities, weight gain, treatment dropout, and relapse following treatment (Bewell & Carter, 2008; Geller et al., 2001; Geller, Drab-Hudson, Whisenhunt, & Srikameswaran, 2004; Rieger et al., 2000).

Clinical Applications

MI can be used to explore and resolve ambivalence regarding a number of disordered eating behaviors and cognitions, including binge eating, compensatory behaviors (e.g., vomiting, laxative use, excessive exercise), dietary restriction, dietary restraint, and overvaluation of weight and shape. MI has been used in treatment-seeking samples as a prelude to action-oriented treatments (e.g., intensive inpatient or day treatment programs, outpatient CBT) in order to increase treatment enrollment and adherence (e.g., Geller, Brown, & Srikameswaran, 2011; Katzman et al., 2010; Treasure et al., 1999). It has even been integrated into the assessment process itself (e.g., Readiness and Motivation Interview; Geller et al., 2001). In addition, MI has been used as a single-session stand-alone intervention for individuals with disordered eating recruited from the community (Cassin, von Ranson, Heng, Brar, & Wojtowicz, 2008; Dunn, Neighbors, & Larimer, 2006). Below we describe some of the key components that tend to be included in MI protocols focused on disordered eating, using some illustrative examples.

Engaging

The core skills of MI (OARS: open-ended questions, affirmations, reflections, summaries) are used initially to engage clients in a conversation about change, and they are equally important throughout the focusing, evoking, and planning processes that make up MI (Miller & Rollnick, 2013). The clinician begins by opening up a dialogue about the client's eating behaviors: "I'd like to find out a little bit more about your eating habits. Can you tell me why you decided to come to the clinic?" The purpose of this dialogue is to explore the client's eating behaviors and to elicit change talk (i.e., self-motivational statements of the reasons to change the behavior). If the client hints at the need for change, the clinician can follow up by asking with interest, "What makes you think you need to change something about your eating?" If a client presents to a treatment program that routinely conducts diagnostic assessments prior to commencing treatment, we recommend that the spirit of MI be incorporated into the assessment process by using a clinical tool such as the Readiness and Motivation Interview (Geller et al., 2001). After all, relying on closed-ended questions can promote disengagement by socializing the client to provide short and succinct responses and by placing the client in a passive role relative to the "expert" clinician (Miller & Rollnick, 2013) rather than encouraging elaboration.

Focusing

The amount of focusing required depends to some extent on the treatment context. For example, little focusing is generally required for a client who voluntarily takes part in a research study examining the impact of treatment on a specific form of disordered eating (e.g., MI for binge eating). In contrast, more focusing would likely be required for a client who presents to an eating disorder treatment program with a variety of maladaptive eating behaviors (e.g., dietary restraint, eating binges, compensatory behaviors), particularly if the client does not present for treatment of his or her own volition. An even greater level of focusing might be required for a client who presents to a primary care physician with a variety of psychological and medical complaints but does not openly acknowledge his or her disordered eating. It is recommended that the client be invited to list any concerns he or she might want to discuss and that the clinician ask for permission to discuss an issue he or she feels is important to address but which is not spontaneously raised by the client (Miller & Rollnick, 2013).

Evoking

Clients with disordered eating rarely present for treatment ready to take action toward a clear and specific goal. In the event that they are ready to take action, the clinician is advised to proceed directly to the planning process (Miller & Rollnick, 2013). More typically, clients with disordered eating feel highly ambivalent about making changes because their eating behaviors serve important and valued functions. MI is particularly helpful for such clients owing to the variety of strategies used to evoke the client's own motivations for change, such as discussing the life areas that have been affected by disordered eating, assessing and bolstering the importance of change and the client's confidence in his or her ability to make changes, and imagining the future with and without disordered eating. The overall goal of the evoking process is to increase the amount of change talk vocalized by the client. This can be accomplished by asking strategic questions that encourage clients to talk themselves into change by articulating prochange arguments (Miller & Rollnick, 2013). For example, the clinician might pose a question such as "How might your health improve if you decide to stop binge eating?" A number of these strategies are described below; however, it is important to note that MI is not a "one-size-fits-all" approach intended for delivery according to a structured protocol. Therefore, the clinician should exercise clinical judgment in selecting the most appropriate MI strategies, their timing, and tailoring the strategies to the unique needs of each client.

Exploring Eating Behavior and Eliciting Change Talk

If the client has expressed a high level of ambivalence regarding improving eating behaviors and has voiced a lot of sustain talk, the clinician should explore the impact that current eating habits have had on certain life areas. For example, the clinician might ask, "I'd like to hear about the ways in which your eating habits have affected different areas of your life, if at all. For example, how have your eating habits affected your physical health?" The client might mention the physical effects of binge eating (e.g., nausea, bloating) and/or medical complications associated with weight loss (e.g., poor concentration, low blood pressure). Some common responses include:

> "I feel really uncomfortable after I've had a big eating binge, and can't really do anything the rest of the night."
> "I've gained weight and I'm afraid I'll develop health problems if I keep this up, like diabetes. I already have high blood pressure."
> "I often feel dizzy when my weight is low and have difficulty concentrating."
> "I would like to have children one day and realize I will need to gain weight in order to get my period back."

If the client provides a vague response such as "My health has deteriorated," the clinician encourages the client to provide examples in order to elaborate on his or her responses. For example, the clinician might ask, "In what ways has it deteriorated?" or "Can you say a little bit more about that?" After summarizing the ways in which the client's eating habits have impacted his or her physical health, the clinician can ask, "How much have your eating habits affected your physical health on a scale from 1 (not at all affected physical health) to 10 (severely affected physical health)?" The clinician then continues on to explore the impact of eating patterns on mental health, finances, and relationships.

After exploring the impact of eating patterns on these life domains, the clinician can summarize by saying: "It seems that you have noticed the greatest effect of your eating habits in the area of . . ., and the least effect in the area of . . . Does this fit with the way you see things? What do you make of this? Have you noticed any other areas of your life that I haven't asked you about already?" Each of these questions aims to encourage the client to vocalize reasons for change, thereby increasing the amount of change talk articulated during the session. If the client continues to vocalize a lot of sustain talk, the clinician might use *amplified* reflection by stating, "Your eating has never caused any real problems for you." The intention implicit in amplified reflection is to overstate what the client has articulated with the express aim of having the client vocalize the contrary side of the argument, that is, change talk (Miller & Rollnick, 2013).

Importance and Confidence Ruler

Before planning for change, the clinician should assess the importance of change from the client's perspective, as well as the client's level of confidence in his or her ability to make changes. As mentioned earlier, individuals who regularly engage in disordered eating often feel that it is important to stop but feel reluctant to start making changes because they are not confident in their ability to succeed, given a history of unsuccessful attempts to improve their eating behaviors. Fear of failure can lead to ambivalence about making changes. Therefore, it is important to bolster the client's confidence that he or she has the ability to stop binge eating before setting out to devise a concrete plan for change. The clinician can initiate this discussion in the following way: "We've been talking a lot about your eating and about the possibility of making some changes. If we had a ruler in front of us, and zero on the ruler was 'not at all important to change my eating' and 10 on the ruler was 'extremely important to change my eating'—where would you put yourself right now?"

If the client rates the importance of change as being a 6, the clinician can then ask, "How did you decide on a 6? And why are you at a 6 rather than a zero?" Some common responses include:

> "I'm worried about my health, so I really need to do something now."
> "I'm going to keep gaining/losing weight if I don't."
> "I feel really terrible about myself when I binge eat, and I can't keep going on like this."
> "I feel isolated because I can't meet my friends around mealtimes."

In addition to determining the importance of change from the client's perspective, this question can also be very effective in eliciting preparatory and mobilizing change talk. Next, the clinician might ask, "And what would it take to move it up just a notch, to a 7 or 8?" Some common responses include:

> "If I knew how to stop binge eating."
> "If I knew I could succeed."
> "If I didn't feel overwhelmed at the thought of gaining weight!"

Such responses lead naturally into a discussion of the client's confidence in his or her ability to change. The clinician can open up this dialogue in the following way: "OK, now we're going to do the same for confidence. If you decided you did want to make changes to your eating, how confident are you that you would be successful? If zero means that you are 'not at all confident' and 10 means that you are 'extremely confident if you set your mind to it'—where would you put yourself right now?" The clinician can then follow up with the same questions asked previously. As mentioned, clients with disordered eating typically provide lower ratings for confidence than for importance owing to their many previous unsuccessful change attempts and the feeling that they have inadequate coping skills to successfully make the changes. When asked about what it would take to move their confidence up a notch, they often respond that it would be helpful to have strategies in place and that their confidence would be bolstered if there were some evidence that they were making small improvements.

Enhancing Self-Efficacy

The importance and confidence ruler exercises can lead naturally into a conversation about self-efficacy. Typically clients acknowledge the importance of changing their eating behavior; however, they often feel pessimistic regarding their ability to make changes, given their extensive history of unsuccessful change attempts. As previously discussed, disordered eating fulfills important and valued functions, and clients often feel as though they do not have sufficient coping resources to manage the anxiety they feel when attempting to change. Increasing the importance of change from the client's perspective is not helpful if the client feels that any change attempt would be futile. Thus, enhancing self-efficacy is a key component of MI for disordered eating. Research by our group has demonstrated that self-efficacy assessed immediately following a single-session MI intervention predicts behavioral change (i.e., reduced binge eating) 4 months later (Cassin et al., 2008).

One way to enhance self-efficacy is to elicit examples from the past in which the client successfully made a change that was important to him or her. The clinician might inquire: "So far, we've been talking a little bit about the idea of making some changes to your eating. Have you previously made changes in other areas of your life?" Some examples might include quitting smoking, cutting down on drinking, or increasing exercise. The clinician can then ask, "What kinds of things did you do back then when you decided to change?" The clinician can enhance self-efficacy by encouraging the client to reflect on whether any of the strategies he or she used in the past might also be helpful in changing the person's eating behaviors. For example, if a client with bulimia nervosa was able to quit smoking after smoking a pack a day for many years, the clinician could respond by saying, "That's really impressive! Not only are cigarettes really difficult to give up, but you would have had to make the decision to not smoke 25 times each day. What did you do back then to ride out the urge to smoke—when you would have previously reached for a cigarette? What obstacles did you face, and how did you overcome them? I wonder if any of those same strategies might also be helpful when you get the urge to binge-eat?"

Another way to increase self-efficacy is to ask the client if there have been times when he or she has had the urge to binge-eat but decided against it. Most clients do not have eating binges every day, so the clinician can inquire: "Have you had days when you wanted to binge-eat but didn't? What did you do differently on *those* days?" In the event that the client is bingeing every day, the clinician can inquire about times that the client delayed binge eating, or resisted the urge to engage in multiple binges in one day. In addition to enhancing self-efficacy, this conversation also provides an opportunity to think about strategies that might improve eating behaviors, which can ultimately be used when developing a plan for change.

Conversely, for clients who are underweight and restrict their eating, the clinician can ask if there have been times where they were able to eat more. Many clients can identify conditions in which eating is easier, such as in the presence (or absence) of certain individuals, at a particular time of day, or when they are feeling more relaxed and focused on their long-term goals.

Developing Discrepancy

The clinician may develop discrepancy between the client's higher values and his or her current behavior by referring back to the life areas affected by his or her eating. For example, if the client expresses concern that his or her physical health is deteriorating as a result of current eating habits—leaving little energy to play with his or her children—or worries about setting a bad example for his or her children, the clinician could say: "You mentioned earlier that setting a good example for your children and having energy to play with them is really important to you. Can you say a little bit about how your eating fits in with that?" The clinician can also ask the client to describe his or her ideal life and then inquire about how the current eating habits fit in with that ideal life. Behaviors often conflict with broader personal values, and cognitive dissonance theory (Festinger, 1957) suggests that when this discrepancy is great enough, it is typically the behavior that changes.

Looking to the Future

Another way of eliciting change talk is to have the client imagine the future with and without disordered eating. For example, the clinician might say: "We've been talking a lot about the idea of making some changes to your eating. How do you hope your future would be different if you decided to change your eating?" This question could next be followed by: "Suppose you don't make any changes, and you continue as you have been or your eating gets worse. How do you see your future if you decide *not* to change your eating?" After summarizing the client's responses, the clinician might encourage him or her to engage in a reflective writing exercise. For example, the clinician might suggest: "These are some questions that you might want to think more about after our meeting. Some people find it helpful to reflect on these questions by writing two hypothetical letters to a good friend: one describing their life in 5 years if eating continues as it is now and one describing their life in 5 years if they are successfully able to normalize their eating." The client can then reflect on the contrasts between these two letters.

Planning

If change talk has increased and sustain talk has decreased throughout the intervention, the focus can then shift toward developing a concrete plan for change. The clinician is advised to seek permission to proceed with the planning process by asking, "Would it make sense to think about how you might go about making changes to your eating?" The clinician can then provide a summary of what has been discussed thus far:

> "We've talked a lot about things related to your eating today. You mentioned that binge eating [or restricting] used to provide you with a sense of pleasure, but now it's causing you a lot of distress. You're worried about the impact it's having on your physical health, and it's also making you feel more depressed and anxious. We've also discussed your confidence in your ability to change your eating, as well as a few things that might move it up a notch, such as having a concrete plan in place and successfully making some small changes. We've also discussed some of the changes you've successfully been able to make in the past (such as quitting smoking), and some of the strategies you used back then that might potentially help you change your eating. What would you like to do about your eating at this point in time?"

If the client engages in more change talk and reconfirms his or her commitment to change, the clinician might ask, "What kinds of things do you think you could do to change your eating?" It is best to use an open-ended question and elicit ideas for change from the client, because self-efficacy will generally be increased if the client is able to generate some of his or her own ideas. If the client is unable to generate any strategies to change his or her eating and asks for a lot of suggestions, the clinician might say: "I can give you some ideas of what some other people have tried, but I really don't know what will work best for you. You are the expert on yourself. Would you like to hear about some strategies other people have found helpful?"

The remainder of the planning phase of MI is very compatible with evidence-based treatments for disordered eating, such as CBT. It can be very helpful to complete a "Plan for Change" worksheet together in session so that the client has a concrete plan in place when leaving the session. The clinician can guide the client through the worksheet by asking the following questions:

"What are the changes you want to make?"

- "To reduce my binges to no more than one per week" or "to not skip any meals on three days of this week."
- "To eat breakfast three times this week" or "to exercise no more than 3 hours this week."

"What are the most important reasons why you want to make these changes?"

The client might then refer back to the "Costs of Staying the Same" and "Benefits of Changing" sections of the decisional balance to complete this section. Possible answers he or she might offer include:

- "To learn more adaptive coping skills to manage my anxiety."
- "To improve my physical health (i.e., increase my energy, improve my concentration)."
- "To improve my relationships with family and friends."

"What are the steps you plan to take in changing?"

These steps might include ideas generated by the client in previous sections of the MI intervention (i.e., strategies that were helpful in changing other behaviors, strategies that were helpful on days he or she was able to make a change, ideas generated when asked how he or she might be able to improve disordered eating). However, they might also include some ideas offered by the clinician with the client's permission (i.e., "Would you like to hear about some strategies other people have found helpful? You are the expert on yourself, so you will have a better idea of which ones might work well for you.").

- "Eat regular meals and snacks every 3–4 hours throughout the day."
- "Develop a list of alternative activities I can engage in when I feel the urge to binge."

- "Avoid grocery shopping or take a grocery list and limited amount of money to the grocery store when the urge to binge is high."
- "Tell a few people (e.g., mom, sister) about my plan."
- "Eat tempting 'forbidden foods' in moderation while out in public rather than keeping binge foods at home and eating them in secret."
- "Eat at designated eating areas (e.g., kitchen, dining room, cafeteria) rather than while distracted (e.g., in front of TV or computer)."
- "Not weighing myself each day."

"What are the ways other people can help you?"

Again, the clinician should first try to elicit some ideas from the client, but he or she can also provide a menu of options based on "what some other people have found helpful."

- "I can tell my mom and sister about my plan so I feel more accountable."
- "I can call my mom, sister, or friend to help distract me if I have the urge to binge-eat/restrict."
- "I can arrange to go out for a walk with my friend or make plans with my sister after work, during the time I would typically binge."
- "I can ask a friend to come over and watch a movie instead of exercising excessively at the gym."

"How will you know if your plan is working?"

Given that self-efficacy typically increases in response to early successes, it is important to set some intermediate-term benchmarks so the client can begin to see that progress is being made. For instance, a client who is currently bingeing daily is unlikely to immediately reduce the frequency of binges to once per week, but he or she will feel more encouraged to continue with his or her commitment to make changes by noting the successes that occur from day to day and week to week.

- "If I monitor my food intake, and the food records show that I am eating three meals and two to three snacks throughout the day, on more days than not."
- "If I am able to eat my meals and snacks in designated eating areas and without distractions in the evenings."

- "If I monitor my binges, and the frequency reduces from week to week."

"Do you anticipate any difficulties? What obstacles might get in the way, and what could you do to overcome them?"

The client might mention some practical barriers, but he or she might also refer back to the "Costs of Changing" section of the decisional balance.

- "Boredom and loneliness—I could plan activities in advance if I don't have anything to do with my time in the evenings."
- "High levels of anxiety—I could call my mom or sister, I could listen to a relaxation CD, I could get out for a walk."
- "Overwhelming urge to exercise excessively—I can plan on phoning a friend and meeting for coffee."

Upon completion of the Plans for Change worksheet (if the client was considering change), the clinician can conclude by saying, "I just want to thank you for being willing to be so open in talking about your eating habits and how they fit in to your life." The concluding remarks will vary depending on whether and to what extent the client is considering change. For example, if a client is considering change, the clinician might say: "I hear that you really want to do something about your eating and that you'd like to get going right away. We talked about things you could do differently, and you think that it would be best to . . . Is that correct? What steps are you willing to take this week?" If the client has exhibited a lot of sustain talk and is not yet considering change, the clinician should honor the client's autonomy. For example, the clinician might say: "I recognize that you're not too interested in changing your eating at the current time, and that is really your choice. You are the person who knows yourself best. If you are thinking more about it at some point in the future, my door is always open, and I'd be happy to talk with you again." The clinician can then conclude by asking: "How has it been to talk about your eating today? We've been talking about a lot of things today, and I hope it's been helpful to take some time to reflect."

Problems and Suggested Solutions

In light of the ego-syntonic nature of many symptoms of disordered eating and the valued and important functions the symptoms serve, MI is generally a helpful approach in addressing ambivalence about change and engaging clients in treatment. The client and clinician develop a collaborative therapeutic relationship in which the client is viewed as the expert on his or her own experience and the therapist seeks to foster the client's autonomy in making changes. In the case of more severe eating disorders such as anorexia, maintaining a collaborative stance can present additional challenges. For instance, a client may have to abide by certain rules in order to remain in a day hospital program and therefore may not have the same ability to exercise his or her autonomy. In the most extreme case, a critically ill client may require involuntary hospitalization for medical stabilization. In these instances, some aspects of treatment such as mandatory weight regain may be considered "treatment nonnegotiables." The use of the MI stance in implementing treatment nonnegotiables is critical. Nonnegotiables need to have a clear rationale, be predictable and implemented consistently, and maximize client autonomy (Geller & Srikameswaran, 2006). Tertiary care eating disorder patients report a clear preference for an MI stance, considering it to be more acceptable and more likely to encourage them to remain in treatment and to follow through with treatment recommendations than would clinicians' use of a directive stance (Geller, Brown, Zaitsoff, Goodrich, & Hastings, 2003). The clinician is thus advised to discuss the treatment nonnegotiables and associated rationales as early as possible in treatment and thereby provide the client with a menu of options in order to enhance his or her sense of autonomy. For example, a client in an inpatient unit who needs to regain weight for medical stabilization may be offered a choice from a selection of meals with the option of drinking a meal supplement as a replacement or, alternatively, may receive nasogastric feeding if he or she is unable to eat or drink a meal replacement. Similarly, a client in a day hospital program who needs to consume a certain number of calories per day for weight restoration may be offered some choice when creating his or her meal plan.

Another issue that often arises in the treatment of disordered eating is working with clients who are in different stages of change with respect to each symptom. For example, the client may feel ready to stop bingeing but ambivalent or even highly precontemplative about reducing dietary restriction and/or compensatory behaviors. Unless contraindicated for medical reasons (i.e., dietary restriction and/or compensatory behaviors are so severe that they require immediate intervention), it can be helpful to meet the client where he or she is at and honor his or her autonomy to work toward personally meaningful treatment goals. This approach can foster a collaborative therapeutic alliance and enhance the client's self-efficacy for making changes, thereby increasing the likelihood that the client will engage in treatment and consider changing other symptoms of disordered eating as well.

Empirical Research

Few studies have examined the impact of stand-alone MI interventions on disordered eating; however, the studies conducted to date suggest that MI can be effective in improving binge eating and psychosocial functioning. In one study, college students with full or subthreshold bulimia nervosa or binge-eating disorder who were randomly assigned to receive MI plus a self-help handbook reported increased readiness for change and higher binge abstinence rates at 4 months (24% vs. 9%) compared to those who received a self-help handbook only (Dunn et al., 2006). In another study, women with binge-eating disorder recruited from the community who were randomly assigned to receive MI plus a self-help handbook reported higher binge abstinence rates (28% vs. 11%) and greater improvements in binge eating, depression, self-esteem, and quality of life over a 4-month follow-up period as compared to those who received a self-help handbook only (Cassin et al., 2008). The findings of these studies are promising; however, it should be noted that both of these studies compared MI to a self-help handbook alone and not to another active therapy.

MI has also been used as a prelude to inpatient, day patient, and outpatient treatment of eating disorders in clinical samples with the aim of increasing readiness for change and treatment engagement, as well as an adjunct to treatment with the aim of preventing dropout and improving remission rates.

An early pilot study reported that individuals with anorexia nervosa and bulimia nervosa participating in a four-session group MI intervention as a prelude to a specialized eating disorder treatment experienced improvements in readiness for change, depression, and self-esteem over the course of treatment (Feld, Woodside, Kaplan, Olmsted, & Carter, 2001). Improvements were not reported in eating pathology over the 6-week period, perhaps because the intervention did not explicitly focus on behavioral changes; however, the majority (90%) of participants enrolled in specialized eating disorder treatment following the MI intervention. Similarly, more recent studies conducted with inpatient samples have reported that MI does not improve eating pathology but does increase readiness for change and treatment engagement. One study conducted in an inpatient population with anorexia nervosa reported that a greater proportion of individuals who received a four-session MI intervention as an adjunct to treatment-as-usual moved from "low" to "high" readiness for change over the study period relative to the treatment-as-usual group, whereas a greater proportion of the treatment-as-usual group dropped out of the study (Wade, Frayne, Edwards, Robertson, & Gilchrist, 2009); however, among the individuals who completed treatment, the MI and treatment-as-usual groups did not differ with respect to eating pathology. Another study reported that inpatients with eating disorders participating in a four-session group MI intervention as an adjunct to treatment-as-usual did not experience greater improvements in eating pathology as compared to treatment-as-usual alone; however, the MI intervention fostered greater engagement in therapy and promoted treatment continuation (Dean, Yonyz, Rieger, & Thornton, 2008).

A randomized controlled trial examining the efficacy of MI in a tertiary care eating disorder population reported that both the MI and control groups reported similar improvements in eating pathology and depression; however, a smaller proportion of individuals in the MI group were rated as "highly ambivalent" at 6-week and 3-month follow-up as compared with those in the control condition (Geller et al., 2011). The improvements noted in the control group might have been at least partly attributable to the fact that participants in both groups completed the Readiness and Motivation Interview (Geller et al., 2001) to assess readiness and motivation for change, and the interview has several ingredients that are similar to single-session MI interventions. Lending some support to this theory, an earlier study reported that adolescents with anorexia who participated in a motivational assessment experienced increased motivation following the assessment, and 80% enrolled in an outpatient CBT program (Gowers & Smyth, 2004). Moreover, those who experienced increased motivation following the assessment gained significantly more weight over a 6-week period.

A randomized controlled trial comparing four sessions of either MI or CBT in a sample of individuals with bulimia nervosa reported that MI was as effective as CBT in reducing the frequency of binge eating, vomiting, and laxative abuse over the first 4 weeks of treatment despite a focus on motivation rather than symptom reduction (Treasure et al., 1999). A subsequent two-stage randomized control trial in which individuals with bulimia nervosa and eating disorder not otherwise specified were randomly assigned to receive four sessions of MI or CBT in Phase 1 as a prelude to eight sessions of either individual or group CBT in Phase 2 reported that the groups did not differ with respect to symptom change or treatment completion/dropout (Katzman et al., 2010). Specifically, all groups reported significant improvements in binge eating, vomiting, and laxative abuse.

Conclusions

MI appears to be particularly well suited for the treatment of disordered eating, given that the symptoms of disordered eating often serve important and valued functions and individuals who engage in disordered eating often feel ambivalent about changing their behaviors (e.g. dietary restriction, binge eating, vomiting, laxative use, excessive exercise) and cognitions (e.g., overvaluation of shape and weight). A recent systematic review concluded that MI holds promise in the treatment of disordered eating, particularly with respect to its impact on readiness for change (MacDonald, Hibbs, Corfield, & Treasure, 2012). It has been noted that the heterogeneity in study design and methodology limits comparisons across studies. However, the bulk of research to date suggests that MI has the potential to increase readiness for change and improve eating pathology and psychosocial functioning (e.g., depression, anxiety, self-esteem, quality of life), particularly in individuals who binge-eat and/or engage in compensatory behaviors. Motivational interviewing has also been shown to increase readiness for change in individuals with anorexia nervosa; however, the studies conducted to date have reported relatively little impact on eating pathology. This finding could be partly attributable to individuals with anorexia nervosa having more severe symptoms (e.g., inpatient and tertiary care populations vs. nonclinical community samples) or to MI being largely delivered in group formats to individuals with anorexia nervosa, making it more difficult to tailor the intervention to the unique needs of each individual.

MI was not intended to be a "solution" to all clinical problems (Miller & Rollnick, 2013). It has proven quite effective in increasing readiness for change and treatment engagement; however, evidence-based "action-oriented" treatments are likely required as an adjunct to MI for many individuals with moderate to severe eating disorders in order to improve eating pathology and psychosocial functioning. Of note, the MI stance and MI techniques are increasingly being incorporated into evidence-based treatments for disordered eating, including CBT and dialectical behavioral therapy. The integration of MI with other evidence-based interventions appears to be a particularly fruitful area of clinical practice and empirical investigation.

References

American Psychiatric Association. (2013). *Diagnostic and statistical manual of mental disorders* (5th ed.). Arlington, VA: Author.

Bewell, C. V., & Carter, J. C. (2008). Readiness to change mediates the impact of eating disorder symptomatology on treatment outcome in anorexia nervosa. *International Journal of Eating Disorders, 41*, 368–371.

Cassin, S. E., & von Ranson, K. M. (2007). Is binge eating experienced as an addition? *Appetite, 49,* 687–690.

Cassin, S. E., von Ranson, K. M., Heng, K., Brar, J., & Wojtowicz, A. E. (2008). Adapted motivational interviewing for women with binge eating disorder: A randomized controlled trial. *Psychology of Addictive Behaviors, 22,* 417–425.

Dean, H. Y., Touyz, S. W., Rieger, E., & Thornton, C. E. (2008). Group motivational enhancement therapy as an adjunct to inpatient treatment for eating disorders: A preliminary study. *European Eating Disorders Review, 16,* 256–267.

Dunn, E. C., Neighbors, C., & Larimer, M. E. (2006). Motivational enhancement therapy and self-help treatment for binge eaters. *Psychology of Addictive Behaviors, 20,* 44–52.

Fairburn, C. G. (1995). *Overcoming binge eating.* New York: Guilford Press.

Fairburn, C., Cooper, Z., Doll, H., O'Connor, M. E., Palmer, R. L., & Grave, R. D. (2013). Enhanced cognitive behaviour therapy for adults with anorexia nervosa: A UK–Italy study. *Behaviour Research and Therapy, 51*(1), R2–R8.

Feld, R., Woodside, D. B., Kaplan, A. S., Olmsted, M. P., & Carter, J. (2001). Pretreatment motivational enhancement therapy for eating disorders: A pilot study. *International Journal of Eating Disorders, 29,* 393–400.

Festinger, L. (1957). *A theory of cognitive dissonance.* Stanford, CA: Stanford University Press.

Geller, J., Brown, K. E., & Srikameswaran, S. (2011). The efficacy of a brief motivational intervention for individuals with eating disorders: A randomized controlled trial. *International Journal of Eating Disorders, 44,* 497–505.

Geller, J., Brown, K., Zaitsoff, S., Goodrich, S., & Hastings, F. (2003). Collaborative versus directive interventions in the treatment of eating disorders: Implications for care providers. *Professional Psychology: Research and Practice, 34,* 406–413.

Geller, J., Cockell, S. J., & Drab, D. L. (2001). Assessing readiness for change in the eating disorders: The psychometric properties of the Readiness and Motivation Interview. *Psychological Assessment, 13,* 189–198.

Geller, J., Drab-Hudson, D., Whisenhunt, B., & Srikameswaran, S. (2004). Readiness to change dietary restriction predicts outcomes in the eating disorders. *Eating Disorders: The Journal of Treatment and Prevention, 12,* 209–224.

Geller, J., & Srikameswaran, S. (2006). Treatment non-negotiables: Why we need them and how to make them work. *European Eating Disorders Review, 14*, 212–217.

Gold, M. S., Frost-Pineda, K., & Jacobs, W. S. (2003). Overeating, binge eating, and eating disorders as addictions. *Psychiatric Annals, 33*, 117–122.

Gowers, S. G., & Smyth, B. (2004). The impact of a motivational assessment interview on initial response to treatment in adolescent anorexia nervosa. *European Eating Disorders Review, 12*, 87–93.

Katzman, M. A., Bara-Carril, N., Rabe-Hesketh, S., Schmidt, U., Troop, N., & Treasure, J. (2010). A randomized controlled two-stage trial in the treatment of bulimia nervosa, comparing CBT versus motivational enhancement in phase 1 followed by group versus individual CBT in phase 2. *Psychosomatic Medicine, 72*, 656–663.

MacDonald, P., Hibbs, R., Corfield, F., & Treasure, J. (2012). The use of motivational interviewing in eating disorders: A systematic review. *Psychiatry Research, 200*, 1–11.

Miller, W. R., & Rollnick, S. (2013). *Motivational interviewing: Helping people change* (3rd ed.). New York: Guilford Press.

National Institute for Health and Care Excellence. (2004). *Eating disorders: Core interventions in the treatment and management of anorexia nervosa, bulimia nervosa, and related disorders*. London: National Institute for Health and Care Excellence.

Rieger, E., Touyz, S., Schotte, D., Beumont, P., Russell, J., Clarke, S., et al. (2000). Development of an instrument to assess readiness to recover in anorexia nervosa. *International Journal of Eating Disorders, 28*, 387–396.

Serpell, L., & Treasure, J. (2002). Bulimia nervosa: Friend or foe? The pros and cons of bulimia nervosa. *International Journal of Eating Disorders, 32*, 164–170.

Serpell, L., Treasure, J., Teasdale, J., & Sullivan, V. (1999). Anorexia nervosa: Friend or foe? *International Journal of Eating Disorders, 25*, 177–186.

Treasure, J. L., Katzman, M., Schmidt, U., Troop, N., Todd, G., & de Silva, P. (1999). Engagement and outcome in the treatment of bulimia nervosa: First phase of a sequential design comparing motivation enhancement therapy and cognitive behavioral therapy. *Behavior Research and Therapy, 37*, 405–418.

Wade, T. D., Frayne, A., Edwards, S-A., Robertson, T., & Gilchrist, P. (2009). Motivational change in an inpatient anorexia nervosa population and implications for treatment. *Australian and New Zealand Journal of Psychiatry, 43*, 235–243.

Wilson, G. T. (1991). The addiction model of eating disorders: A critical analysis. *Advances in Behavior Research and Therapy, 13*, 27–72.

Wilson, G. T. (2005). Psychological treatment of eating disorders. *Annual Review of Clinical Psychology, 1*, 439–465.

Wilson, G. T., & Fairburn, C. G. (2007). Eating disorders. In P. E. Nathan & J. M. Gordon (Eds.), *Guide to treatments that work* (3rd ed., pp. 559–592). New York: Oxford University Press.

CHAPTER 15

• • • • • •

Conclusions
and Future Directions

Hal Arkowitz
William R. Miller
Stephen Rollnick

Until recently, most research and practice in motivational interviewing (MI) had been on problem drinking, substance use problems, and health-related concerns. Several reviews have supported its efficacy for these problems (e.g., Hettema, Steele, & Miller, 2005; Lundahl & Burke, 2009). A goal of the first edition of this book (Arkowitz, Westra, Miller, & Rollnick, 2008) was to demonstrate the potential value of MI for other clinical problems, including anxiety, depression, gambling, and eating disorders. This book examines developments that have occurred since then.

When the first edition appeared, publications in the area were somewhat sparse, and for the most part the research presented was preliminary, often consisting of single-group studies and case reports. Since then, researchers have used MI for different problems and with stronger research designs. The chapters in this book illustrate these advances.

MI can be used in a variety of ways, reflecting a flexibility absent in other therapies. For example, MI has been used to motivate people to seek psychotherapy for their mental health problems and as an adjunct to other therapies to address resistance when it arises. It has been used as a pretreatment to other evidence-based therapies and even an integrative framework within which other therapies are conducted.

Most often, MI has been used as part of a treatment approach that includes several other therapeutic elements. In fact, most chapters in this book elucidate this type of approach. However, these uses make it difficult to evaluate the specific contribution of MI to outcomes. In order to determine this, we need studies that compare a group given the treatment including MI and another given the treatment without MI.

Many refer to one use of MI as a "stand-alone" therapy. But the concept of "stand-alone" becomes blurred because a common part of MI in the planning process is to collaboratively develop and carry out an active treatment to address the target problems. If the client cannot come up with a plan, the therapist may offer a menu of options from which the client can choose, including cognitive-behavioral therapy (CBT). In some cases treatment in the action stage continues using MI as a framework, while in others the therapy is delivered without MI. Thus, MI is commonly used in conjunction with other treatments, as illustrated throughout this volume. It is only "stand-alone" when used alone to increase motivation for change or to engage in another therapy.

The data presented by the authors in this volume suggest that MI and MI-related procedures can positively influence the way mental health treatment is provided. Nevertheless, much still remains to be discovered about when and how MI can improve client engagement, retention, and outcomes.

The Diffusion of MI

Among the many things yet to be understood with regard to MI is why it has diffused so rapidly. Since the publication of the first book on MI (Miller & Rollnick, 1991), the number of studies based on it has grown exponentially, with over 200 randomized clinical trials in print and many more in progress. Adoptions spread rapidly through the addiction field, where MI was first applied, and then into health care and health promotion, corrections, social work, and most recently dentistry and education. This volume represents yet another set of applications of MI, as part of treatment in the service of mental health.

One source of MI's appeal is that it directly addresses motivational problems that have long vexed the helping professions and yet have received insufficient attention in the psychotherapy literature.

Often clients were blamed for being "unmotivated," "noncompliant," "resistant," and for "not following through" on what their caregivers prescribed. In the addiction treatment field, practitioners' attitudes sometimes went as far as refusing to treat people with life-threatening conditions until they were sufficiently "ready." The helper's heart knows that there is something wrong with this picture. One contribution of MI has been a realization that enhancing motivation for change is an important part of the therapist's job. Rather than waiting for sufficient suffering to render the person "ready" for treatment, or dismissing clients because they are "unmotivated" or "noncompliant," instead it is possible to evoke motivation for change. That makes it possible to treat a broader range of people and to do so earlier than might otherwise occur. This is a particularly timely development in mental health, making it possible to engage some who are not receiving treatment or who are reluctant to accept a particular needed treatment.

The MI approach also entails a welcome shift in therapeutic perspective. Rather than trying to fill a deficit and install missing motivation, the therapist evokes motivations that are already present in the client. It is a matter of calling them forth rather than creating them. When people are suffering, the problem is not usually a lack of motivation for—but rather ambivalence about—change: They want it, and they don't want it. MI is about resolving that ambivalence in the direction of change. The practice of MI offers a pleasant relief for clinicians from the alternative of "wrestling" with clients about change. It is quite a burden and a significant source of professional frustration to perceive that it's up to you as the therapist to make your clients change. In such a scenario, you are the champion of change, but you must overcome the dragons that guard your client's status quo. This is a very difficult battle to win. MI reframes the helper's work from wrestling to dancing. Working with client motivation becomes no longer a power struggle or contest of wills, but instead a collaborative endeavor.

Another reason for the rapid and continuing dissemination of MI and its expansion to new areas of practice is that it often achieves at least modest success in relatively few sessions (Burke, Arkowitz, & Menchola, 2003; Hettema et al., 2005). Burke and colleagues (2003) found that the average number of MI sessions that clients received in the studies they reviewed was two, and the maximum was four. These brief treatments yielded substantial therapeutic effects. In Project MATCH (Project MATCH Group, 1997, 1998), clients receiving 4 sessions of an MI-based treatment (MET; motivational enhancement therapy) did as well as with 12 sessions of other well-established therapies (CBT and 12-step approaches), though a comparison of MI with four sessions of these other approaches would be needed to determine if indeed MI works faster. Similarly, in the United Kingdom Alcohol Treatment Trial (UKATT Research Team, 2005) comparable outcomes were found with three sessions of MET versus eight sessions of family-involved behavior therapy. The majority of MI interventions discussed in this book are also rather brief, ranging from one to four sessions. The question of whether there is a "dose effect" for MI such that longer treatments will yield even larger effects is an intriguing one. There is evidence, at least, that a single session of MI is less effective than two or more sessions (Rubak, Sandbaek, Lauritzen, & Christensen, 2005).

Another, more speculative, reason for MI's rapid dissemination is that it helps bring the humanistic spirit back to the field of psychotherapy. MI is strongly based in client-centered therapy (Rogers, 1959) and retains its humanistic spirit and style, with a strong emphasis on the healing power of the therapeutic relationship. By contrast, manualized CBT emphasizes technique over relationship (Miller & Moyers, in press). In this book and in the field in general, MI is often used in combination with CBT, suggesting that the two approaches are compatible. Several studies (Burns & Nolen-Hoeksema, 1992; Carlin, 2014) have shown empathy and some components of MI to be causal factors in the outcomes of CBT. Thus, in addition to bringing humanism back to the field of therapy, there is evidence to suggest that, in doing so, we may enhance the effectiveness of CBT and possibly other therapies.

Over the past 10 years, Arkowitz has taught an MI clinical-research practicum to students in a graduate program that emphasizes CBT. The practicum is very popular, and the humanistic spirit of MI excites most students who take it. The course evaluations have reflected their excitement about MI's emphasis on the uniqueness of people, getting to know and understand them in depth, and building a therapeutic relationship based on caring and compassion.

The rapid dissemination of a complex treatment method also brings problems. Diffusion can result in a diffuse product. Clinicians invariably adapt the method to their own style, practices, and model of human nature. Adaptation is a natural part of the diffusion process (Rogers, 2003). Questions then arise as to what adaptations are feasible without losing the essence or efficacy of the core method. Poor fidelity in MI delivery can undermine efficacy (Miller & Rollnick, 2014).

Furthermore, practitioners often learn a new practice informally on their own, perhaps through reading or learning about it from colleagues, and misunderstandings can abound. We have witnessed clinicians practicing and trainers teaching "motivational interviewing" that was far from the spirit and methods of MI as we understand it. Variations in the key elements of MI such as accurate empathy may alter outcomes (Moyers & Miller, 2013). If what the clinicians do is respectful of people in distress and is effective, in one sense it doesn't matter whether it's MI. Calling an intervention something that it's not, however, can create confusion for people who want to learn it and for interpreting research on the treatment (Miller & Rollnick, 2009).

There is substantial variability in the effectiveness of MI across clinicians and settings. Even within a highly controlled clinical trial, clients' outcomes vary widely, depending on the clinician who delivers the MI (Project MATCH Research Group, 1998). In addressing a particular problem, MI seems to work in some trials and not others, and its efficacy can even vary by site within a multisite trial (Carroll et al., 2006). This variability is not unique to, but is certainly characteristic of, MI in studies to date. This raises the question of what accounts for these differences in effectiveness among clinicians and sites (Miller & Rollnick, 2014). Answers to this question may help us to better understand the true nature of the effective ingredients of MI and of psychotherapy in general.

One might expect that a brief intervention like MI would be differentially effective for clients who have less severe problems. Research published to date, however, has yielded little evidence that this is so, and some studies suggest the opposite—namely, that the response to MI is greater with increased problem severity (e.g., Handmaker, Miller, & Manicke, 1999; McCambridge & Strang, 2004; Westra, Arkowitz, & Dozois, 2009). Larger between-group effect sizes have been observed for MI in studies with clients having more severe symptoms (Bien, Miller, & Boroughs, 1993; Brown & Miller, 1993) than with those whose symptoms are less severe (Miller, Benefield, & Tonigan, 1993). The applicability and flexibility of MI across a wide spectrum of severity and problem areas appears to be a further appeal of this approach.

What Is Essential to the Efficacy of MI?

Every psychotherapy contains superstitious elements, components that are believed to be important but that are, in fact, optional, inert, or perhaps even detrimental. The challenge is to separate the beliefs of progenitors and practitioners from the realities of clinical outcomes. This is best done not by armchair debate or individual case experience but, rather, through scientific methods that are designed specifically to test hypotheses and control for human biases. What components or processes of a psychotherapy are truly the "active ingredients" in facilitating change?

In this regard, clinical science is at a relatively young stage in understanding how and why psychotherapies work. Beyond studies to support the efficacy of specific methods for particular problems, attention has been given to hypothesized general factors that may promote change across a wide range of therapies (e.g. Arkowitz, 1997, 2002). Of proposed general factors, the therapeutic relationship (Lambert & Barley, 2002) and empathy (Bohart, Elliott, Greenberg, & Watson, 2002; Miller & Moyers, in press; Moyers & Miller, 2013) have received the most attention and have been shown to have substantial effects on the outcomes of treatment, regardless of the type of therapy employed.

MI is an interesting hybrid in that some of its hypothesized "active ingredients" overlap with what are often regarded as general factors. Accurate empathy, for example, has from the beginning been regarded as a foundational skill in MI (Miller, 1983). Empathy is also often regarded as a "common" or "nonspecific" factor, both of which are misnomers (Miller & Moyers, in press). It is unclear how "common" empathy is in practice in that therapists vary widely in this skill, and to dismiss such factors as "non-specific" merely implies that we have not done our homework to specify, study, and teach them as important determinants of treatment outcomes. Research to date indicates that both relational and specific factors affect the efficacy of MI (Miller & Rose, 2009).

Is It MI Yet?

Some years ago in a television commercial, a child watched the parent stirring a cooking pot and asked eagerly, "Is it soup yet?" We have faced a similar challenge in training clinicians through successive approximations of the clinical method of MI. The same issue arises whenever we are asked to provide fidelity checks for MI interventions being offered in clinical trials. Practitioners do their best to practice what we preach, and the question then becomes "Is it MI yet?"

It is perhaps easier to recognize what is *not* MI (Miller & Rollnick, 2009). Painful early experience taught us that clinicians could adopt specific techniques from MI but entirely miss the essence of the method, from our perspective. They had the words but not the music. They were emitting MI-consistent responses, and yet it was not MI. In a study of training, Miller and Mount (2001) found that after a workshop clinicians had incorporated a few MI-consistent behaviors (such as reflective listening) into their existing stew of practice habits, but the change was too small to make any real difference to their clients. Nevertheless, they believed that they had learned and were practicing MI.

This state of affairs led to a description of the underlying spirit of MI as consisting of partnership, acceptance, compassion, and evocation (Miller & Rollnick, 2013). These four characteristics of the MI spirit in turn clarify what MI is not. It is not about an expert telling people what they should or must do. It is not about "getting in the face" of clients to "make them see" a reality that is different from their own. MI is not about installing things that the person lacks or tricking people into doing what they don't want to do. It is not "confrontational" in the usual sense of that term, although MI is all about helping people to explore possibly difficult and painful realities and come face to face with their choices. This "spirit" of MI is not amorphous. Observers listening to counseling tapes can reliably rate its presence (Moyers, Martin, Catley, Harris, & Ahluwalia, 2003), and better client outcomes are predicted by these global ratings, above and beyond the practice of MI-specific behaviors (Moyers, Miller, & Hendrickson, 2005).

Miller and Rollnick (2014) specified three conditions that should be present for an intervention to be regarded as MI:

1. The treatment should clearly contain the components that are theoretically or empirically related to the efficacy of MI. In the four-process formulation of MI (Miller & Rollnick, 2013), the processes of engaging (client-centered relational skills), focusing (a clearly defined change goal), and evoking (eliciting and strengthening client change talk) should all be present for an intervention to be considered MI.
2. Providers should be trained to an adequate and specified criterion of proficiency in MI before treating trial patients.
3. The fidelity of treatment should be documented by reliable coding of practice throughout the study and reported in a manner that permits comparison with skill levels in other trials.

Of the more than 200 published clinical trials of "MI," only a small fraction would meet these three criteria.

Why Does MI Work?: Three Hypotheses

Studying what components of MI are crucial to its efficacy points to a more fundamental question of why this approach works at all. As MI has evolved, various hypotheses have emerged to explain its impact. Interestingly, they lead to somewhat different prescriptions about how MI should be practiced. All assume the presence of the MI spirit.

The first of these posits that people literally talk themselves into change. To the extent that people voice change talk, they tend to move in the direction of actual behavior change. Conversely, to the extent that clients argue against change, they are likely to continue on as before. From this dichotomy it follows that the counselor should seek differentially to evoke and reinforce change talk but also counsel in a way that minimizes resistance and client arguments against change. This formulation was the original premise of MI (Miller, 1983), also reflected in Miller and Rollnick's books on the subject (1991, 2002, 2013). This might be termed a *technical* hypothesis of MI, emphasizing the importance of differentially eliciting change talk (Miller & Rose, 2009).

A second account of how MI works might be called a *relational* hypothesis (Miller & Rose, 2009; Norcross & Lambert, 2011). In this perspective, MI works primarily because of the underlying humanistic spirit in which the counselor provides the accepting and affirming client-centered atmosphere described by Carl Rogers (Rogers, 1980; Truax & Carkhuff, 1967). It is this quality of the counseling relationship that is therapeutic, and clients naturally move in the direction of positive change when counselors provide this facilitative atmosphere. This is essentially the underlying theory of nondirective client-centered counseling (Rogers, 1959). Research on the efficacy of client-centered therapy is consistent with this view (e.g., Elliott, Greenberg, & Lietaer, 2004).

A third explanation of MI could be called a *conflict resolution* hypothesis. In this view, it is important for the counselor to thoroughly explore *both* sides of the client's ambivalence: reasons to change and reasons to stay the same (Engle & Arkowitz; 2006; Greenberg, Rice, & Elliott, 1993). This differs from the first (technical) hypothesis in asserting that it is essential for the client to voice and explore counterchange motivations: the good things about the status quo as well as the downsides of change. In this perspective, counseling would be incomplete (and ineffective) if it failed to evoke from the client these counterchange as well as prochange arguments. The assumption is that when clients equally explore *both* sides of their dilemma in an empathic and accepting atmosphere, they naturally tend to resolve their ambivalence.

In this sense, a conflict resolution hypothesis overlaps with the relational hypothesis but departs from a purely client-centered perspective in the intentional and strategic evocation of both sides of the ambivalence.

These three causal hypotheses do lead to potentially conflicting and testable predictions about the relationship between MI process and outcomes. There is research evidence that relational components such as empathy do promote behavior change (Bohart et al., 2002; Burns & Nolen-Hoeksema, 1992; Miller & Baca, 1983; Miller, Taylor, & West, 1980; Moyers & Miller, 2013; Valle, 1981). There is also clear evidence that in-session change talk does predict subsequent behavior change and that the amount of counterchange or sustain talk voiced during an MI session is inversely related to change (e.g., Amrhein, Miller, Yahne, Palmer, & Fulcher, 2003; Miller et al., 1993; Moyers et al., 2007). Both experimental and correlational research have shown that the balance of client change talk and counterchange (sustain) talk is clearly influenced by MI-consistent practice (Glynn & Moyers, 2010; Keeley et al., 2014; Moyers & Martin, 2006; Moyers, Miller, et al., 2005; Romano & Peters, in press; Vader, Walters, Prabhu, Houck, & Field, 2010). There is also evidence that this technical component of MI adds efficacy beyond that accounted for by its client-centered relational components (Lincourt, Kuettel, & Bombardier, 2002). In a randomized clinical trial (Sellman, Sullivan, Dore, Adamson, & MacEwan, 2001), MI significantly reduced heavy drinking relative to a control condition whereas nondirective reflective listening did not.

The conflict resolution hypothesis differs in the importance given to eliciting and thoroughly exploring clients' counterchange motivations. A decisional balance (DB) intervention thoroughly and equally explores the pros and cons, whereas MI differentially evokes prochange statements. DB was originally developed to help people make difficult decisions without any attempt to influence the direction of choice (Janis & Mann, 1977). However, DB also has been used sometimes with the intention of promoting change in a particular direction, based in part on the finding in transtheoretical research that people report considering the pros and cons of change while in the contemplation (ambivalent) stage (Prochaska, 1994; Prochaska, Norcross, & DiClemente, 1994). The fact that ambivalent people mull over the pros and cons is not surprising, but this is not evidence that doing so helps them move out of ambivalence. From the perspective of MI research reviewed above, intentionally evoking and exploring both pros and cons would be expected to exacerbate rather than resolve ambivalence.

A comprehensive review of research on clinical outcomes (Miller &

Rose, in press) found that commitment to change *decreases* when ambivalent people are given a DB intervention. For those who had already decided to change, DB appeared to enhance commitment by evoking change talk that justified their decision. Thus, we do not recommend a DB intervention that strategically evokes and explores counterchange motivations when people are ambivalent and the goal is change. DB remains an appropriate clinical tool with the purpose for which it was developed—to help with decision making when clinicians want to avoid influencing the direction of choice (Miller & Rollnick, 2013).

Combining MI and CBT

Given the prominence and effectiveness of CBT for a wide range of clinical problems, it is worthwhile to consider how MI might be integrated or combined with CBT. Such a combination or integration has much to recommend it. Most work in CBT assumes that the person is motivated to change and thus usually starts with work in the action stage. With very few exceptions (e.g. Leahy, 2002), CBT does not specifically address issues of motivation, resistance, or ambivalence. Perhaps, through the addition of MI to CBT, more clients will remain in CBT and cooperate with the tasks of therapy, leading to potentially better outcomes.

One of the clearest ways that MI and CBT may be combined is to use MI as a pretreatment to CBT. The work of Westra and Aviram (Chapter 4, this volume) points to the potential of an MI pretreatment to enhance client engagement and treatment efficacy of subsequent CBT for anxiety disorders. Connors, Walitzer, and Dermen (2002) similarly found positive effects for an MI pretreatment for alcoholism followed by a multifaceted therapy that included many aspects of CBT. They also found that the MI pretreatment was more effective than another pretreatment (a role induction interview) that had been shown to be effective in earlier studies. The amount of MI pretreatment can be tailored to the client's degree of readiness to engage in CBT. For example, Amrhein et al. (2003) found that two-thirds of clients responded well to one session of MI, but the remaining third showed reversal of gains when pressed to complete the process in a single session.

MI can be used not only as a pretreatment to CBT but also as an adjunct that can be employed when ambivalence occurs throughout the course of CBT as well. Problems related to low motivation and resistance can arise at any point during therapy. When such problems do arise, the therapist may switch to MI for part of a session or for one or more sessions as necessary to resolve the resistance and increase the motivation to change (see Boswell, Bentley, & Barlow, Chapter 2, this volume). Finally, MI can be used as an integrative framework within which CBT can be conducted. Such an integrated psychotherapy was developed for the COMBINE study, a multisite trial of treatments for alcohol dependence. The Combined Behavioral Intervention began with motivational enhancement therapy and then proceeded to a menu of CBT modules delivered within the overall clinical style of MI (Miller, 2004)). Trial results showed that patients receiving this psychotherapy or a medication (naltrexone) or both had significantly better outcomes than those receiving placebo medication without psychotherapy (Anton et al., 2006).

Much of what is written about CBT speaks to the content of specific techniques. However, there is little written and much to learn about the *style* of conducting CBT. That is, much of the focus in the CBT literature is on *what* to do rather than *how* to do it. There is surprisingly little in the CBT literature on how to cultivate and maintain a positive and collaborative working relationship throughout therapy. It may be that the MI spirit can form a relational context for CBT that may enhance the outcome of treatment. However, it should be emphasized that the MI spirit is not unique to MI and, in itself, is not MI. Thus, using the MI spirit to conduct CBT is not really an integration of the two approaches. That would occur when the spirit as well as the processes and methods of MI were employed. These different uses of MI with CBT may hold promise for increasing engagement and outcomes in CBT, and perhaps in other therapies as well.

It may be that such a style is particularly important with angry, reluctant, and ambivalent clients (Karno & Longabaugh, 2005). Here, preserving autonomy, evoking the client's ideas about what might help or how you can help, and eliciting feedback may prove to be particularly critical to engaging such clients in treatment. As just one illustration, clients are often highly ambivalent about doing exposure therapy (see Zuckoff, Balán, & Simpson, Chapter 3, this volume). With such clients, high doses of empathy and validation, developing discrepancy, and rolling with resistance may be crucial to navigating these impasses.

Much more remains to be discovered about the manner of conducting CBT that contributes to good (and poor) outcomes. Process research in CBT would be particularly important in explicating the relationship principles that facilitate engagement with CBT. One study found that the therapist quality of empathy strongly predicted drinking outcomes in CBT for alcohol problems (Miller et al., 1980). Marcus, Westra, Angus, and Stala (2007) studied experiences of clients who were in CBT for generalized anxiety disorder (GAD). They found that good-outcome clients consistently described the therapist as a "guide" in the service of achieving their goals and explicitly contrasted this with an expected more directive style. One client remarked, "She [the therapist] was a teacher, but not a director." Another noted that "I thought it [therapy] would be more opinion-based, but it was more about me than her." Rollnick, Miller, and Butler (2008) have described this guiding style of MI as intermediate between a directing-authoritarian style and a following-passive style. Combining or integrating the MI spirit and methods into CBT may hold promise for contributing to more positive engagement and outcomes.

Measurement and Mechanisms in MI

An important problem in MI research to date has been the frequent lack of clear specification of the treatment being delivered and tested (Burke et al., 2003). It is not sufficient to defer to a manual or describe the intended intervention. Even with careful training and supervision, the implementation of MI can be highly variable. Documentation of what was actually delivered is thus essential. The gold standard for doing so is routine recording of MI sessions and systematic coding of sessions. Several coding systems have been developed for this purpose (Lane et al., 2005; Madson & Campbell, 2006; Madson, Campbell, Barrett, Brondino, & Melchert, 2005; Miller & Mount, 2001; Moyers et al., 2003; Moyers, Martin, Manuel, Hendrickson, & Miller, 2005). Such coding also permits informative analyses of the relationships between treatment processes and outcomes (Moyers, Miller, et al., 2005).

Despite the existence of good coding systems for MI sessions, the mechanisms of MI's efficacy are still insufficiently understood (Romano & Peters, in press). Motivation for change is a complex latent construct, with many different dimensions that can be measured. Change talk (and its opposite, sustain talk) is one such variable that mediates the relationship between MI and behavior change but still accounts for a relatively small proportion of variance. Problem or risk perception (Miller & Tonigan, 1996) and hope (Snyder, 1994; Yahne & Miller, 1999) are other often cited components. Another promising lead is a self-report measure of motivation for therapy, including intrinsic motivation, developed by Pelletier, Tuson, and Haddad (1997) based on Deci and Ryan's (1985) self-determination theory.

Ambivalence is another motivational construct and a key concept in MI. A measure of the "decisional balance" of the pros and cons of change is one operational definition of ambivalence (Ma et al., 2002; Miller & Rose, in press; Velicer, DiClemente, Prochaska, & Brandenburg, 1985). McConnaughy, Prochaska, and Velicer (1983) developed a measure of stages of change derived from the transtheoretical model called the University of Rhode Island Change Assessment. While it doesn't measure ambivalence directly, some of the early stages of change are likely associated with it. Further research is needed to understand and measure the construct of ambivalence.

Remaining Questions

There are many other questions and issues relating to MI that need to be addressed. Below, we have listed some of the main ones that have occurred to us. The list is by no means exhaustive. In fact, it is typically the case in research that answering one question raises many more, so this list is just a beginning to stimulate the thinking of researchers and practitioners about MI.

• *How effective is MI for problems other than substance abuse and health-related problems?* Research conducted and reviewed by contributors to this book suggests that MI may be effective for a wide variety of clinical problems. It remains for randomized trials and other rigorous research to answer this question in areas where MI has not been adequately tested. It is gratifying to note how many of the chapters already use strong research designs. Nevertheless, the question posed here is not as simple as it seems. As discussed above, MI is often used in combination with other treatment components. This may occur as part of a manualized treatment (Boswell, Bentley, & Barlow, Chapter 2, this volume) or in the course of the planning and execution stage of MI. Because of this, it is often difficult to examine the contribution of MI to outcomes.

• *How effective are different ways of using MI?* The chapters in this book illustrate the flexibility of the MI approach. It has been used as a pretreatment or complete treatment. It has also been used in combination with other treatment methods and could be used in a "shifting" manner in which the therapist conducting a different type of therapy shifts into MI when problems relating to resistance arise. Further, it may be that MI can serve as an integrative framework into which other therapy methods could be incorporated. MI can be used in groups (Wagner

& Ingersoll, 2013) as well as individual consultations. These different uses of MI need to be further developed and evaluated in well-designed research with various populations and clinical problems.

- *When is MI enough?* Head-to-head comparisons of MI with more intensive *bona fide* treatments such as CBT have often found little or no difference in outcomes (e.g., Babor & Del Boca, 2003; UKATT Research Team, 2005). In this sense, MI may serve as a "minimum treatment" comparison, much as a placebo is used in pharmacotherapy research. Such comparative studies may clarify when a briefer MI intervention is sufficient and may help to identify characteristics of clients for whom more intensive treatment is needed. Of course, failure to respond to a less intensive treatment does not guarantee that a more intensive treatment will be effective. Those who do not respond to a less intensive intervention such as MI can then be randomized to various levels of further treatment.

- *Is MI better than a waiting list?* Waiting lists are common in overburdened treatment systems; yet, placing patients on a waiting list implies that they are not expected to change, and thus the practice may be pernicious. Harris and Miller (1990) found in a randomized trial that problem drinkers immediately given a single session and self-help materials showed change comparable to that for clients assigned to outpatient treatment, whereas those placed on a waiting list showed no change. It is worth evaluating whether an immediate brief intervention such as MI will yield change for a significant proportion of clients, thus decreasing the waiting list and again further specifying the characteristics of those who need additional treatment.

- *Does MI impact other outcomes?* Beyond evaluating the impact of MI on target symptoms, research can determine whether it improves other factors such as treatment retention, adherence, working alliance, change in associated problems, and maintenance of change over time. These questions can be asked in comparative as well as additive research designs.

- *Is MI more effective for some people than for others?* Some results from Project MATCH suggested that anger predicted positive outcomes for MI. This finding needs to be replicated. In addition, other individual differences (e.g. reactance, expectations for change) need to be examined as well to determine how personal characteristics might interact with treatment to influence outcomes. Also, as we discussed earlier, some studies suggest that those whose problems are more severe do better than those with less severe difficulties (e.g., Handmaker et al.,

1999; McCambridge & Strang, 2004; Westra et al., 2009). Clients who are already in the "action" stage and ready for change may be slowed down by spending too much time on evoking rather than moving on immediately to the planning process. This observation suggests a need for studies that better match clients to appropriate processes within MI.

• *What characteristics of the therapist are associated with high effectiveness in the use of MI?* Clearly, therapists vary widely in their effectiveness when using MI. What accounts for these differences? Empathy appears to be one key skill, not only in MI but in clinical outcomes more generally (Moyers & Miller, 2013). Efforts to date have identified no trait-related, educational, or sociodemographic variables that predict therapists' ability to *learn* MI (Miller, Yahne, Moyers, Martinez, & Pirritano, 2004).

• *How effective is MI for different populations?* Is MI differentially effective for different age groups? It is unclear what age or developmental level may be necessary for MI to be effective. Efficacy with adolescents is well established; the picture is less clear with younger children, where intervention with parents and caregivers may be more important. Similarly, what cognitive capacities are required for responding to MI among elderly or neuropsychologically impaired people? Preliminary research with MI for brain-injured populations has been encouraging (Bombardier & Rimmele, 1999; Rimmele & Bombardier, 1998). A meta-analysis (Hettema et al., 2005) found that ethnicity predicted the efficacy of MI in outcome studies, such that the effect size with minority samples was double that for white "majority" samples.

• *How effective is MI in couple, family, and group therapy formats?* What impact does MI have on outcomes when treatment is delivered not to just one but to multiple clients (Wagner & Ingersoll, 2012)?

• *Would longer MI treatment lead to better treatment outcomes?* Most studies of MI have involved relatively brief contact of one to four sessions. As discussed earlier there is evidence that one session of MI is less effective on average than two or more, but it is unclear what length or intensity of MI is optimal, and for whom.

• *What is the role of problem-related normative feedback in MI?* The defining difference between MI and motivational enhancement therapy (MET) is the addition of individual assessment feedback relative to norms. This "check-up" format has been used to address alcohol (Hester, Squires, & Delaney, 2005; Miller, Sovereign, & Krege, 1988), cannabis (Martin, Copeland, & Swift, 2005), and family issues (Morrill et al., 2011; O'Leary, 2001; Slavert et al., 2005; Uebelacker, Hecht,

& Miller, 2006; Van Ryzin, Stormshak, & Dishion, 2012). Assessment feedback is not an integral part of MI but may add motivational impact. It is worth exploring how such feedback interacts with the relational and technical components of MI to influence change. Is there a role for such feedback in other problems such as anxiety, mood, or eating disorders?

• *What is the best way to train people in MI?* Early studies (e.g., Miller & Mount, 2001; Miller et al., 2004) found that the widely used format of introductory workshops to teach MI has only a minimal impact on participants' subsequent practice. There is a large and rapidly growing literature on how to help clinicians develop proficiency in MI. Coaching and feedback based on observed practice appear to be important in the acquisition and maintenance of MI skills.

• *Can it be beneficial to train clients in MI for certain problems?* Clinically, Arkowitz has trained clients in MI as a way of dealing with problems involving spouses or problem children. In this use of MI, the focus is not on increasing change talk and motivation to change but rather training people in MI as a way of relating to others. In many cases of marital distress and child behavior problems, spouses and parents try to get the other person to change what they consider to be wrong by using confrontation, persuasion, or coercion. That is, they focus on the "righting reflex." Often this approach results in a demand–withdraw pattern in which the other person becomes even more defensive or withdraws entirely from the interaction (Christensen, Eldridge, Catta-Preta, Lim, & Santagata, 2006; Eldridge, Sevier, Jones, Atkins, & Christensen, 2007). Teaching partners or parents to use MI methods in these contexts may help avoid such difficulties and enable the people to interact in a more constructive manner (e.g., Smeerdijk et al., 2014).

Conclusions

We hope this second edition of our book will continue to stimulate innovations and extensions in the use of MI. The chapters in this book represent creative and flexible uses of MI and its application to a variety of clinical problems.. The amount of controlled research on the effectiveness of MI with different problems, populations, and in different formats (e.g., as a pretreatment or in an integrative framework) is small but growing rapidly. We hope that this trend will continue, and it appears that it will. If this book serves as a catalyst for such research and practice, then we will have accomplished our goals.

References

Amrhein, P. C., Miller, W. R., Yahne, C. E., Palmer, M., & Fulcher, L. (2003). Client commitment language during motivational interviewing predicts drug use outcomes. *Journal of Consulting and Clinical Psychology, 71,* 862–878.

Anton, R. F., O'Malley, S. S., Ciraulo, D. A., Cisler, R. A., Couper, D., Donovan, D. M., et al. (2006). Combined pharmacotherapies and behavioral interventions for alcohol dependence. The COMBINE study: A randomized controlled trial. *JAMA, 295,* 2003–2017.

Arkowitz, H. (1997). Integrative theories of change. In S. Messer and P. Wachtel (Eds.), *Theories of psychotherapy: Origins and evolution* (pp. 227–288). Washington, DC: American Psychological Association.

Arkowitz, H. (2002). An integrative approach to psychotherapy based on common processes of change. In J. Lebow (Ed.), *Comprehensive handbook of psychotherapy: Vol. 4. Integrative and eclectic therapies* (pp. 317–337). New York: Wiley..

Arkowitz, H., Westra, H. A., Miller, W. R., & Rollnick, S. (Eds.). (2008). *Motivational interviewing in the treatment of psychological problems.* New York: Guilford Press.

Babor, T. F., & Del Boca, F. K. (Eds.). (2003). *Treatment matching in alcoholism.* Cambridge, UK: Cambridge University Press.

Barlow, D. H., Farchione, T. J., Fairholme, C. P., Ellard, K. K., Boisseau, C. L., Allen, L. B., et al. (2011), *Unified Protocol for Transdiagnostic Treatment of Emotional Disorders: Therapist guide.* New York: Oxford University Press.

Bien, T. H., Miller, W. R., & Boroughs, J. M. (1993). Motivational interviewing with alcohol outpatients. *Behavioural and Cognitive Psychotherapy, 21,* 347–356.

Bohart, A. S., Elliott, R., Greenberg, L. S., & Watson, J. C. (2002). Empathy. In J. C. Norcross (Ed.), *Psychotherapy relationships that work: Therapist contributions and responsiveness to patients.* New York: Oxford University Press.

Bombardier, C. H., & Rimmele, C. T. (1999). Motivational interviewing to prevent alcohol abuse after traumatic brain injury: A case series. *Rehabilitation Psychology, 44,* 52–67.

Brown, J. M., & Miller, W. R. (1993). Impact of motivational interviewing on participation and outcome in residential alcoholism treatment. *Psychology of Addictive Behaviors, 7,* 211–218.

Burke, B. L., Arkowitz, H., & Menchola, M. (2003). The efficacy of motivational interviewing: A meta-analysis of controlled clinical trials. *Journal of Consulting and Clinical Psychology, 71,* 843–861.

Burns, D., & Nolen-Hoeksema, S. (1992). Therapeutic empathy and recovery from depression: A structural equation model. *Journal of Consulting and Clinical Psychology, 92,* 441–449.

Carlin, E. (2014). *The effect of a motivational interviewing relational stance on symptomatic improvement, dropout, and the Working Alliance in Cognitive Therapy for Depression.* Unpublished doctoral dissertation, University of Arizona, Tucson.

Carroll, K. M., Ball, S. A., Nich, C., Martino, S., Frankforter, T. L., Farentinos, C., et al. (2006). Motivational interviewing to improve treatment engagement and outcome in individuals seeking treatment for substance abuse: A multisite effectiveness study. *Drug and Alcohol Dependence, 81,* 301–312.

Christensen, A., Eldridge, K. A., Catta-Preta, A. B., Lim, V. R., & Santagata, R. (2006). Cross-cultural consistence of the demand/withdraw interaction pattern in couples. *Journal of Marriage and Family, 68*(4), 1029–1044.

Connors, G. J., Walitzer, K. S., & Dermen, K. H. (2002). Preparing clients for alcoholism treatment: Effects on treatment participation and outcomes. *Consulting and Clinical Psychology, 70,* 1161–1169.

Deci, E. L., & Ryan, R. M. (1985). *Intrinsic motivation and self-determination in human behavior.* New York: Plenum.

Eldridge, K. A., Sevier, M., Jones, J., Atkins, D. C., & Christensen, A. (2007). Demand–withdraw communication in severely distressed, moderately distressed, and nondistressed couples: Rigidity and polarity during relationship and personal problem discussions. *Journal of Family Psychology, 21*(2), 218–226.

Elliott, R., Greenberg, L. S., & Lietaer, G. (2004). Research on experiential psychotherapies. In C. R. Snyder & R. E. Ingram (Eds.), *Handbook of psychological change: Psychotherapy processes and practices for the 21st century* (pp. 493–539). New York: Wiley.

Engle, D., & Arkowitz, H. (2006). *Ambivalence in psychotherapy: Facilitating readiness to change.* New York: Guilford Press.

Glynn, L. H., & Moyers, T. B. (2010). Chasing change talk: The clinician's role in evoking client language about change. *Journal of Substance Abuse Treatment, 39,* 65–70.

Greenberg, L. S., Rice, L. N., & Elliott, R. (1993). *Facilitating emotional change: The moment-by-moment process.* New York: Guilford Press.

Handmaker, N. S., Miller, W. R., & Manicke, M. (1999). Findings of a pilot study of motivational interviewing with pregnant drinkers. *Journal of Studies on Alcohol, 60,* 285–287.

Harris, K. B., & Miller, W. R. (1990). Behavioral self-control training for problem drinkers: Components of efficacy. *Psychology of Addictive Behaviors, 4,* 82–90.

Hester, R. K., Squires, D. D., & Delaney, H. D. (2005). The drinker's check-up: 12-month outcomes of a controlled clinical trial of a stand-alone software program for problem drinkers. *Journal of Substance Abuse, 28,* 159–169.

Hettema, J., Steele, J., & Miller, W. R. (2005). Motivational interviewing. *Annual Review of Clinical Psychology, 1,* 91–111.

Janis, I. L., & Mann, L. (1977). *Decision making: A psychological analysis of conflict, choice and commitment.* New York: Free Press.

Karno, M. P., & Longabaugh, R. (2005). An examination of how therapist directiveness interacts with patient anger and reactance to predict alcohol use. *Journal of Studies on Alcohol, 66,* 825–832.

Keeley, R. D., Burke, B. L., Brody, D., Dimidjian, S., Engel, M., Emsermann, C., et al. (2014). Training to use motivational interviewing techniques for depression: A cluster randomized trial. *Journal of the American Board of Family Medicine, 27*(5), 621–636.

Lambert, M., & Barley, D. E. (2002). Research summary on the therapeutic relationship and psychotherapy. In J. Norcross (Ed.), *Psychotherapy relationships that work* (pp. 17–36). New York: Oxford University Press.

Lane, C., Huws-Thomas, M., Hood, K., Rollnick, S., Edwards, K., & Robling, M. (2005). Measuring adaptations of motivational interviewing: The development and validation of the behavior change counseling index (BECCI). *Patient Education and Counseling, 56,* 166–173.

Leahy, R. L. (2002). *Overcoming resistance in cognitive therapy.* New York: Guilford Press.

Lincourt, P., Kuettel, T. J., & Bombardier, C. H. (2002). Motivational interviewing in a group setting with mandated clients: A pilot study. *Addictive Behaviors, 27,* 381–391.

Lundahl, B., & Burke, B. L. (2009). The effectiveness and applicability of motivational interviewing: A practice-friendly review of four meta-analyses. *Journal of Clinical Psychology, 65,* 1232–1245.

Ma, J., Betts, N. M., Horacek, T., Geoorgiou, C., White, A., & Nitzke, S. (2002). The importance of decisional balance and self-efficacy in relation to stages of change for fruit and vegetable intakes by young adults. *American Journal of Health Promotion, 16,* 157–166.

Madson, M. B., & Campbell, T. C. (2006). Measures of fidelity in motivational enhancement: A systematic review. *Journal of Substance Abuse Treatment, 31,* 67 73.

Marcus, M., Westra, H.A., Angus, L., & Stala, D. (201). Client experiences of cognitive behavioural therapy for generalized anxiety disorder: A qualitative analysis. *Psychotherapy Research, 21,* 447–461

Madson, M. B., Campbell, T. C., Barrett, D. E., Brondino, M. J., & Melchert, T. P. (2005). Development of the Motivational Interviewing Supervision and Training Scale. *Psychology of Addictive Behaviors, 19,* 303–310.

Martin, G., Copeland, J., & Swift, W. (2005). The adolescent cannabis checkup: Feasibility of a brief intervention for young cannabis users. *Journal of Substance Abuse Treatment, 29,* 207–213.

McCambridge, J., & Strang, J. (2004). The efficacy of single-session motivational interviewing in reducing drug consumption and perceptions of drug-related risk and harm among young people: Results from a multi-site cluster randomized trial. *Addiction, 99,* 39–52.

McConnaughy, E. A., Prochaska, J. O., & Velicer, W. P. (1983). Stages of change in psychotherapy: Measurement and sample profiles. *Psychotherapy:Theory, Research and Practice, 20,* 368–375.

Miller, W. R. (1983). Motivational interviewing with problem drinkers. *Behavioural Psychotherapy, 11,* 147–172.

Miller, W. R. (Ed.). (2004). *Combined Behavioral Intervention manual: A clinical research guide for therapists treating people with alcohol abuse and dependence* (COMBINE Monograph Series, Vol.1. DHHS No. 04-5288). Bethesda, MD: National Institute on Alcohol Abuse and Alcoholism.

Miller, W. R., & Baca, L. M. (1983). Two-year follow-up of bibliotherapy and therapist-directed controlled drinking training for problem drinkers. *Behavior Therapy, 14,* 441–448.

Miller, W. R., Benefield, R. G., & Tonigan, J. S. (1993). Enhancing motivation for change in problem drinking: A controlled comparison of two therapist styles. *Journal of Consulting and Clinical Psychology, 61,* 455–461.

Miller, W. R., & Mount, K. A. (2001). A small study of training in motivational interviewing: Does one workshop change clinician and client behavior? *Behavioural and Cognitive Psychotherapy, 29,* 457–471.

Miller, W. R., & Moyers, T. B. (in press). The forest and the trees: Relational and specific factors in addiction treatment. *Addiction.*

Miller, W. R., & Rollnick, S. (1991). *Motivational interviewing: Preparing people to change addictive behavior.* New York: Guilford Press.

Miller, W. R., & Rollnick, S. (2002). *Motivational interviewing: Preparing people for change* (2nd ed.). New York: Guilford Press.

Miller, W. R., & Rollnick, S. (2009). Ten things that motivational interviewing is not. *Behavioural and Cognitive Psychotherapy, 37,* 129–140.

Miller, W. R., & Rollnick, S. (2013). *Motivational interviewing: Helping people change* (3rd ed.). New York: Guilford Press.

Miller, W. R., & Rollnick, S. (2014). The effectiveness and ineffectiveness of complex behavioral interventions: Impact of treatment fidelity. *Contemporary Clinical Trials, 37*(2), 234–241.

Miller, W. R., & Rose, G. S. (2009). Toward a theory of motivational interviewing. *American Psychologist, 64,* 527–537.

Miller, W. R., & Rose, G. S. (in press). Motivational interviewing and decisional balance: Contrasting responses to client ambivalence. *Behavioural and Cognitive Psychotherapy.*

Miller, W. R., Sovereign, R. G., & Krege, B. (1988). Motivational interviewing with problem drinkers: II. The Drinker's Check-up as a preventive intervention. *Behavioural Psychotherapy, 16,* 251–268.

Miller, W. R., Taylor, C. A., & West, J. C. (1980). Focused versus broad spectrum behavior therapy for problem drinkers. *Journal of Consulting and Clinical Psychology, 48,* 590–601.

Miller, W. R., & Tonigan, J. S. (1996). Assessing drinkers' motivation for change: The Stages of Change Readiness and Treatment Eagerness Scale (SOCRATES). *Psychology of Addictive Behaviors, 10,* 81–89.

Miller, W. R., Yahne, C. E., Moyers, T. B., Martinez, J., & Pirritano, M. (2004). A randomized trial of methods to help clinicians learn motivational interviewing. *Journal of Consulting and Clinical Psychology, 72,* 1050–1062.

Morrill, M. I., Eubanks-Fleming, C. J., Harp, A. G., Sollenberger, J. W.,

Darling, E. V., & Cordova, J. V. (2011). The marriage check-up: Increasing access to marital health care. *Family Process, 50,* 471–485.

Moyers, T. B., & Martin, T. (2006). Therapist influence on client language during motivational interviewing sessions. *Journal of Substance Abuse Treatment, 30,* 245–252.

Moyers, T. B., Martin, T., Catley, D., Harris, K. J., & Ahluwalia, J. S. (2003). Assessing the integrity of motivational interventions: Reliability of the Motivational Interviewing Skills Code. *Behavioural and Cognitive Psychotherapy, 31,* 177–184.

Moyers, T. B., Martin, T., Christopher, P. J., Houck, J. M., Tonigan, J. S., & Amrhein, P. C. (2007). Client language as a mediator of motivational interviewing efficacy: Where is the evidence? *Alcoholism: Clinical and Experimental Research, 31*(Suppl,), 40S–47S.

Moyers, T. B., Martin, T., Manuel, J. K., Hendrickson, S. M. L., & Miller, W. R. (2005). Assessing competence in the use of motivational interviewing. *Journal of Substance Abuse Treatment, 28,* 19–26.

Moyers, T. B., & Miller, W. R. (2013). Is low therapist empathy toxic? *Psychology of Addictive Behaviors, 27,* 878–884

Moyers, T. B., Miller, W. R., & Hendrickson, S. M. L. (2005). How does motivational interviewing work? Therapist interpersonal skill predicts client involvement within motivational interviewing sessions. *Journal of Consulting and Clinical Psychology, 73,* 590–598.

Norcross, J. C., & Lambert, M. J. (2011). Psychotherapy relationships that work, II. *Psychotherapy, 48*(1), 4–8.

O'Leary, C. C. (2001). *The early childhood family check-up: A brief intervention for at-risk families with preschool-aged children.* Doctoral dissertation, University of Oregon, Eugene.

Pelletier, L. G., Tuson, K. M., & Haddad, N. K. (1997). Client Motivation for Therapy Scale: A measure of intrinsic motivation, extrinsic motivation, and amotivation for therapy. *Journal of Personality Assessment, 68,* 414–435.

Prochaska, J. O. (1994). Strong and weak principles for progressing from precontemplation to action on the basis of twelve problem behaviors. *Health Psychology, 13,* 47–51.

Prochaska, J. O., Norcross, J., & DiClemente, C. (1994). *Changing for good: A revolutionary six-stage program for overcoming bad habits and moving your life positively forward.* New York: Avon.

Project MATCH Research Group. (1997). Matching alcoholism treatments to client heterogeneity: Project MATCH post-treatment drinking outcomes. *Journal of Studies on Alcohol, 58,* 7–29.

Project MATCH Research Group. (1998). Therapist effects in three treatments for alcohol problems. *Psychotherapy Research, 8,* 455–474.

Rimmele, C. T., & Bombardier, C. H. (1998). Motivational interviewing to prevent alcohol abuse after TBI. *Rehabilitation Psychology, 43*(2), 182–183.

Rogers, C. R. (1959). A theory of therapy, personality, and interpersonal relationships as developed in the client-centered framework. In S. Koch (Ed.),

Psychology: The study of a science: Vol. 3. Formulations of the person and the social contexts (pp. 184–256). New York: McGraw-Hill.

Rogers, C. R. (1980). *A way of being.* Boston: Houghton Mifflin.

Rogers, E. M. (2003). *Diffusion of innovations* (5th ed.). New York: Free Press.

Rollnick, S., Miller, W. R., & Butler, C. (2008). *Motivational interviewing in health care: Helping people change.* New York: Guilford Press.

Romano, M., & Peters, L. (in press). Understanding the process of motivational interviewing: A review of the relational and technical hypotheses. *Psychotherapy Research.*

Rubak, S., Sandbaek, A., Lauritzen, T., & Christensen, B. (2005). Motivational interviewing: A systematic review and meta-analysis. *British Journal of General Practice, 55,* 305–312.

Sellman, J. D., Sullivan, P. F., Dore, G. M., Adamson, S. J., & MacEwan, I. (2001). A randomized ontrolled trial of motivational enhancement therapy (MET) for mild to moderate alcohol dependence. *Journal of Studies on Alcohol, 62,* 389–396.

Slavert, J. D., Stein, L. A. R., Klein, J. L., Colby, S. M., Barnett, N. P., & Monti, P. M. (2005). Piloting the family check-up with incarcerated adolescents and their parents. *Psychological Services, 2,* 123–132.

Smeerdijk, M., Keet, R., de Haan, L., Barrowclough, C., Linszen, D., & Schippers, G. (2014). Feasibility of Teaching Motivational interviewing to parents of young adults with recent-onset schizophrenia and co-occurring cannabis use. *Journal of Substance Abuse Treatment, 46,* 340–345.

Snyder, C. R. (1994). *The psychology of hope.* New York: Free Press.

Truax, C. B., & Carkhuff, R. R. (1967). *Toward effective counseling and psychotherapy.* Chicago: Aldine.

Uebelacker, L. A., Hecht, J., & Miller, I. W. (2006). The family check-up: A pilot study of a brief intervention to improve family functioning in adults. *Family Process, 45,* 223–236.

UKATT Research Team. (2005). Effectiveness of treatment for alcohol problems: Findings of the randomised UK alcohol treatment trial (UKATT). *British Medical Journal, 331,* 541–544.

Vader, A. M., Walters, S. T., Prabhu, G. C., Houck, J. M., & Field, C. A. (2010). The language of motivational interviewing and feedback: Counselor language, client language, and client drinking outcomes. *Psychology of Addictive Behaviors, 24*(2), 190–197.

Valle, S. K. (1981). Interpersonal functioning of alcoholism counselors and treatment outcome. *Journal of Studies on Alcohol, 42,* 783–790.

Van Ryzin, M. J., Stormshak, E. A., & Dishion, T. J. (2012). Engaging parents in the family check-up in middle school: Longitudinal effects on family conflict and problem behavior through the high school transition. *Journal of Adolescent Health, 50*(6), 627–633.

Velicer, W. F., DiClemente, C. C., Prochaska, J.O., & Brandenburg, N. (1985). Decisional balance measure for assessing and predicting smoking status. *Journal of Personality and Social Psychology, 48,* 1279–1289.

Wagner, C. C., & Ingersoll, K. S. (2012). *Motivational interviewing in groups.* New York: Guilford Press.

Westra, H. A., Arkowitz, H., & Dozois, D. J. A. (2009). Adding a motivational interviewing pretreatment to cognitive behavioral therapy for generalized anxiety disorder: A preliminary randomized controlled trial. *Journal of Anxiety Disorders, 23,* 1106–1117.

Yahne, C. E., & Miller, W. R. (1999). Evoking hope. In W. R. Miller (Ed.), *Integrating spirituality into treatment: Resources for practitioners* (pp. 217–233). Washington, DC: American Psychological Association.

Index

The letter *f* following a page number indicates figure, the letter *t* indicates table.